Stacy Jones

Bee-line therapia and repertory

Stacy Jones

Bee-line therapia and repertory

ISBN/EAN: 9783742815620

Manufactured in Europe, USA, Canada, Australia, Japa

Cover: Foto ©Lupo / pixelio.de

Manufactured and distributed by brebook publishing software (www.brebook.com)

Stacy Jones

Bee-line therapia and repertory

Bee-Line

Therapia and Repertory.

BY

STACY JONES, M. D.

SECOND EDITION.

———————

PHILADELPHIA:
BOERICKE & TAFEL,
1899.

PREFACE.

The use of a Therapia and Repertory, such as hereby presented, is self-evident, and therefore needs no apology, or comment.

I would beg leave, however, to suggest that in using it the physician should especially consult the sections on CAUSE, conditions of AGGRAVA-TION and AMELIORATION; and also on PAIN as to kind, and INFLAMMATION as to appearance, &c.; as the indications from these sources generally hold good alike in all parts of the body; and if we can get three legs to the stool of affilia-tion, we will have a pretty sure base for a success-ful prescription.

In this second edition of the Repertory, will be found several captions introduced that were not in the first: Notably a section on Aggravation and Amelioration in general; one on Person (see PER-SONALITY) as distinguishing the peculiar phy-sique of the patient; and another on the various kinds and uses of Suppositories.

The indications for the remedies are much more full and specific in this edition; so that the Book is now aptly styled, A Bee-Line Therapia and Repertory.

THE AUTHOR.

Bee-Line Therapia and Repertory.

ABDOMEN.—

Appendicitis: Aco. ATROP. ECHIN θ. *Lyc.*
"Dios θ 60 drops in hot sweetened water, and
Castor oil purge." "*Ferr p. and Kali m
alt.*" "Leading remedy Mer iod." Persistent vomiting Nat s. 3x, ½ hour, in water.
(See Hot water. Turpentine. Yeast. Poultice)

Ascites.—Apoc. Ars. Aur 3x trit. Chin. Croton.
See Dropsy.

Colic—Enteralgia: Injections of hot water; or
still better, *hot coffee.* Hot fomentations.
(See Bandage. Celery. Hot water. Ice.
Chloroform. *Coffee.* Lard. Onion. Sulphur. Turpentine. *Yeast.*)

Administer in hot sweetened water, Collin θ 10
drops. Dios. θ 60 drops. Pass. θ 60 drops.
Meli 2x Mag p 3x, 5 gr. Acetate of morphia
1 gr in water 1 ounce, adult, a teaspoonful,
¼ hour. Paregoric, adult, a teaspoonful in
hot water, ¼ hour.

Bent double with pain, Cimi. COLO—Relieved
by eating, Bovis.

Drum tight—"Bursting," Carb v. Chin.
Colch. ROBIN.

Frantic with pain, Aco. Cham. Coff. Meli 2x.
(See Pain)

5

Cold, Mer. Pul. *Verat a.*

Navel drawn in, PB. *PB ac* 3x trit.

Urging to urinate, Cep.

Vomiting, Ipe. *Nat s.* Tart e. *Verat a—*Bitter, *Bry.* Cham. *Nat s—*Sour, *Iris v.* Nux v. *Robin.*

Relief by lying on the stomach, Bry. Stan: or pressure upon the seat of pain, *Colo.* Mag p; or tight bandage, Fl ac. *Mag p.* Nat m.

Baby's Colic: CHAM *θ* 1 drop, ¼ hour, in hot water. *Coff.* "Sips of table coffee." MAG P 3x, 5 grs, ¼ hour, in hot water. "Mer d 1x, 1 gr, one dose. *Lob i* 1x, drop doses in hot water. Sour baby, *Robin—*vomiting breast milk in thick curds, Æth. (See Celery. Lard. Onion— See Infant.)

Bilious Colic: "Paregoric." See Colic—with vomiting.

Hepatic Colic: See Liver—Gall stone lodged.

Renal Colic: See Urinary Organs — Stone lodged.

Lead Colic—Painter's Colic: *Alu* 30. Nux v. Op. PB 200. Chloroform 10 drops, ½ hour; on sugar. Dios *θ* 60 drops in hot sweetened water. "Alum powder, adult 10 grs, in mucilaginous liquid, 2 hours, until relief; on the third day, if bowels not open, take an aperient" *Milk diet.*

Hæmorrhoidal Colic: Æs. COLLIN. Nux v.

Menstrual Colic: See Female—Menses painful.

Worm Colic: CHENOPOD ANTH. 2x in hot water, ¼ hour. "Mer. d 1x, 1 gr, one dose." *Santo* 2x. Stan. TEREB.

Enteritis: "Ferr p and Kali m"—Of infants. Aco. Bell. *Lyc.*

6

Hot fever. ACO. *Ars.* Bell—Steaming hot, *Bell.*

Cold sweat, Ars. Mer.

Lying quiet—Faint on rising, Bry.

Restless, ACO. Ars. Canth.

Straining at stool, Mer. c.

Urging to urinate, Cep.

Meteorism, Lyc. Uran n. Tereb. (See Hot water. Turpentine. Yeast. Poultice.)

Flatulence: *Carb v.* China, *Collin. Fl. ac.* Lyc. Robin—Hot flatus, Aco. *Alo.* Cham. Pho—Incarcerated, Carb v. China. Grap. Lyc. See Abdomen—Bloat.

Hernia—Strangulated: Aco. Apis. Nux v. *PB.* Morphia ⅓ gr, hypodermic; during sleep the rupture reduces itself. "During *taxis,* have patient cough violently." "Hold patient, clear of the bed by the feet." "Grasp with thumb and finger of each hand tightly between the tumor and the body; and lift up strongly; this repeated a few times insures success." Administer strong coffee, copious draughts, and bathe the rupture with the same; presently gas will escape and the tumor vanish. (See Coffee. Cold Water. Dry Cup. Ether.)

Inguinal Glands: Swollen, Aur. *Clem. Dul.* Hep. Mer. *Sil.* Sul—Hard, Aur. *Clem.* Dul—Painful, Dul. *Mez.* Thuj—Sore, Grap. Mer—Suppurating, Aur. *Hep.* Mer. Nit a. Sul.

Intussusception—Bowel obstruction: *Coal oil* 15 drops, 2 hours, 4 doses; then inject glycerine if needful. Olive oil, 2 ounces, 2 hours, 3 days. "Opium, adult, ½ gr, 4 hours, 3 days, or longer. This directly arrests the most dangerous symptoms, and finally brings about free operation of the bowels." "Place patient on right side, propped up at angle of 45 degrees, and, adult, inject into the bowel, ½ gallon of warm water, containing 1 ounce of strong decoction of tobacco; keep patient in this position, 20 minutes, with external pressure on anus, then place the person in bed. Sleep will ensue, and on waking the bowels be moved." Yeast, give to drink a teacup-full, and inject a quart; repeat if necessary.   Inject warm brine large quantity slowly.   Hold patient inverted.

Fever guard, Aco. Bell.

Fecal vomit, Op. PB.

Writhing pain, GEL *0*. PB ac., 3x trit. Nux v. (See *Dry Cup*)

Mesenteric Glands affected: See Atrophy.

Pendulous abdomen: Cro. *Iod*. Plat. Sep. *Stap*.

Peritonitis: Hot fomentations.   Turpentine stupes.   (See Aconite.)

Hot fever, Aco. Bell. Canth—Steaming hot, Bell.

Cold sweat, Ars. Mer. Verat a.

Quietude, Bry.

Restlessness, *Aco. Ars*. Bell. Canth.

Meteorism, Lyc. *Tereb*.

Retention of stool or urine, Colo. Mer c.

Tenesmus rectal, Colo. Mer c—vesical, Canth. Colo. Mer c.

Vomiting, *Ars*. Bell. *Verat a. Verat v*.

Purulent effusion, *Mer c*. Sul.

"Pot-Belly :"—See Abdomen—Bloat.

—Children, *Bar c*. CALC. Cina. Stap.

Girls at puberty, *Lach*.

—Women, Plat. SEP.

Tympanitis—See Bloat.

—In Typhoid, Ars. Crotal. EUCA. Lach. TEREB.

Typhilitis :—See Appendicitis. *Same treatment.* See indications under Enteritis.

Pains, Sensations, Conditions, of Abdomen :

—In general, *right* side, see Liver—*Left*, see Spleen—Near above the groin, see Ovary.

Bearing down pain, or pressure, Agar. Alo. *Bell.* Caul. *Cham.* Cimi. LAPPA. LIL T. Nit a. Plat. *Pul.* SEP. Nat m. *Nux v.* Sec.

Bruise-like soreness, *Apis. Arn.* Cimi. Ferr. *Mer c*—Hurts when stepping, Arn. Alo. Lil t. See Tenderness.

Bloat (Meteorism).—Carb v. Chin. Colch. Lyc. Robin—See Tympanitis.

—Sudden bloat (Hysterical). Arg n. *Asa.* Cic. *Val.* ZN.

Bubbling, Berb. Lyc.

Burning, *Ars.* Carb v. *Canth.* Lach. Pho— Burning and gnawing, Kreo—Burning and stinging, Apis.

Clawing. Clutching, BELL. Dios. Ipe.

Coldness, *Æth.* Ars. AMB. *Calc.* Colch. PUL.

Constriction as by a band, ARG N. Con. Lyc— Taking the breath, *Coc.*

Cramp. CUP AC. Dios. Nux v. (See Ice.)

Creeping, like ants, Plat. ZN.

Cutting, Ars. BELL. Colo. Ipe. KAL C. Op. *Verat.* ZN.—Crosswise, BELL. Chin. CIMI. Ipe.

Empty feeling, PHOS. Pod. *Sep.* Sul a.

Gurgling, ALO. Asa. Dios. LYC, *Pul.* Sul.— As liquid from a bottle, Jat.

Hardness, Bar c. Calc. Mer.

Heat, ALO. CUP M. Kali c. SIL—At the navel, Sul a.

9

ABORTION.

Heaviness—Pul. Sep.

Jumping, life-like, CRO. Cann s.

Movement like a wave rolling, Thuj—Like a worm, Mer. Spig.

Numbness, *Sang.* Tarent C.

Pressure like a stone, *Bry.* Mer. *Nux v.* Pul—Like a plug at the navel, Ana.

Pricking like needles, Agar.

Quivering, life-like, Sabin.

Rumbling and other noise, Alo. DIOS. LYC. Pass θ. Ph ac.

Soreness, Aco. Bell. Cup. Sep—of the navel, Thuj in and ex—Oozing blood, Crotal 200.

Stinging, APIS. Mer. Thuj.

Stitches, Aco. BRY. Cimi. KAL C. Nat m. SUL.

Sunken, "Caved in," CAL P—Retracted, PB. Pod.

Tenderness all over, Aco. APIS. Bell. Bry. MER C.—Cannot bear pressure of clothing, Calc. *Lach.* Lyc. Nux v.

Throbbing, Æs.

Trembling, Ig. IOD. LIL T. Rhus.

Weak, empty feeling, PHO.

ABORTION.—See Female—Pregnancy.

ABRASION.—See Skin.

ABSCESS.—(See Alcohol. Onion.)

To abort an abscess, in early stage, apply Camphor spirits and Lime water, equal parts, mixed.

To hasten "to head," administer Guai ix, and apply Lard and Flour mixed.

To prevent suppuration, Cham θ. IOD. Mer. PHO.

To promote suppuration, when inevitable, HEP.
Lach. Mer.

To soothe the pain. See Calend. Clay. Hydrogen—Ichthy. Poultice.

To open without the knife. See Potash.

To open without pain. See Anæsthesia—
Local.

—Among the tendons, Mer. MEZ. Sil.

—Burning, Aco. *Ars.* Bell.

—Blue, Ars. *Lach.* Sil.

—Stinging, *Apis*, Mer. Pul.

—Throbbing, Bell. HEP. Mer.

—Mammary,—See Female—Breasts.

ACETANILIDE. (Antifebrin).—Odorless—Soluble in 200 vol. of water: 19 vol. of ether: 4¾
vol. of Alcohol—Antiseptic, Hemostatic, Stimulant, Desiccant, Analgesic—A perfect substitute
for Iodoform.

All Surgical Cases, Wounds: Acetan full
strength powder. Checks formation of pus
at once. No danger even to an infant.

All cases, acute or Chronic, requiring local
*treatment: Eruptions of all Kinds: Itching
and Burning of the Skin: Erythema,
Prickly heat, Ivy poison, Psoriasis, Tinea,
Sycosis, Suppurating sores, Old ulcers:*
Acetan alone, or with Boric acid and Bismuth combined in equal parts: or Ointment, 5 : 20 grains in Petroleum 1 ounce;
spread upon lint and apply.

Conjunctivitis. Acetan laverment: 2 per cent
solution in alcohol, diluted, to suit the case.

Otorrhœa: Acetan powder, dust in the ear,
morning and evening. "Cure in 5 days."

ACIDITY.—See Stomach.

ACNE.

ACNE.—See Face.

ACONITE.—In all cases of *internal* inflammation, apply flannel cloths wrung out of hot water containing Acon θ, a teaspoonful to the pint of water.

Earache: The same on cotton in the ear.

Toothache: On cotton to the gum.

ADENITIS.—See Gland.

AFTER-BIRTH.—See Female—Labor.

AFTER-PAINS.—See Female—Child-bed.

AGALACTIA.—See Female—Breast.

AGGRAVATION.—

As to Food—Worse:

Cold food, Alu. Arg n. *Ars.* Hep. *Lyc.* Kreo. *Nux v. Rhus.*

Ice Cream, ARS. BELLIS P. Pul. Verat a.

Warm food, *Bry.* Lach. *Pho.* Ph a. Pul. Sul.

Bread, Bry. Pul.

Bread and butter, Carb v. Pul.

Cabbage, Bry. Lyc. Pet.

Fat, Carb v. Cyc. Ferr. *Pul.* Tarax.

Onions, Thuj.

Oysters, Lyc. Sul a.

Potatoes, ALU. Sep.

Soup, Alu.

Sour food, Ant c. Lach.

Sweets, Arg n. Ig.

Veal, *Ip.* Kali m. Nit a.

As to drink.—Worse:—

Cold drink, ARS. *Canth.* FERR. *Nux v. Rhus.* Sul.

Hot drink, BRY. Caps. Carb v. Nat s. Phyt.

Coffee, Canth. Caust. *Cham.* Ig. *Nux v.*

Tea, Ferr. Selen. Thuj.

Milk, *Æth*. Calc. Chin. Con. Nit a. Sep. SUL.

Beer, Kali bi.

Brandy, APO C. Ig. Lach. Nux m. NUX V. Op.

Wine, ANT C. Ars. Nux v. Ran b. ZN.

As to Sound.—Worse :—

Noise in general, Aco. BELL. Coff. Nux v. THERID.

Music, Nat c. Nux v. Sep.

Talking, Ars. Cact. NUX V. Sep. ZN.

Running water, Canth.

As to odor—Worse :—

Strong odors, Aco. Aur. BELL. Coff. COLCH. IG. Nux v.

Odor of tobacco, IG. NUX V. Pul. Spig. *Spong*.

As to weather—Worse :—

Cold weather, Aur. DUL. Nux v. RHOD.

Cold *wet* weather (catarrhal and rheumatic ailments), Am c. CALC. DUL. MER. Phyt. ·RHOD. Thuj.

Hot, sultry weather, BRY. Caps. COLCH. Hyo. Nux v.

Hot *damp* weather, Alo. CARB V. Gel.

Stormy weather, Am c. Rhod. Rhus—Wind storm, Cham. PLAT. Rhod.

Before a thunder storm, Agar. Pet. RHOD. RHUS.

As to time—Worse:--

During the day, Arn. Sep. Sul.

Every other day, China.

Before breakfast, Calc. Cro. Iod. Stap.

After breakfast, Cham. Pho. Nux v. ZN.

Before dinner, Pho. *Sep. Sul.*

AGGRAVATION.   As to Heat.

After dinner, ARG N. Cedron. Ig. NUX M.
ZN.

10 a m, Nat m—11 a m, Arg u. Sep. Sul—12
m, Arg n. *Cedron*. Nux m. Val—3 p m, *Bell*.
Thuj—4 p m, Hep. Hell. LYC.

Towards evening, *Colch*. *Pul*. Sep. Sul. ZN.

Night, Ars. MER. Rhus. Sil. Sul—After midnight, ARS. Bell. Rhus. SUL. Thuj.

Monthly. See Female—Menses.

New moon, *Alu*. Am c. Caust. CALC. SIL.

Full moon, *Alu*. CALC. Grap. SIL.

Spring, Amb. Calc. *Lach*. Lyc. Rhus.

Autumn, Aur. *Colch*. *Mur*. Rhus.

Winter, Aur. Dul. Nux v. *Rhus*.

As to heat—Worse :—

.Warmth in general, Apis. Bry. DIG. Glo.
IOD. PUL. Sec.

Warmth in bed, Aur. MER. Pul. SUL. Tart e.

Sun blaze, Agar. *Ant c*. Bry. *Glo*. Lach.
Therid.

As to cold—Worse :—

Cold in general, ARS. Aur. Dul. *Hep*. Rhus.
Sil.

Uncovering *Hep*. Nux v. *Rhus*. *Rumex c*. Sil.

As to rest—Worse :—

Repose in general, Aur. Con. FER. *Ph a*.
Rhod. RHUS. Sul. Val—" Sunday the worst
day," Sep.

Lying down, Ars. Dig. LYC. Nat m—On the
back, Ars. PHO. NUX V—On the left side,
Aco. Cact. *Phos*. Pul—On the right side,
Mer—After sleep, Apis. LACH. Verat a.

Sitting, Ferr. Helon. PLAT. Pul. RHUS. Sep.
VAL.

Standing, ALO. Con. LIL T. Plat. SUL.

14

As to motion—Worse :—
Motion in general, Aco. BRY. CHIN. Colch.
Led. Mer. SPIG.

First motion after rest, Con. Lyc. *Rhus.* Sep—
Motion and pressure, *Phyt*—Dread of exer-
cise, Nux v.—Downward motion, Borax.

Rising up in bed, ACO. BRY. Coc. Dig. Sul.

Ascending hill or stairs, Ars. CALC. IOD.
Spo. SUL.

Descending hill or stairs, Borax. Ferr. STAN.

Rocking or swinging, BORAX. Carb v. COC.
Pet.

Talking fatigues and excites pain, SUL.

As to touch—Worse :—
Sensitive to contact, *Asa.* Arn. CHINA. Hep.
SPIG.

The slightest touch painful, *Aco.* Asa. Bell.
CHIN. HEP. Nux v. SPIG.

AGUE.—(See Chill, Heat, Sweat.)
" First a Podo purge, adult, 1 gr. at bed time,
then Ipe. *low,* then the indicated remedy."
" Quinia, *hypoderm,* 5 to 10 grs. before
the chill. In 150 cases treated in this way,
only one relapsed." CHINOIDINE, 2 gr.,
pill, 3 hours. Gels θ 5 drops, 3 hours.
EUCA θ 30 drops, 3 hours. Sulph θ 10 drops,
3 hours: and Sulph ointment to spine, well
rubbed in daily. *Polyporus, Pambolano* θ,
Tarent C.

Treatment in Cold Stage, see Amyl. Camphor.
" Chloroform 10 drops in milk, before the
chill, arrests the ague."

Chronic Ague, Ars iod. Lach 200. Nat m 200.
"Corn shuck tea"—with jaundice, Iod.
Pambo θ—Enlarged spleen, Chin. Diadem.

Nat m. URTICA *θ*. (See Bandage. Coffee. Hot water. Onion. Salt. Sulphur.)

Relapsing Ague. BELL.

Ague Chill. Time :—
6 a m, Verat a.
7 to 9 a m, Eup per.
10 to 11 a m, Nat m.
3 p m, Apis.
4 to 8 p m, Lyc.
11 a m, or p m, Cact.

Ague Chill Begins :—
In hands and feet, Gel.
In lips, fingers, and toes, Bry.
In the back, CUP M. Nat m. Sul.
Between the shoulders, Caps.
On the right side, Bry. Mer.
On the left side, Caust. Carb v.

During Ague Chill :—
Blue lips and nails, Nux v.
" Dead cold " fingers, Sep.
Fiery red face, Ig. FERR.
Cough, Bry. Rhus.
Nettle rash, Apis.
Pain in the back as if *broken*, Eup per.
Desire to be held down, Lach; or have hands held, Gel.
Chill relieved by warmth, Ig.
Short chill and long heat, Ipe.
Every stage well marked, Chin.
One stage wanting, Ars.

During Ague Heat :—
Burning hot skin, Aco. BELL.
Hot breath, Aco.
Hot vertex, Sul.
One red cheek, Cham.
Cough, Aco.

Drowsiness, Ant c.

Headache, Bell. NAT M. Nux v.

Vertigo, Carb v. Gel. NUX V—Extreme, even
to insensibility, Sep.

Throbbing carotids, Bell.

Restlessness, extreme, Aco. ARS. Gel. Rhus.

Nettle rash, Hep. Ig. Rhus.

Must be covered, Hep., NUX V.

During Ague Sweat:—See Sweat.

AIR INDOORS PURIFIED.—Place in the room
a small basket, or porous box, containing fresh
charcoal and *quick lime.* Renew once or twice
a week. The charcoal imbibes the foul vapor
emanating from the body, and the lime absorbs
the Carbonic acid exaled from the lungs.

"To sweeten a musty room, dip a bundle of
phosphorus matches into warm water, and suspend it in the room; this produces ozone,
which purifies the air." (See Disinfectant.)

ALBUMINURIA.—See Urinary organs.

ALCOHOL.—*Local sweat, Itch, Erysipelas, Bed
sore, Ulcers, Open Cancer, Wound, Compound
fracture :* Apply Alcohol pure, two or three
times a day; or when necessary, first apply it
pure, and later diluted with water equal parts.
Keep the surface macerated with it on cotton, or
cloth covered with oil-silk, held in place by
bandage.

Pain of abscess, felon, burn, scald, bruise: Apply
by compress, alcohol *ice*-cold.

Diphtheria. Sore throat : Gargle with Alcohol diluted one-half with water; and adult,
take 1 teaspoonful every two or three hours:
Child ⅓ or ½, the quantity according to age.

Scarlet fever. Typhoid fever. Sponge with

A*   17

tepid water, containing a little Alcohol, morning and evening.

X **ALCOHOLISM.**—Avenasat, 30 to 60 drops, at bed time.

Pass ө 60 drops at bed time. Strych 2x, 2 gr, 12 hours. Strophantus ө 7 drops, 6 hours. Moschus 3x, 5 gr, 6 hours. "To 1 oz of Acetic acid, add 1 pint of water, and in this steep ½ oz of ground Quassin, and of this give 1 teaspoonful in a little water every time the craving is felt, and the thirst for liquor will soon cease." Flavor with spirits, all food and drink taken, and the craving will turn to loathing. Drink milk. See hot water.

"Dead Drunk": *A wine glass full of dilute vinegar.* A teaspoonful of Laudanum. Injection of coffee.

Effects of "a spree": APOC ө in water. Nux v 2x. Ran b. ZN P.

Ailments resulting from Inebriety :—Headache, Agar, Cimi, Nux v.

Dyspepsia, Caps ө 10 drops in water, before meals.

"Shakes" Tremor, Caps ө 60 drops in milk.

Vomiting, Ars. *Caps.* ө Nux v.—from beer, Kali bi.

Insomnia, "IPE. FL. EX. 10 to 20 drops from a spoon with no water, direct patient to be perfectly quiet for 5 minutes after taking it. This will produce sleep when all other means seem to fail. It may be taken in whisky." See Delirium Tremens.

ALOES.—*Wound Pain:* Aloes pulv. ex: removes the pain at once: and the powder renewed occasionally heals the wound with little or no scar.

Pimples: Glycerole of Aloes.

ALUM.—*Local Itching, Burn, Scald, Ulcerated Mouth, Unhealthy gums, Ulcerated throat, Relaxed throat, Palate down, Otorrhœa, Ozæne, Leucorrhœa, Falling of the Womb, Chronic Catarrh of the bladder, Bronchorrhœa:* Alum water 5 to 10 grains of the Alum powder to an ounce of water—Use as a wash, gargle, injection, or spray.

Falling of the Womb: Support with sponge soaked with Alum water.

Ophthalmia, Purulent Ophthalmia, Conjunctivitis: Use as an eye wash, Alum water; made with Rose-water, instead of plain water; or apply Alum curd.

Granulated eyelids: Alum pencil.

Nose-bleed: Snuff pulverized Alum; or Alum water.

Bleeding wound: Dust it with Alum powder. (Rice flour is a good styptic. Mix with lint and apply.)

Bleeding socket after tooth extracted. Cold in the jaw after tooth extracted: Dampen a small roll of cotton, roll it in Alum powder, and plug the cavity with it.

Internal Hæmorrhage. Menorrhagia. Diarrhœa and Vomiting. Chronic Bronchitis. Diphtheria. Croup: Alum whey—Made by stirring 2 drachms of Alum powder, into a pint of boiling milk, the curd strained off, and the whey sweetened—To an adult, a wine glass full several times a day.

AMAUROSIS.—See Eye—Sight.

AMELIORATION.—

As to Food—Better :—

When eating, *Ana.* Ig. Lach., *ZN.*

AMELIORATION. As to Drink.

After eating, Hep. Iod. Pho. Sep. Spon.
Cold food, Bry. Pho. Pul.
Warm food, Ars. Lyc. Nux v.

As to Drink—Better :—
After drinking, Lob-i. Spo.
Cold drink, Bry. Caust. Pho. Sep.
Warm drink, Ars. Lyc. Nux v.
Coffee, Cham. Colo.
Tea, Carbol a. Dig.
Milk, *Ars*. Mez. Ruta.
Wine, Aco. Con.

As to Time—Better :—
During the day, Aco. Ars. Mer. Rhus. Sul.
  Thuj—Every other day, China.
Before breakfast, Cham. Con. *Nat m*.
After breakfast, Calc. Cro Fl ac. Iod. Stap.
After dinner, Nat m. Sep. Sul.
Towards evening, *Arn. Chel. Kal bi*. Lob i.
At night, *Arn*. Sep. Sul.

As to Heat—Better :—
Warmth in general, ARS. Aur. *Kal c*. Nux v.
  Rhus. Sul.
Warm in bed, Bry. Caust. Led. Lyc. Nux v.
Warm wraps, Ars. *Hep*. Kal c. *Sep. Sil*.

As to Cold—Better :—
Cold in general, Fl a. *Iod*. Lyc. *Pul*.
Cold application (cold water), *Allo*. Alu. *Apis*,
  ASAR. Cal. fl.
Cold weather, winter, Bry. *Lyc*.

As to Rest—Better :—
Repose in general, Bry. Colch. Led. Nux v.
Lying down, Am m. Bry. Nux v—After sleep,
  Pho.
On the back, Bry. Calc. Ig.
On the side, Nux v.

20

AMENORRHŒA.

Right side, Lyc. Nat m. *Pho.*
Painful side, *Bry.*
On the stomach, Alo. Am c. *Stan.*
Sitting, Bry. Colch.' Cup m. Nux v—Bent,
    Kal c—Erect, Dig. Sam. Tart e.
Standing, Bell. Pho.

As to Motion—Better :—
Motion in general, Aur. *Con.* Dul. *Ferr.* Lyc.
Rhus—Continued motion, Caps. Con. *Ferr.*
Pul. Rhus—Of the affected part, Caps. Dul.
Ferr., Pul. *Rhus*—Change of position, Ig.
Rhus.
Riding in a carriage, Nit a.
Running, dancing, Ig. Sep.
Stretching, Rhod. Sec—Yawning, Stap.

As to Contact—Better :—
Pressure upon the affected part, Con. Ig. *Mag
    p.* PB. *Stan.*
Rubbing, stroking, Calc. Canth. PB. Pho—
Rubbing the side, Pod—The Back, Nux v—
Hands together, Tarent c.
Scratching, Asa. Calc. Cyc. Mur a. Pho.
Touching the part, Asa. Calc. Thuj.

AMENORRHŒA.—See Female. Menses, suppressed.

AMPUTATION DRESSING.—See *Acetan.* Alcohol. *Calend.* Eucalyp. Salicyl. Potash.
—Stump pain, Cep *0. Hyper.* See Aloes.

AMYL NITRITE.—*Pain Neuralgia, Angina
pectoris, Asthma, Spasm, Seasickness, Unbearable Labor pains, Obstetric operations, Dysmenorrhœa, Opium Stupor:* Inhale Amyl gently;
or take 2 or 3 drops in liquor, at short intervals.
Ague: to break the chill, inhale Amyl until the
face reddens; the chill will then break into a
sweat.

21

ANÆMIA.

Epilepsy: To ward off the attack, snuff Amyl at the moment of warning.

Opium poisoning: Amyl 20 drops, on handkerchief to the nose. In a few seconds the patient will "Come to."

ANÆMIA.—*Acet a.* Cal p. *Ferr. Helon.* Kali p.— Profound, Pic ac.

ANÆSTHESIA. — More prompt, *less nausea,* quicker recovery; by shutting off the circulation in the extremities, upper and lower; by tight bandage, at groin and arm-pit.

"Never untoward symptoms if Amyl nit, 3 to 6 drops, be added to the ounce of Chloroform."

A mixture about as safe as Ether, is (A, C. E.) Alcohol 1 part, Chloroform 2 parts, and Ether 3 parts, by measure: Used much the same as Chloroform.

With Chloroform, commence gently, permit free access of air.

"With Ether, admit no air, push vigorously." (Keep *flame* from *Ether* vapor.)

In all cases watch the *breathing* and *pupil.* A few short inspirations, or holding the breath awhile is sure to be followed by a deep inspiration; *then* withhold the cone for fear of overdose.

When the pupil dilates the patient is insensible—stop a while—proceed with caution. One hour is the limit of safety.

In case of danger. Admit fresh air—draw forward the tongue. Clear the throat—*Forcibly dilate the anus*—Invert the patient.

Hypnotism: "Have patient, while in easy sitting, or reclining position, steadfastly gaze at a shining object, as for instance the bulb of a thermometer, placed a few iuches from the eyes, and a little above range, *requiring a convergent squint to fix the sight upon it.* In five minutes, or less, the pupils will dilate, eyelids tremble, and then sleep will ensue, with insensibility to pain. An operation may be performed, or *labor progress* without consciousness. In order to waken the patient blow your breath upon the eyelids, or rub them with your thumbs, or apply heartshorn to the nose."

Local Anæthesia: Aniline oil. Piper m θ. (See Alcohol. Chloroform. Cocaine. Ether. Ice. Turpentine.)

ANEURISM.--*Cal p, 3 to 6x.* Dig. *Fl ac. 12 to 30x.* Lyc--Of the aorta, Spo. "Ergot, 1 to 2 grs. in solution; or Ham θ dilute, 20 drops, inject behind or near the vessel."

ANGINA PECTORIS.--See Heart.

ANKLE.--See Limb--Leg, foot.

ANTHRAX.—See Carbuncle.

ANTIDOTE.--

In general: Olive oil, gill doses. Sugar and water mixed, thick. White of egg. See *Emetic.*

Acids in general: Powdered Magnesia, Soda or Chalk in warm water.

Alkalies in general: Vinegar. Lemonade. Sour Milk. ("Need not induce emesis.")

Vegetable poisons: Camphor θ 10 to 30 drops, in Sugar water. Vinegar. Emetic, see.

Phosphorus poisoning: Turpentine, ½ oz. in coffee—*no oil* or grease of any kind.

Arsenic: Lime water and milk equal parts. Dialyzed Iron, teaspoonful dose. Peroxide of

ANTISEPTIC.

Iron, a teaspoonful. Iron rust stirred in sugar
water. White of egg.

Atropia or Belladonna: Bromide of Potash,
adult 8 gr, ½ hour. Opium tincture 30 to 60
drops, ¼ hour, until effect apparent. Emetic,
see.

*Acetate of Lead, Corrosive Sublimate. Blue
Vitriol, and other Soluble Salts:*—Baking
Soda, adult 50 grains, dissolved in water. (See
general advice at head of this Caption.)

Opium or Morphine: Cocaine 1x. 1 gr, ¼ hour.
Nux v 0, 1 drop, 5 minutes. Permanganate of
potash, ¼ grain for every grain of Morphine.
Strong coffee. VINEGAR 4 OUNCES. *Dilate
the Anus.* (See Amyl. ICE.)

Strychnine or *Nux vomica:* Chloral hydrate 1
drachm, in teacupful of water, adult, take of
this a teaspoonful, ¼ hour. IODINE TINCT-
URE 30 drops, in a teaspoonful of whisky,
"unfailing."—Camphor 5 grains dissolved in
mucilage.

Sinking, "*death-door*" *condition,* from poisoning, or from any cause:—Hydrogen perox 1
vol. 10 drops in water, ¼ hour. Cocaine 1x,
1 gr, ¼ hour.

ANTISEPTIC.—See Wound. See Amputation.
ANUS AND RECTUM :—

Ascarides :—See Worms.

Fissure :—*Cal fl.* Grap. Nat m. Nit a. *Pæon int.
and ex. Thuj int. and ex.* Collodion applied,
though severe for a moment, directly soothes
and heals. (See *Acetan.* Coca. Glycerine.
Hamamel. Iodoform. *Silver*—See Ointment—
See *Suppository.*)

Fistula : Calc. *Fl ac.* Sil. Thuj int. and ex. *Essence of Turpentine inject.* Dilute tincture of

Iodine inject. (See *Acetan*. Cocaine. Iodoform. *Suppository*.)

Piles: Æs 2x. Collin *ᵛ* 10 drops, 6 hours. *Nux v* and *Sulph*. Thuj int. and ex. "For inflamed protruding piles, there is nothing that gives more speedy relief than the application of the broad leaf plantain reduced to a pulp, and kept bound to the parts by compress, and renewed as occasion requires." Raw Onion pulp applied is excellent.

Bleeding, ACO. Bell. Ham. Ip. Pho.

Burning, *Ars*. Calc. *Caps*. Lach.

Itching, *Aco*. Nux v. Pul. *Sul*.

Exceedingly sensitive, intolerant of touch, *Aco*. Aur. Bell. MUR A. Nit a—Ulcerated, Sil—Walking insupportable, Caust. Ph a.

With sense of weight in the anus, *Allo*. Collin —Worse when stools are loose, Ig.

Apply Bismuth, or Calomel ointment; or Calomel powder dry—(See Borax. Cocaine. Hot Water. Mullein oil Ham. Lime. Sulph. Onion. Soda. Solar Cautery. Thuj. Ichthyol. Tann.—See Ointment—See Suppository.)

Proctitis: (Oozing and urging at the anus.) *Colch*. Collin. Lach—Oozing bloody slime, Nit a.

Paralysis of sphincter: (Incomplete closure of the anus):—Alo. Bell. Gel. Ham. Hyo—Anus stands open in diarrhœa, Apis, Pho.

Prolapsus of the rectum:—Æs. Cal. iod. *Indig*. 2x. Ferr iod—With every stool, Chel 2x. *Ig*. *Pod*—Anus dark and bloody, Mer— Stools costive, Grap. Mez. *Nux v*. Lyc. (See Turpentine.)

Stricture: Borax. Pho. (See Coca—See Suppository.)

Tenesmus: *Caps.* Mer c. Rheu. *Mag p.* See Bowel—stools, with.

Pain. Sensation. Condition of Anus and Rectum:—

Aching, Æs. Ig. PB. *Sep.* Sul—After eating, Nux v—After stool, Alu. *Grap.* Sil. Sul.

Beating like little hammers, Lach.

Bleeding, *Aco. Lach.* Mer. ZN—Oozing bloody slime, Nit a.

Burning, Am c. Ars Berb. *Caps.* Nat m—With diarrhœa, Alo. Ars. *Iris v.* Mer—With constipation, *Grap.* Nit a. Sep. *Sul.*

Constriction or tight Closure, Alu. Collin. Lyc. Nat m—Spasmodic, Nux v. Op. PB. (See Suppository.) Cramp, Cinni. Kali bi. Kreo.

Cutting pain, Ars. *Lach.*, Nit a. Nux v. Sil.

Dampness, Ana. *Carb a.* Carbol a. Sil. Sul.

Dryness and Pricking, Æs. Agar. Collin.

Fulness and pressure, Æs. Lil t.—Like a plug, Ana. Alo. Sep.—With urging to stool constant, Lil t.

Heat, Æs. Alo. *Con.* Mer c.

Irritation in rectum and vagina constant, Sabin.

Itching, ACO. Æs. Grap. Lyc. *Spig.* Ratan. *Slag. Sul*—With burning, Alu. Carb v—With tingling, *Aco. Urti*—Preventing sleep, Teucr. "Stop drinking coffee"—(See Itching—*Local*—Pruritus.)

Numbness, Aco.

Soreness, Smarting, Æs. Berb. Caust. Ig. Pæon int. and ex. *Sul. Thuj int and ex*—For hours after hard stool, Am m. Grap. Ig—

Relieved by cold water applied, Alo. Alu. Apis.

Stitches, *Cro.* IG. Lyc. Nit a. SEP—When coughing, Lach—During stool, Grap—After eating, Nux v.

Stricture. See Cocaine. See Suppository.

Throbbing, Apis, Mer.

Tingling, *Aco.* Urti. Teuc.

Urging constant *not* to stool, Lach

Ulcer, Grap. *Hydras int. and ex.* Pæon in and ex. Nit a. Sil. *Thuj in and ex.* (See Cocaine. Ham. Silver. See Suppository.)

Warts around the Anus, Nit a. *Thuj int. and ex.*

APHONY.—See Chest—Voice

APOPLEXY.—

Early stage, insensibility, ACO. Gel θ. Glo 3x. Amyl by inhalation. Injection of table tea.

Involving the lungs, "breathless," Bacill 30, 200., Helo h. 200.

Inability to swallow, Bell. Hyo. Lach.

Face red, Aco. Bell. Coc—Blue, Bell. Lach— Drawn to the right, Lach—To the left, Bell.

Mouth frothing, Hyo—Wide open, Nux v.

Limbs rigid, Op Nux v.

Twitching, Hyo. Op.

Involuntary passages, ARN. Bell. Hyo.

After effect, Caust. PB. ZN.

Guard—Hell. *Nux v.* Pho. *Temperance.*

APPARENT DEATH.—From *anæsthesia*, or other cause, hold patient suspended by the feet a few seconds. Same for *new born babe.*

Forcibly dilate the anus. (See Hot water. Ice.)

From coal gas:—Supply of fresh air. "Snap the end of a wet towel against the bare breast and stomach."

APPARENT DEATH.

From Convulsions:—See Hot water.

From Hæmorrhage:—Hot sand bag to back of the head. Ligature of limbs at axilla and groin. Hydrogen perox. 1 vol. 10 drops in water, 5 minutes. (See Hot water.)

From Drowning:—Glo 2x solution, hypoderm. Lach. Tart. e. (See *Salt.*) Suspend patient, head down for 8 or 10 seconds, then place on the back, and press the chest for 2 or 3 seconds, then *suspend* again—and thus proceed—Recovery even after an hour.

From Freezing: Rhus. Sponge all over with Bicarbonate of Soda, rich solution, in cold water. The same treatment as for burn or scald. (See Hot water.)

From Lighting: Nux v. See Cold water—Blindness from lightning, Pho.

From sun-stroke: Camp. GLO. 2x. Therid. *Quinin,* hypoderm.

From fall or blow: Arn. Hyper. (See Hot water.)

☞ To discriminate between real and apparent death; bind a cord tightly around the middle finger, above the first joint; if the tip of the finger assumes a *dark reddish* hue, life is not extinct. Place the end of patient's finger in the flame of a candle until a blister forms: then open the blister; if it contains liquid, the patient is *not* dead. Pinch the pupil of the eye between thumb and finger until closed; and if it does not return to its round shape, death is real. In case of real death, a wound made by the prick of a pin *stands open*.

When there is a suspicion that life is not totally extinct, the body should be placed in a *warm* room, with wrappings about the feet. Nature in her time, perhaps, after several days, may restore to life.

APPENDICITIS :—See Abdomen.

APPETITE :--See Stomach.

ARM :--See Limb.

ARM-PIT :--See Limb--Arm--*under*.

ARNICA :—*Ailments from Injury:* Wring flannel out of hot water, containing Arnica θ a tablespoonful to the pint, and apply.

Bee-sting, Boil, Carbuncle, Sore nipple: Arnica θ dilute, apply; or Arnica oil. (See Ointment.)

Deafness: Arnica tincture dilute, drop in the ear.

ARSENIC POISONING :—See Antidote.

ARTHRITIS :—*Benzo ac. Lith lac.* (See Gout--Rheumatism.)

ASCARIDES :—See Worms.

ASPHYXIA :--See Apparent Death.

ASTHENOPIA :—See Eye—*sight.*

ASTHMA :—See Chest--*Respiration difficult.*

ASTIGMATISM : — Lil t. Physos. See Eye—*sight.*

ATHEROMA :—Pho—See Seaton.

ATROPHY, MARASMUS :—(See Diet F—See Olive Oil.)

Old wrinkled look, Arg n. Calc. Oll-j θ, Sars.
Good appetite, Calc. Iod. Stap.
Cough, *Ars iod.* Calc. Pho. *Stan iod.*
Large head, open fontanelles, Calc. Sil. Sul.
Head sweat in sleep, *Calc.* Mer Sil.
Hot vertex, Sul.
Dry—parchment-like skin, Ars.
Undigested stools, Chin. Pho.

ATROPIA POISONING.

Cold damp feet, Calc.
Progressive Muscular Atrophy, Pho. *PB.* Physos. Nux v. (See Person.)

ATROPIA POISONING :—See Antidote.
AVERSION :—See Stomach.
AXILLA :—See Limb—Arm, *under.*
AZOTURIA :—Caust. Con. Gel. Nat m.
BABY'S SORE MOUTH :—See Mouth.
BACK :—(See Belladonna.)

Backache :—(See Pains, sensations and conditions of the Back.)

Constant pain in the back, without aggravation or amelioration, *Cann I.* Hemp extract ¼, ½ gr, 12 hour.

Pains extending up into the head, Kalm. Phyt. Sil—Beneath the right shoulder-blade, *Chel*—Down the thighs, Cimi—Into the bladder, Berb—Into the groin, Cann I—Pubes, Sabin—Across the shoulders, causing to stoop, Cann I—Across the hips, *Cimi.* Berb. Ox a—*Deep seated spine pain*, Agar. Alu Ox a. Pic a.

Better lying perfectly still, BRY—On the back, Nat m. Rhus—On the stomach, Acet a—Moving, RHUS Ruta—Continual motion, Cal fl. Rhus—After passing urine, Lyc.

Worse from motion, jar, misstep, *Agar.* BELL. BRY. Berb. Sil. Thuj—At night, Mer. Rhus. Phyt—Lying down, BELL—Sitting, Berb. Rhod. *Rhus.* ZN—stooping, Æs—Turning in in bed, NUX V.

From fall or hurt, Arn. Con. Hyper—Stone in the kidney, Bell. Berb. BURSA θ. Lyc. URTI θ.

With hot urine, Canth—Urinary tenesmus, Canth. Nux v—High fever, Aco. *Bell.* TART E —Cold sweat, TART E—Trembling, Agar. Cic.

Lumbago: — See Remedies *indicated* under **Backache**; especially Bell. *Bry.* Nux. *Rhus. Tart e.*

"Collodium, Iodine tincture, and Ammonia water, in equal parts mixed and applied, with Camel-hair brush: Constitutes an instantaneous remedy for *Lumbago.*" (See Pain—See Lard. Sulphur. Turpen.)

Curvature Dorsal:—Bacil 30—200. *Calc. Cal p.* Lyc. *Sil.* Sul—See Veratrum.

Spinal Irritation:—*Agar. Alu.* Bell. Cimi. Pho. *Sil*—Congestive, Alu. *Gel.* Sec. *Ustil.* Vert v. (See Belledon. Ether. Veratrum.)

Softening of the Spine :—Alu. Pic ac.

Spina Bifida:—Cal p. Sil—See Veratrum.

Pain, Sensation, Condition of Back :—

Aching, Agar. Cimi. *Eup per.* Ran b—As after stooping a long time, Dol. Pul. Rhus—As if broken, *Eup per.* GRAP. Kal c. Ova t. Nux v—Would break, BELL. Eup per. Ox a.

Bubbling, Berb. Tereb.

Burning along the spine, Alu. *Carb a.* Pic a. *ZN*—Between the shoulders, Bry. *Lyc.* Pho Under the shoulder blade, Ran b—In the small of the back, Bar c. Sep. Sul—Over the loins, Tereb—As if hot iron thrust through the spine, Alu.

Bruise-like pain, Arn. Berb. *Eup per.* Nux v. Rhod. *Rhus. Ruta.* Sul.

Coldness, Sec. Sil. Sul. Verat a—Between the shoulders, Ars. Agn. *Am m. Sep*—As from cold wind, Cact—Chills ran up and down the back, *Gel.* Spo. *Sul.*

Dragging down, Alston v. Nat m—From the shoulders, Lil t.

BALANITIS.

Heat, Con. Mer. Sul—low down, Berb.

Pressure low down in the spine, Arg n. Ox a—
Like a weight, Pet. Sep. Sul—The limbs
cold and heavy, Pic ac.

Numbness, Aco. *Berb*. Spo.

Rubbing as of one spine upon another, Sul.

Shrugs, involuntary, Mygal.

Stiffness, Berb. Rhus—"Stiff as a board,"
Phel—Stiff between the shoulders, Am m.
Chel—Hard rigid muscles, Cimi.

Stitches, Alu. *Kal c*. Sul—Beneath the right
shoulder, Chel.

Sprained feeling, *Cimi*. Pet. *Sul*.

Tenderness of the spine, *Agar. Chin s.
Cimi*. Hyper. Ox a. *Pho. Sil*. Tarent c.

TELL—With trembling, Cic. Ox a. ZN.

Weak "Lame back," Con. Lach. Sep—"Bell
plaster "—"Gives out," ÆS. Berb. Nux v.
Sul—Cannot sit up, ZN—Walking bent, Sul
—Weak knees, COC — Trembling limbs,
Apis, ZN.

Weary, tired back, Apis, Nat m. Rhus. Sul.

Lowest point of the spine:—

Bruise-like feeling, Ruta. Sil.

Burning, Val.

Itching, Ox a.

Stinging, Sil.

Tenderness, Cist. Sil.

Painful sitting, Pet—Standing, Val.

Tetter around the seat bone, BOVIS. Pet.
Nat m.

BALANITIS :—Thuj—See Male.

BALDNESS :—See Head—hair.

BANDAGE :—

Speedy labor—No flooding:—Put the bandage on

early: secure it firmly with strong safety
pins: as labor advances renew the tightening.

Flooding after Labor, or *Miscarriage*, *Congestion of Lungs and Heart*, *Ague Chill at the
Onset:*—Bandage limbs tightly at groin and
arm-pit: keep the blood in the extremities.

Diarrhœa:—Bandage the lower abdomen tightly.

Epileptic fits, prevention:—Wear a buckled strap
around the waist, or ankle, and draw it quickly
tight at the first warning of the fit.

Colic: Tight bandage around the waist.

Hiccough: Tight girth, just below the point of
the breast bone.

Pneumonia, *Pleurisy*, *Pleurodynia:*—Apply a
firm tight bandage of adhesive plaster all
around the region of the Chest in which is the
seat of pain and over this a roller bandage.

In case of extensive pneumonia, it may sometimes be necessary to bandage from waist to
arm-pit. This gives entire relief to the
muscles of the Chest, and throws the whole
labor of respiration upon the abdominal
muscles.

" *Inward weakness*," *Dragging down sensation*,
Falling of the womb, or *Bowel:*—The one essential thing needed—Extra of medicine—is
abdominal and dorsal support—Secure a good
Brace.

BARBER'S ITCH :—See Face.

BARRENNESS—STERILITY :—Alet θ. Borax.
Con.

Seek cause and treat accordingly.

BASEDOW'S DISEASE :—Natrum sali.

BEARD :—On Lady's face. See face.
—Falling out, Calc. Grap. Nat m. See Face.

BED-ROOM AIR KEPT PURE:—See Air, purified.

BED-SORE:—See Skin.

BEE STING:—Led. The whole system power-fully affected. Olive oil, adult 1 oz.
> Apply *Arnica θ.* Tobacco juice. Urine. Moist-ened Salaratus. Ice. (See *Salt.*)

BELCHING:—See Stomach.

BELLADONNA:—"*Lame back," Spine pain. "Pain in the side* ": Bell plaster.
> *Breasts threatening to gather:* Bell. plaster, with hole for nipple.
> *Rigid os:* Bell. Ointment.
> *Ophthalmia. Pain in the eye ball:* Introduce into the eye as often as needful, Atropia solu-tion, (2 gr to 1 oz water) a drop or two at time.
> *Suppurative Keratitis:* "Bell. fl. ex. 1 part, to 8 parts Rose water; use as a Collyrium, and fleck Calomel into the eye."

BENZOIN:—*Ganglia, Tendinous swelling, at the back of the wrist:* Benzoic Ointment, 5 grains of the Acid to 1 ounce vaseline.
> *Freckles, Eruptions on the face:* Benzoin, spirit-uous solution, in 20 parts Rose water, ap-ply several times a day.
> *Toothache in hollow tooth:*—Saturate Cotton with Compound tincture of Benzoin, and pack it in the hollow tooth.
> *Sore nipples:* Wipe the nipple dry, after the child has nursed, then with Camel hair brush, apply four or five coats of the Compound tincture of Benzoin. This forms an artificial skin. It burns a little at first, but soon affords relief.

Chapped Skin, Chafing, Cuts, Wounds: Coat with Compound Tincture of Benzoin, or apply the same on a soft rag.

" *Bronchial affections. Obstinate winter cough, Hawking, Catarrh of the Throat. Chronic Sore Throat:* Compound Tincture of Benzoin, adult, take a teaspoonful, beaten up with milk, three or four times a day."

BETTER:—See Amelioration—See Pain, better—See the special affections, or organs.

BILIARY CULCULI:—See Liver—Gall stone.

BILIOUSNESS:—See Liver—See Stomach.
Prominent remedies, Chel. *Eup per.* Euony. *Homar* 3x. POD. Mer. Sang. See Lemon.

BILIOUS FEVER:—See Fever—Bilious.

BIRTH MARK:—See Skin.

BISMUTH SUBNIT:—*Burn, Scald, Chap, Eczema:* Bism. 5 per cent in Lanolin or vaselin apply.

Chancre—Chafing, Eczema, Erythema, Erysipelas, Bed sore, Sore mouth, Noma, Sore nipple, Wound: Bism pulv. ext: Cover the parts well, renew as often as needful.

Offensive feet:—Bism pulv. well rubbed in daily.

Pain and Swelling of Testes: Bism pulv. in water, paste thick as cream, apply.

Nasal Catarrh ("Catarrh Snuff"): Bism powder 6 oz: Morph sulph 2 grs: Pulv. Gum Arabic 2 drachms: Mix thoroughly: Snuff freely of this several times a day.

BITE:—
Human, Lach.
Animal, Hyper, int. and ex. Pæon, int. and ex. (See Lime. Vinegar.)
Mad dog—See Hydrophobia.

BLADDER.

Snake, ACO. Cedron *θ* Hoang *θ* LACH. Pæon. Plantago *θ*. Sisyrinchium *θ* drop doses in water, and the same on cotton apply to the bite. Alcoholic liquor to intoxication. OLIVE OIL, ½ oz, ½ hour. Iodine Tincture, adult 6 drops, 3 hours, in water. IODIDE OF AMMONIA, adult, 3 drops, ½ hour, in water. Potash permang 2 gr, in water 1 drachm, hypoderm. *Spirits of Ammonia, 60 drops, hypoderm.* Pour *gun powder* on the bite, and touch it with a lighted match. This is an almost painless Cautery, and excellent guard against infection. Put your mouth to the wound, and suck out the poison; if there is no sore in the mouth or on the lips, you may thus save a life, and do yourself no harm.

"The remedy that never fails in case of *snake bite*, (and perhaps our best hope in case of mad dog bite) is to procure half dozen fowls, pluck the feathers *and skin* from the fleshy part of one, and apply the raw surface to the bite: the first fowl will die in 10 seconds, the second in 2 minutes, the third in 6 minutes, the fourth in 10 minutes, the fifth will become giddy but not die. The poison is *now* extracted! Patient saved."

Spider: Lach. Plantago. INDIGO IN STRONG SOLUTION APPLY: this destroys the venom even of a Tarantula. Soda moistened and applied is excellent. (See Salt. See Ointment.)

Mosquito: Apis. Am c. LED. Apply Arnica *θ*. *Ledum θ*. Lemon juice. (See Ointment.)

BLADDER:—See Urinary Organs.

BLEAR-EYE:—See Eye—phlegm.

BLEEDING, IN GENERAL:—Cocaine 2x. *Ipe. pure*, 2 gr ¼ hour. *Ipe θ 3 drops*, 3 minutes.

36

Tereb *θ* in milk 5 to 10 drops, ¼ hour. VINEGAR dilute 1 gill, ¼ hour.

Introduce the fumes of boiling vinegar upon the bleeding part; inhale the fumes if bleeding from nose or lungs. Tight cordage of the limbs at gorin and axilla.

Hæmorahagic Diathesis: COCAIN 2x. Crotal 200. FERR. MILL. PHOS. Sec. Tereb., TRILL. USTIL.—Active, MELI.—Passive, HAM. (See Organs affected.)

Bleeding Growth: Cal p. Ergot 1x. Ham *θ*. Thuj in. and ex. Chloroform on lint; or absorbent cotton apply. (See Iron—Solar Cautery.)

Bleeding Wound: Pho. Shot bag pressure. (See Alum. *Chloroform.* Hot Water. IRON. VINEGAR.)

Bleeding from Socket After Tooth Drawn:— See Alum.

Bleeding from the Navel: Crotal 200. Plaster of Paris plug. Ham *θ* on cotton apply. (See Alum. Iron.)

BLENORRHŒA :—See Gonorrhœa—Gleet.

BLEPHARITIS :—See Eye—Lids inflamed.

BLINDNESS :—See Eye-Sight.

BLISTER : See Skin.

BLOAT :—See part affected—See Dropsy.

BLOOD DISEASE :—See Ichthyol.

BLOOD POISON : ECHIN. See Cause.

BLOOD BOIL :—See Skin—Boil.

BLOOD TUMOR ON SCALP :—Cal fl. Sil. It disappears without treatment.

BOIL :—See Skin.

BOLD HIVE :—See Skin—Hive.

BONE :—Disease in general, Bacill 30-200. Cal fl. Fl ac. Therid.

BORAX.

Caries: ASA. AUR. Cal p Fl ac. LYC. Mer.
Pho. SIL. Sul. (See Hydrogen. Lactic acid.)

Necrosis: ARS. AUR. Pho. SIL. Therid.

Exostosis. — Tumor: Aur. Cal fl. HEC L.
Kali iod. Pho.

Node—Lump: Aur. MEZ. Nit a. Sil. STILL—
Gouty node, Ant c. Cal c. *Led and Rhod.* Lyc.

Rickets—Softening: Asa. CAL C. Mer. SIL.

Ostitis: Asa. Mer. Sil Stap. Sul.

Periostitis: Asa. Mer. *Phyt. Ruta.* Sil.

Pain. Sensation. Condition of Bone.
Fracture pain., Cal p. Ruta. SYMPH.

Nightly pain, Aur. *Mer.* Kal iod. Phyt. Mez—
In the shin bone, Dul. Lach.

Band like, binding, Nit a. Pul. Sul.

Bruise-like, Coc. Hep. Ruta.

Burning, Mez. ZN.

Gnawing, *Bell.* Kal iod. Ruta.

Jerking, Asa. *Chin.* Sul.

Loosened, as from the flesh, *Rhus.* Thuj.

Numbness, Fl a.

Pinching, Verb.

Scraping, as flesh from bone, Chin. Ph a.
Rhus.

Swelling, Asa. Cal c. Ph a. Sil. Stap. Sul.

Tenderness, *Asa. Eup per.* Hep. *Led.* Pho.
Tell.

BORAX:—*Baby's Sore Mouth:* Borax dissolved in
glycerine, or mixed in honey, apply.

Local Itching. Itching Piles: Borax and Lard.
1 part to 3, mix and apply. On sponge in vagina or vulva; on bougie in urethra.

Pimple: Borax 1 part, and Rose water 100 parts;
mix; lave.

Eye Wash: Boracic acid 2 drachms to water 1

pint; or Boracic acid 5 grains in water 1 ounce
a few drops in the eye several time a day.

Noises in the Ear: Boracic acid 10 grains, in
water 1 ounce. Mix; drop a little in the ear
three times a day

Otorrhœa: Sponge out the ear with warm water,
and swab dry, then saturate a piece of cotton
with glycerine and squeeze it until only moist;
dip it into pulverized Boracic acid, and insert
it into the ear, daily. "Cure in 12 days."

Dandruff. Eczema. Eruptions: Boracic acid,
saturated solution, in boiling water, apply
three or four times a day—do not make an
ointment of it.

Gonorrhœa: Male—Inject twice a day, a solution of Boracic acid, 5 gr. to 1 oz. water. *Female*—Use 10 to 15 gr. to the oz. of water.
Saturate a sponge, tied to a stick, with this,
and therewith cleanse the part thoroughly
once a day. This is much better than using a
syringe for women. "This treatment does not
fail to cure in from 10 to 15 days."

BOWELS:—

Cholera: ARS 2x. CUP M 2x. VERAT A 1x.
Camp θ 5 drops, 5 minutes, on sugar. "Cup
m 2x trit. 1 grain: in 10 minutes repeat; in 20
minutes again; and in 30 minutes again;
Cure!" "Chloroform 10 drops, 10 minutes:
or adult, a tablespoonful in 4 tablespoonfuls of
water. One dose cures." "Ice water all the
patient will drink. Cure even in collapse."
"Blister behind the ear, and along the jugular
to collar bone. This arrests all the symptoms
at once."

Hot and thirsty, Aco θ.

Cold, blue, Carb v., *Camp.* Laur. *Sec.* Verat a—

But will not be covered, Camp. Sec.
Cold sweat, *Ars.* Tab. *Verat a.*
Collapse, *Laur. Kal p.*
Liquids gurgle in the throat, Cup m. Laur.
Urine suppressed, *Ars.* Canth. Tereb.
Guard. Take Cap m. Carry Gum Camphor
about the person—See Sulphur. (See *Camphor.* Collodion.)

Cholerine: Ipe. *Ph ac.* Pod.

Cholera Morbus: *Ipe.* and *Pet.* IRIS V.
Verat a.
Persistent *nausea*, Ipe.
Violent retching, *Verat a*—Sour vomit, Iris v.
Cold sweat, *Verat a.*
Cramp, Cup m. Nux v. *Verat a.*
Violent thirst, Ars.
Milk white tongue, Ant c.

Cholera Infantum—" Summer Complaint":
(See Infant) Ferr p. *Ipe and Pet.* IRIS V.
" Resorcin 1 to 3 grain dose excellent."
Verat a See Diet. D. E. Z.
Restlessness, thirst, Aco. Ars.
Drowsiness, starting in sleep, Bell.
Stupor, shrieks, Apis—Fixed stare, Æth.
Moaning, rolling the head, *Bell.* POD.
Gagging, Æth. POD.
Vomiting milk in thick curds, Æth.
Head sweat in sleep, Cal c—Hot head sweat,
Cham.
Cold sweat on the forehead, Verat a.
Sour Stools. See Gum Arabic. See Diet. Z.
Urine suppressed, Apis. Ars. (See Coffee—See
Diet. K. Z.)

Constipation: " *Alu* 200 and *Opi* 200 alt. 3
hours." COLLIN θ 10 drops, 6 hours. Nat m 2x
trit., 5 grains, 6 hours. " Cascara Segrada, 1

ounce; Glycerine 2 ounces; Water 1 ounce. Mix;
Adult, 1 teaspoonful, every 4 hours for 2 days,
then three times a day, until stools loose, then
reduce the doses gradually, and lengthen the
intervals between them, until the cure is effected." " Aloes, 1 pervule, 3 times a day."
"Podophyl 2 pervules, 3 times a day." Headache and pain in the anus after stool, Hydras
0. 1 drop before breakfast for a week. (See
Elm. Ichthyol).

Headache and piles, ÆS. Hydras. Nit a.

Drowsiness—dizziness, Op.

Flashes of heat. Hot vertex, Sul.

Dry, harsh skin, ALU. GRAP.

Flatulence, rumbling, LYC. Nit a.

Burning anus after stool, Sul.

Ineffectual urging, Lyc. *Nux v.*

Stool hard dry, as if burnt, Bry.

Small hard balls, Op. PB.

Putty like stools—straining, Plat.

Aperients: " Sugar of Milk, 3 teaspoonfuls in
½ teacupful of hot milk, or hot water, taken
one hour before breakfast, will move the bowels in two hours." " Irisin, adult, 5 grs.; insures a painless passage, without being followed by costiveness."

A cup of yeast is pleasant, safe and sure.

" Aloes 6 Parvules at bed time." " Podoph.
6 Parvules at bed time." Glycerine enema,
1 drachm. Introduce a pledget of cotton
saturated with Glycerine into the rectum.
(See Castor Oil. See Lard See *Suppository*.)

Diarrhœa:—CHINA ARS Cuprum ars. Iris v.
IPE and PET. MER C 3x trit. ŒNOTH 0
10 drops, 4 hours. "Codein ½ to 1 gr, 12 hours."
" Nine-tenths of all ordinary cases of Diar-

rhœa, also *Lientery*, may be cured with Compound tincture of Cinchona 2 parts; and Tincture of Opium 1 part, mixed; Adult, 5 drops. Every hour or two." "Cinnamon tea." "Nutmeg tea." Hot Lemonade. *Hot boiled milk.* (See Alum. Bandage: Charcoal. Lemon.)

Day time diarrhœa, *Ipe and Pet.* Nat m.

Early morning, Bry. Pod. *Sul.*

Night, Chin. Pul. Sul.

Alternating with constipation, *Ant c.* Nux v. Pho. Pol.

Catarrhal, "Camp diarrhœa," DUL. *Ipe and Pet.* Lept. Nabal θ—"From *bad water*, Essence of Ginger."

Consumptive, *Arg n.* Bap. Chin. Ferr. PHO.

Chronic, Ars. DUL. IPE and PET. ŒNOTH θ 10 drops 6 hours. Pho. Pod Sul.

Adiposa. (Fat in stool). Adult cured by taking olive oil. 1 gill. 4 times a day.

Fever—Thirst, Aco. Ars.

Dry tongue—No *thirst.* Apis.

Pallor, Ars.

Cold hands, blue, Apis. Cup m.

Clammy sweat, Ars—Profuse, Verat a.

Chilliness, Mer.

Pain—Colic, Ip. Dul. *Gambo.* Mer. *Verat a.*

Painless, Ph a. Pod.

Nausea, Ip.

Vomiting, Ip. Iris v. Verat a.

Stools gushing, Croton—Noisy flatulent, Alo. Ph a.

Undigested, Bry. Chin. Ferr—Watery, Ars. Apis. Cal c. Chin. Croton—Whitish, Cal c. Mer. Ph a.

Dysentery: In general, IPE and PET. COLO

and MERC. MER C 3x trit. ŒNOTH b θ 10
drops, 4 hours. See (Hot water. Starch)
"First," ACO 2x.

High fever, Aco. Bell. Euca.

Nausea and vomiting, Ipe.

Prostration extreme, Ars. Rhus.

Stool *very* bloody, *Arn.* Bap. Ip. *Mer c*—
shreddy like scrapings, Arg n. Canth. Colch
—Red like washings, Rhus.

During stool, Colic, Colo—Rumbling, Alo—
Painful tenesmus, Bell. Caps *Mer c*. MAG. P.
Nux v.

After stool, faintness, Alo—Burning anus, Ars.
Bap—Prolapsus ani, Mer. Pod—Great relief,
Nux v.

Urine scanty hot, or suppressed, Bell. Canth.
Merc—Stranguary, Canth. Caps.

Hæmorrhage of the bowel: Am c. Arn. CO-
CAINE 3x. Ham. *Ipe*. Pho. Charcoal powder
20 gr. 2 hours, in milk. See stools bloody—
See BLEEDING.

Intussusception — Bowel obstruction. — See
Abdomen.

Stools Costive:—

Dry hard, as if burnt, Bry—Crumbling, Am.
m. *Mag m. Nat m.* Nux v—In *balls*, like
sheep dung, Chel. *Op. PB.* Sep—Scanty
hard hurting the anus, *Alu. Grap.* Lyc.
Nit a. Nux v. Sul. ZN.

Hard dry long slender, Pho.

Partly digested, Cal c. Hep.

Bowels loose:—

Acrid, corroding the anus, Ars. *Cham.* Mer.
Sul.

Black, Ars. LEPT. Mer. Verat a—First part

black the rest white, Æs—Black liquid, *Ars.*
Kal bi. verat a—In Typhoid, Ars. Ph a.

Bloody, *Arn.* Apoc. *Bap.* Caps. Carb v. Ferr p.
Mer c—Nearly pure blood, Arn. Bap. Mer c
—Blood and slime, Arn Apis. Carb v. IPE
AND PET. *Mer c.* With fever, Aco. Bell.
Bap—In Typhoid fever, Am c. ALU. Lach.
Nit a. TEREB. *Sec 200*—Like charred straw
in Typhoid, LACH—Putrid blood, Kal p.
Lach.

Burning liquid, Ars. Iris v. Nat m—" Hot water," *Ars.* *Cham.* Dios θ. Iris v.

Changeable, no two alike, Pul.

Clay color, Pod. Rheu.

Fermenting, Arn. Ipe.

Frothy, Kali bi, Mag c.

Gurgling, gushing, Gambo. CROTON. Elat.
Pod. PHO. Thuj—Noisy flatulent, *Arg n.*
Alo. Ph a. Thuj.

Green slime, Ars. Bell. *Cham.* Colo. Dul. IPE.
Mag c. Mag p. Mer c—Green with white
masses, Mag c—Green like chopped spinach,
Aco. Arg n. MAG P—Green and sour, Hep.
POD. RHEU. Sul—Green liquid, *Cham.*
Dul. Pod. Mag c. Verat a.

Odorless, Hyo. *Paull s.* Rhus.

Oily, Iod., Thuj—Greasy shine, Caust.

Putrid odor, *Ars.* Asa. *Carb v.* Cham. Kal p.
Lach. Pod. Sul.

Rice water gush, Colch.

Red slime, Arg n *Canth.* Grap. *Rhus.* Sul—
Red like washings of the intestines, Rhus.

Skinny-shreddy-like scrapings of the intestine,
Arg n. *Canth. Colch.* Colo. Nit a. Mer c.

Sour, *Calc.* Cham. Mag c. *Rheu. Hep. Nat p.*

Sticky adhesive, Sul—Sticking like paste to

the anus, Plat—Adhering like mud to the
chamber vessel, *Grap.* Mer pro.

Undigested, Ars. *Chin. Ferr.* Ferr p. Hep. Ol
—undigested and watery, Ph a. Pod. Sul a—
undigested and hard, Cal c. Grap—Painless
undigested, Ars. Chin. *Ferr.* Hyo. Ph a.
Pod—With great thirst, Sang. Sec.

Watery, Ars. Apis. Croton. Pilo—Watery gush,
Croton. Elat. (See *Liquid.* Black, Burning,
Green, White, Yellow)—Watery in Typhoid,
Ars. Ph a.

White, Aco. Bell. *Cal c. Hep.* Mer. Ph a. *Pod*
—With red urine, Aco—Gray-white, DIG.
Pho—Containing white grains, Cina. Pho—
White slime, like jelly, *Alo.* Colch. Hell.
Pod—White liquid, Pho. Ph a.

Wormy, Ant c. Cina. Mer c. Spig. Stan.
Teucr.   (See Worms.)

Yellow (orange or saffron) color, Borax. CHEL.
Colo. Sil. Sul—Yellow liquid, Apis. Chin.
Hyo. Dul.

Involuntary stool: In general, *Alo.* Ars. Carb v.
op. Rhus. Sec—At night, Rhus—In sleep, *Arn.*
Mos. Hyo.

Unnoticed, full form, in bed, *Alo.* Tarant C.

Jelly like mass drops, ALO. Colch. Hell.

Constant oozing, Apis. Pho.

In Typhoid, *Ars.* Hyos. *Mur a.* Op. *Ph a.*
Rhus.

From fall on the back, Hyper.

From fright, Op. Gel.

When passing urine, Mur a: or wind, Alo.

Call to stool urgent: *Alo.* Dul. Mer. *Pod.*

After taking food or drink, *Alo.* Chin. *Colo.*
Staph.

" Drinks go right through," *Arg n.* Croton.

"Morning rush," Apis. Bry. *Pod.* SUL—
Driving from bed, Alo. Rhus. SUL.
With every motion of the body, *Apis.* Bry.
Pho.

During stool:

Backache, Pul.
Bleeding anus (stool hard), Alu. Grap. Lyc.
Nat m.
Bleeding womb, Iod.
Burning anus, ARS. Croton. Canth. CAPS.
IRIS V. Mer. Sul.
Chilliness, MER. Mez. PUL. Verat a.
Cold sweat, Tart e Verat a.
Great prostration: ARS. Alo. *Gambo.* Pod.
Sec. Verat a.
Fainting, Gambo, Kali bi. *Nux m.*
Tremulous weakness, Con.
Gagging, Arg n. *Pod.*
Griping, Bap. CHAM. COLO. *Gambo.* Mer.
Verat a.
Pain in the thighs, Rhus.
Prolapsus ani, IG. INDIG 2x. *Pod.* Mer—stool
hard, Grap. Ig. Lyc. Mez.
Stitches in the anus, Ig. Grap. Sep.
Tearing in the anus, Alu. Nit a.
Weight like a plug in anus, Ana. *Alo.* Sep.
Tenesmus, straining, *Aco.* Bap. Canth. *Caps.*
Colch. Gambo. MER C. MAG P—"Never
get done," Mer c—Straining in vain, Ambr.
Lyc. NUX V—When straining the desire
for stool ceases, Ana—Stool partly expelled
recedes, Sil—Afraid to strain lest something
within should break, Apis: or prolapsus
occur, Ig—Must stand to have a passage,
Caust—*Cannot strain*, Alu. Ana. Sep.

Vomiting, Ant c. Cup m. *Ipe. Iris v.* Verat a—
Sour vomit, Iris v.

BRAIN:—See Head.

BREAST:—See Female.

BREATH OFFENSIVE:—Arn. Cham. Mer—In the morning, Nux v. Pul—After dinner, Cham. Sul—Sour, Nux v. Sul. (See Charcoal. Myrrh. Potash.)

BRIGHT'S DISEASE:—See Urinary Organs.

BROMINE:—See Iodine.

BRONCHITIS:—See Chest.

BRONCHOCELE:—See Chest.

BRONCHORRHŒA:—See Chest.

BRUISE, CONTUSION:—Arn. Hyper. (See *Arnica.* Calendula. Hama. Lead. *Ointment*).
To remove discoloration. See Starch.

BUBO:—See Syphilis.

BUNION:—See Limb—Leg, *foot.*

BURN OR SCALD:—Ars. Canth. Rhus. Urti.
External: *Coat of varnish. Milk dressing.* Bat of cotton. Oil of Peppermint, removes the pain at once. (See Alcohol. Alum. Cold water. Glycerine. Lard. *Lime.* LEAD. SODA. Vinegar. See *Ointment.*)
Powder burn:—Into beaten white of egg, stir in flour, until to consistency of mush. Cover the part with this. "Perfect success."
From inhalation of steam. "Apis first, then Kal bi." Milk gargle.
Slough, Hep. Sil. (See Charcoal. Clay. Thuj.)

BURSA:—Sil. (See Benzoin.)

CALENDULA:—*Contusion, Wound, Laceration, Gangrene, Suppuration excessive or unhealthy, Ulcerated Nipple:* Calendula tincture, diluted one half, or less with water, on cotton, apply. Calendula oil.

CALF.

CALF:—See Limb—Leg.

CAMPHOR:—*Abscess, Carbuncle:* To abort in early stage: Camp. spirits, and Lime water, equal parts, apply. "*Menthol*—ethereal solution—20 to 50 per cent., applied by camel-hair brush, will abort a *Boil* or *Carbuncle*, and assuage the *Itching* of *Eruptions*."

Sprain: Wrap the part in flannel, or absorbent cotton, saturated with Camphor spirits.

Mumps, shifted to the Testes: 'Pour Spirits of Camphor into a basin, and place the scrotum therein, and bathe and rub well in, over the lower abdomen, and region of loins and thighs. "In 30 minutes the pain and swelling will vanish."

CANCER:—*Acet a.* ARS. Carbol a Euca. Hydrast. *θ* in and ex. *Iod.* PHYT. *θ* in and ex. *Sil.* THUJ in. and ex.

Removal without the knife: Inject Mer c. (1000 solution) into the tumor twice a week.

Inject Glacial acetic acid, 10 drops in solution.

Inject pure Alcohol twice a week. Blister the tumor, and sprinkle it daily with a mixture of Arsenious acid 1 part; Morph. sulph. 1 part; and Calomel 8 parts; and Pulverized Gum Arabic 48 parts. This is a *painless* caustic. See Cocaine. (See Chromium. Resorcin)

Relapse prevented after excision: Carbol a 2x. 1 drop. 3 times a day.

Open Cancer: *Ars.* Condu. Ichthyol Hydrocot. Lapis. Sil. Thuj—*Dust it daily with Ars 2x tril*—Castor oil a good dressing.

Reported cure by application, three times a day, of fresh ergot, ground to an impalpable powder. The ulcer being thoroughly

48

cleansed before each application. (See
Acetan, Alcohol, Carbol a, Chlorine, Iodo-
form, Ichthyol, Hydrogen, LIME, SUL-
PHUR, THUJ in. and ex.)

Bleeding: Pho. (See Iron. Lime. Logwood)

Breast: Not open, Con. Iod. PHYT—Open,
Chimaph θ 10 drops, 5 hours. *Cal iod 2x.*

Nose: Ars. Aur. Calc. *Sil.* Sul.

Tongue: Condu. KALI CYANICUM 200. Mur a.
Thuj.

Stomach; Ars. Bacill 30-200. Condu 1x—Acid
vomit, Robin.

Liver: Cholesterin 200.

Womb: Ergot. Iod. Ova t 1-2x. Thuj.

Pain subdued: Ars. Trif p θ. *Salicylate of
sodium* 10 grains, 6 hours. CINNAMON θ full
doses. CITRIC ACID, 1 drachm in water 8
ounces. apply with camel-hair brush, or on
pledget of lint. *Lemon juice* apply.

Felor obviated: See Chlorine. Logwood. Potash.

Epithelioma: See Ichthyol. Resorcin. Lactic
acid. Thuj.

Rose Cancer: Mullein oil in. and ex.

CARBOLIC ACID :—*Baldness:* "Carbolic acid 95
per cent solution, swab on, and rub in; a second
application in two weeks if necessary. If the
baldness is very extensive, cultivate only about
2 or 3 inch square patch at a sitting; after about
2 or 3 weeks, downy fuzz will show. Oil of cade
may be used instead of carbolic acid with like
effect."

Otorrhœa: Inject into the ear daily, of a mixture
of Carbolic acid 1 drachm; Glycerine 1 ounce;
and water 5 ounces. This does not create the
slightest irritation, and is promptly curative.
The same by *lavement,* compress, gargle or in-

B* 49

CARBUNCLE.

jection, for *Anthrax, Gangrene, Ulceration, Unhealthy Suppuration, Offensive discharges and odors, Dandruff, Erysipelas, Burn, Scald, Throat affections, Leucorrhœa, Chronic Nasal Catarrh:* Taking at the same time Carbol ac 2x, alone or in alternation with Iod or Sulp.

Nasal Catarrh: Put Carbolic acid 12 drops into an ounce bottle, and snuff the fumes thereof, 5 minutes at a time, 6 times a day. "Cure."

Fever in general, Hyperæmia, Hyperexia, Hectic fever. All diseases attended with elevation of temperature or delirium; Scarlet Fever, Yellow Fever, Typhoid Fever, Puerperal Fever, Pyæmia, Septicæmia, Trichinosis, Asthma: Carbolic acid 2x, in drop doses in water; alone, or in alternation with *Ammonia,* in some of its preparations or compounds.

Chronic Diseases in general. Also acute when the tongue is coated with a dirty white fur, Chronic Gastric catarrh, Chronic rheumatism, Chronic cough, Smallpox, preventive of pitting: Carbolic acid 2x, drop doses in water; alone; or in alternation with Sulp.

Scrofula in all forms. Syphilis, Cancer, Pott's disease, Hip disease, Malaria, "Liver complaint:" Carbolic acid 2x, 1 drop in water; alone; or in alternation with Iod 2x.

CARBUNCLE :—See Skin.
CARCINOMA :—See Cancer.
CARDIALGIA :—See Stomach—pains.
CARIES :—See Bone.
CASTOR OIL :—Adult, ½ to 1 ounce. Infant 1 to 3 drachms. Unlike other purgatives; Castor oil allows of being lessened in dose, when the

CATALEPSY.

patient who resorts to it does so regularly. For infants it is the best of all purgatives. An Enema may be prepared by the combination of 2 or 3 ounces of Castor oil with some mucilaginous liquid. *Appendicitis, Typhlitis, Constipation from indurated fæces—Irritation of the bowels—Calculous affections;* For these ailments Castor oil is particularly valuable. A drop of the oil of cinnamon added to the dose masks the taste. A peppermint drop taken before and after the dose, also masks the taste.

CATALEPSY. (Motionless fit.) CANN I. Cic. Cinni. Cup m. Mag p. NUX M θ 2 Drop doses. Stram.

CATAMENIA :—See Female—Menses.

CATARACT :—See Eye—Sight.

CATARRH :—See the several organs.

CATARRHAL FEVER : See Fever—catarrhal.

CATHETER :—If in passing the catheter there is a difficulty, try with the patient standing slightly bent forward; if this fails, give a grain of opium, and after an hour try again. If the urine is too thick to flow, even by catheter, inject 16 to 20 grs. of pepsin dissolved in a little water, and in an hour the urine may flow by catheter.

CAUSE :—

Blood poison: from animal matter, ARS. Carb v. ECHIN. LACH. Kal p. PYROGEN (See Ichthyol. Resorcin)—From diphtheria, Ars iod. Kal p. *Pyrogen*—Impure vaccine, Bacill 30-200. Melandrinum Sil. THUJ—Urine retained, Canth. TEREB—Venomous bite, see bite—Cut of dissecting knife, Ars. LACH. (See *Ichthyol*. Resorcin.)

Drug poison: (Drug cachexia) in general,

CAUSE.

Nux v—*From Arsenic*, ZN—*From Bella-donna*, ZN—*From Cantharis*, Apis—*From Copper*, Sul. Verat a—*From Copaiva*, Benz a—*From Iodine*, Apis—*From Iron*, Pul. Sul.—*From Lead*, Kal iod. Op. Sul—*From Mercury*, Arg n. AUR. Carb v. Hep. Iod. KAL IOD. Lach. Mez. Pod. Phyt. NIT A. Stap. Sul—*From Opium*, Avena. Nux v. Pass ZN—*From Quinia*, ARN. Apis. ARS. Carb v. Caps. FERR. NAT M. Pul. Lach. Sul. Verat a—*From Thuja*, Stap—*From Turpentine*, Apis—*Rhus poisoning*, Rhus 200. Ana 200. Sang.

"*Change of life.*" Lach. See Female.

Check of perspiration: Aco. Bell. Cal c. Cham. China, Sil. Sul—Sudden check, *Aco. Bellis p. Rhus*—Inducing dropsy, Bry. Hell—*Check of foot sweat*, Bar c. SIL.

Check of catarrhal discharge, Bry. Cal c. Kal c. Kal iod. NUX V.

Check of menstrual flow, Cyc. grap. *Pul 30.* Verat a. (See Female—Menses, suppressed.)

Check of gonorrhœal discharge, Benz a. Tereb. Thuj.

Cold damp weather, Bellis p. Dul. Rhus. (See Aggravation.)

Cold floors, thin slippers, Dul. Led—feet swollen and tender, Led.

Cold, chilling rain, Bellis p. Cal p. RHUS. Sep —*Sea bathing*, Cal c. *Rhus.* Sep—*Working in water*, Cal c—*Getting feet wet*, Dul. Pul. Sil.

Exhausting drains; Avena. Aur. Carb v. CHINA. Cal c. *Pho.* PH A. Nat m—Seminal, *Ana.* Avena, *Agn.* Arg m. Aur mur. *Bacill 200. Bellis p.* Cal c. Con. PLAT. Ph ac. TARANT C. ZN.

Exposure to Chilling Wind, Aco.—*Hot rays of*

the sun, Bry. Glo. Hyo. (See sunstroke. See Aggravation)—Extreme heat or cold, Glo. Lach.

Emotions; in general, Ig—*Of anger*, Aco. *Cham.* Colo. Pet—*Depressing news*, Gel—*Fright*, Aco. Glo. *Ig. Op.* Stram. Verat a—*Fear remaining after fright*, Gel. *Op—Stage fright*, Ana 30. Cubeb. *Gel—Grief*, Colo. IG. Ph a. Stap—*Suppressed grief*, Hyo. *Ig.* Ly. Ph a. 1x —*Homesickness*, Caps. Ph a—*Indignation*, Colo. Stap—*Jealousy*, Hyo. Lach—*Mortification*, Ig. Colo. Stap—*Scorn*, Bry. Cham. Nux v—*Vexation, Aco.* Ars. *Cham.* Colo. *Ig. Nux v.* Plat. Stap. Verat a. (See Mind.)

Eruptions, suppressed, failing to appear, or receding : Alo 200. Amb. Apis. Bacill 30–200. BRY. Caust. Cic. CUP M. Dul. *Hydrocl.* IPE. Ph a. Stram. SUL. THUJ. ZN—*Hives suppressed*, Ars. Apis. Pul—*Tetter driven in*, Alo. Amb. Dul—(Suppression of eruption, may be the cause of Angina pectoris, Asthma, Blindness, Deafness, Hydrocephalous, Ossification of heart valve, Enlargement of the Liver, and other glands, Indurations, and many other affections.)

Growth too rapid, Ph a—*Getting too fat.* See Obesity.

Indigestion. See Stomach—See Aggravation *as to food.*

Injury mechanical : (See Arnica. Hot water. Lead.)

—Bruise, Arn. Calend. Ham. Rhus—Of bone, Ruta. Symph—Of gland, Con.

—Crush, or pinch, Hyper.

—Cut, surgical or other, Cep. *Hyper. Stap.*

CELERY.

—Fall on the back, HYPER. Bell. Con. Sil—On the head, Arn. Bell. *Cic.* Glo.

—Gun powder, Glycerine, or Vinegar dilute apply.

—Gun shot, Hyper.

—Puncture—Stab. Cic. LED—Festering, Hep. Nit a. Sil.

—Splinter, needle-nail, Hyper. LED.

—Sprain, Led. *Rhus.* Ruta. *Symph*—Sprain of the back, *Hyper.* Rhus—Stomach, Ruta— From lifting, Cal c. Carb v. *Rhus*—Unhandy work, Arn. *Cimi.*

—Sting. Arnica apply—See Bee Sting.

Loss of sleep, Cimi. Ig. Nux v.

Malaria, Ars iod. Nat m. See Ague.

Mental worry, Cimi. Gel. Kal p.

Mind over tasked, Æth. Cimi. Cup m. Kal p. Nux v. ZN p.

Muscles over tasked, Arn. in and ex. Gel. Rhus. SUL 200.

—*Groups of muscles,* as with typewriters, musicians, etc., Gel. Arnica oil.

Pus formation, Hep. *Iod. Pyrogen.* Sll.

Spirituous Liquor. See Alcoholism—See Aggravation.

Tobacco, Apo c. Ars. Bell. IG. Pul. *Nux v.* PLANTAGO 200. Thuj—Chewing especially, Ars. Aurum mur.

Worms: Cina and Ig. Ant c. Mer. Stan.

CELERY:—*Exhaustion of Pregnancy or Labor,— Debility or Languor from any cause, Dysmenorrhœa, Hysteria, Neuralgia, Sciatica, Suppression of Menses, Baby's Colic :*—Celery tea, strong and hot with cream and sugar if preferred; adult a tablespoonful several times a day; Baby, to suit the age.

CEPHALAGIA:—See Head—Pain.
CEREBRO-SPINAL MENINGITIS:—See Fever—Spotted.
CHAFING:—See Skin.
CHANCRE:—See Syphilis.
CHANGE OF LIFE: See Female.
CHAP—: See Skin.
CHARCOAL:—*For sweetening stomach and breath—Augmenting fat. Diarrhœa. ·Dyspepsia. Heart burn. Water brash :* Charcoal powder adult 10 grains, before meals, in a little water or milk.

Gangrene. Putrid sore, or ulcer: Keep the part covered or filled with Charcoal powder. Or apply Yeast poultice mixed with Charcoal powder; renew it frequently.

CHEST:—
Aphonia:—See voice—lost.
Asthma: Apom 2x. *Ars iod.* ARS and IPE. "Fowler's Solution of Arsenic, drop doses in water, every hour; or, 3 to 5 drops in water *after* meals." Carbol a. Glo 2x. *Ipe 0 drop doses.* Jaboran *0*, 4 drops, 6 hours. *Kal iod* pure, adult 3 to 5 grs. 6 hours, in water or syrup; persevere "*Kola nut, 5 gr doses, specific.*" Mullein oil 1 to 5 drop doses according to age. Naph. *Natrum nit.* pure, 2 grs. in water, 2 hours. *Pilo 1x.* Pulmo v 1x trit. 5 grs. ¼ hour. RESORCIN 1 gr. in water. SILPHIUM *0*, adult 15 to 20 drop doses.

Hot gin. Strong Coffee. Pillow of yellow pine shavings. Fumes of burning saltpetre paper, or Stramonium leaves, inhale. "Ice-pack to the neck, over the pneumogastic nerve. Instant relief."

(See *Amyl.* Coffee Ether. Hydrogen. Iodine
Turpen. Vinegar)

Burning in the Chest, Ars.

Chest seems lined with velvet, Tart e

Coldness, Ipe. *Lob i.*

Cold sweat, Ars. Verat a.

Hot head, sweat, Cham—general sweat, Sam.

Choking, Ip. *Lob i*—with phlegm, Blatta or.
Grindel, Ipe. *Kal s* 3x., 5 gr. 2 hours. Sam.
TART E—Raising great quantity of frothy
liquid, *Silphium.*

Croupy hoarseness, Aco. Spo. Pho.

Fear of death. Great restlessness, Aco. ARS.

Loud wheezing, Ars. Sam. Verat v *θ*

Panting, Pho. Pass *θ*—From the least exertion,
Bry. Plantago.

Rapid *irregular* breating, *Pass θ.*

Palpitation, Amb. Ars, Grindel.

Nausea, vomiting, *Ipe. Lob i.* Nux v.

Vertigo, Aco. *Lob i.*

From Indigestion, flatulence, *Asa.* Cham.
NUX V.

—Suppressed eruption, Ars. Dul. Sul

—Lung paralysis, Bacill 200. Helo h 200.

—Fall on the back, Hyper.

—Old age, Con.

—Hysteria Amb. *Lob i. Pass θ.* Plat.

Worse in foggy weather, Hyper.

At night, Aco. *Ars.* Sam. Spo. *Thuj*—wakes up
smothering, Ars. *Lach.* Spo. Sam. Sul. Thuj.

—Morning early on waking, Kal iod. Lach.

—Every other day, Ars. *China.*

Asthma of Millar: "Crowing Asthma"—See
Croup—false.

Bronchitis:—Always a cough—See Cough.

Acute or subacute bronchitis, Am. bro 2x.

Am iod 2x. *Ammon caust.* pure, 3 drop doses at the onset. *Cact* 1x. Euca. Meli 1x. Mullein Oil, 3 drop doses on sugar. STICTA 1x. 5 drops, 2 hours. Hot water, frequent sips, allays cough.

Early stage—Hot fever, *Aco. Bell.* Mer. Pho.

Chill and heat mingling, Cham. *Mer.* Nux v.

Restlessness—Thirst, Aco. Ars.

Cough *violent*, Bell. Mer—with *stitches*, Aco. Bry—Crying after coughing, Bell.

Rattling, Ipe. Tart e. Verat a—Hoarse rattling, CHAM. *Hep.* Pul. Sul.

Wheezing, Hep.

Vomiting, Ip. Tart e.

Suffocation, Ipe. *Tart e.*

Tightness across the chest, PHO.

Tough ropy sputa, Hep. *Kali bi.*

Sweat profuse, Mer. Tart e—Cold, Ars. Verat a.

Sopor—Pallor, Tart e.

Lung œdema, Ars. Pho.

Same for *Bronchial Catarrh, Acute—Catarrhal Fever.*

Chronic Bronchitis: *Am bro* 2x. *Am iod* 2x. Ars iod. BAP. DROS θ 20 drops, 6 hours. Kali m. MYOSOTIS θ 5 drops, 3 hours. *Senega. Squil.* STAN IOD 2x. STIBI ARS. 2x.

Same for *Chronic Pneumonia,* and Chronic Bronchial Catarrh. (See Alum. Benzo Iodine. *Sulph.* Turpen) "The Hectic fever of Chronic Bronchitis, comes on toward *noon,* that of Phthisis toward evening."

Bronchorrhœa: See Cough—KAL BI. Pilo. Stan. *Stan iod. Stibi ars.* (See Alum. Benz a.

Bronchial Catarrh, Acute—*Catarrhal Fever*— See Bronchitis, *Acute.*

Bronchial Catarrh, Chronic—See Bronchitis Chronic.

Cough: AM BRO 2x. AM IOD 2x. *Bry*. Pho. Stan iod 2x. Stibi ars 2x. STICT. Still *0* drop doses on sugar. Mullein oil, 1 to 5 drops on sugar according to age. "The Universal cough remedy Phell. 2x." "Opium, deodorized tincture, adult, drop doses on sugar, after each paroxysm of coughing. Sure to relieve." Sips of hot water allay cough. (See Diet B. Hydrogen. Lemon.)

Barking, BELL. Nit a. Spo. *Stram*.

Choking, CINA. Spo. See Cough—*with suffocation*.

Convulsive, Amb. *Bell*. Dros. *Rum c*. Sep. Verat a.

Deep, Mang. Sep. Stan. VERAT A—As from the stomach, Bry. Nux v. SANG. VERAT A.

Hacking, ALU. Cep. Dros. Hep. IOD. Pho. SANG—Morning hack, Alu.

Hoarse, *Aco*. Bell. Cep. *Spo*. Stan.

Hollow, Bell. Ig. *Verat a*—Deep hollow in shocks, VERAT A. Pass *0*.

Racking, Aco. Bry. *Mer*. Nit a. *Rhus*. Stan.

Rattling, Hep. Ip. Tart e—"As if the lungs were jelly," Lyc.

Splitting, CEP. Calc. *Meli*. Rhus.

Tearful, *Cep*. Ferr p. Nat m.

Cough occurring:—

After eating or drinking, with vomiting of food, *Bry*. Ferr p. Tart e—After dinner, Stap.—After sleeping, Apis, Lach.

At night in bed: Bell. CON. HYO. Ig. MER. *Pul*. Spo. SUL—Warm in bed, Mer. Nux v —In sleep, Cham. Lach — Racking night

cough, with foul breath, Mer—Relieved by
sitting up in bed, Bry. Hyo. Pul—More
after midnight, Cal c. Hep. Hyo. *Nux v
Rhus* — From 3 to 4 a m, Am c. *Kal c.*
Nux v.—From sunset to sunrise, Aur.

In the morning; Arn Bry. Cal c Hep. *Kal bi.*
Nux v—With gagging, *Cina*, Sep—Morning
hack, Alu—Morning till night, *Ferr.* Mang.
Stap.

In the evening: Cal c. Ig. *Pul.* STICTA—
After lying down, Con. *Rum c.* Ig. Nat m.

When uncovered, or any part of the body ex-
posed to cold air, Hep. Rhus. RUM C.

—Coming out of cold air, into a warm room,
Bry—Reverse, Pho.

Cough Relieved by :—

Food, Iod. Spo.

Drink, Spo—Of cold water, Alu. *Caust. Cup m.
Kal c.*

Lying down, Mang—On the back, Aco.

Sitting up in bed, Bry. Hyo. Pul. Spo.

Cough occasioned by :—

Cold cutting wind, Aco Hep.

Cold air, Rum c—Even when head or face uncovered, Hep Rhus. Rum c.

Drinking, Aco. Bry. China. Dros. Kal bi.
Pho. SQUIL — Warm drink, Ferr — Cold
drink, Hep.

Eating. Bry. Hyo—The least morsel, Kal bi—
Cold food, Hep.

Heart affection, LAUR.

Laughing, Arg m. CHINA. Dro. *Pho.* Rhus.

Lying on the right side, Mer—On the left,
Pho.

Pressure upon the throat, Lach.

Relaxation of the palate, Alu. Hep. *Kal bi*—
Mustard seed tea gargle.

Reading, or reflecting, Nux v.

Singing, Alu. Stan—(See Talking).

Smoking, Stan iod 3x.

Seasoning (Salt, pepper), Alu.

Sweet-meats, ZN.

Stopping still, in midst of a walk, Ig.

Stranger entering the room, Pho.

Thinking about the cough, Bar c.

Talking, CHIN. Lach. Nux v. *Pho.* Rhus.
RUM C—Even attempting to speak, Cimi.

Tickling, Aco. Arn. *Cham. Caust.* Carb v.
Ipe. Lach. Lyc. Pho. RUM C. SANG—
Tickling dry spot in the throat, *Stan iod* 3x—
Tickling low down, Ph a. *Verat a*—As from
loose skin, Alu—As from hairs, Sil—As from
feather dust, *Bell.* Calc. LYC. Sul—Crawling tickling, *Carb v.* Con. *Sang.* Sul—Creeping in the stomach pit, Bry.

Worms, *Cina.* Ant c. Mer c. *Stan.*

Cough attended with:

Belching, Amb.

Bruised feeling, Apis. Arn. Nux v. Verat a.

Burning in the chest, Arg n. Caust. Mer.
Seneg—Burning between the shoulders, Bry.

Blue face, Coral. *Cup m. Ipe.* Hyo. Kal p.
Lach. Verat a.

Escape of urine, CAUST. *Nat m,* Pul. SQUIL.
Verat a.

Foul odor from the lungs, CAPS. Cist. Kal p.
Sali ac.

Gagging, *Cina.* Dro. Kreo. Sep.

Gaping, Tart e.

Grasping at the throat, Aco. KALI M 1x.
Naj—At the genitals (Child), Mer. ZN.

Headache—head shock—Bell. *Bry.* Mer. *Nux v. Nat m.* Sang.

Hand to the Chest, Bry. Dro. Pho.

Hip pain, Caust.

Hoarseness, Carb v. *Caust. Cham.* Dul. Hep. *Pho.* Lach. Nit a. *Sang n* 3*x.*

Loss of taste and smell, Pul. Sul.

Palpitation, Calc.

Rattling phlegm, Cact. Hep. IPE. Kal bi. Sul. *Stan iod.* TART E—None raised, CAUST. Ip. *Tart e.*

Retching, Carb v—(See Gagging).

Soreness in the Chest, Arg m. Ars. Apis. Borax. *Caust.* KAL IOD. RUM C. *Pho.* Sul. STAN IOD.

Sore throat, Apis. *Bell.* Lach. *Mer.* SANG.

Spasm, *Cup m.* Lach. Laur.

Stitches, in the Chest, *Aco.* Arn BRY. Pho. *Mer.* Sul—In the left side, Lach. Lyc—In the right side, Bry. Borax. Chel. Mer—Extending through to the back, *Mer.* Sil. *Sul*—Between the shoulders, Carb v.—In the throat, Hep. Nit a—In the anus, Ig. Lach.

Sweat,—*Ars.* Mer. *Tart e.* Verat a—Cold sweat on the forehead, Verat a.

Smothering—suffocating—ARS. Cact. Cup m. Hep. IP. Kal bi. *Laur. Sam.* TART E. Verat a—Must sit up to get breath, *Aco.* Ars. Hep. *Sam.* Tart e.

Trembling, Pho. Tart e.

Tightness of the chest, Aco. *Ars.* Bry. PHO. Sul.

Vomiting, or inclination to vomit, *Alu. Bry.* Dro. Ferr p. Pho. IPE. TART E. Verat a— Of food, *Bry. Ferr p.* Nux v. Pul—Incessant vomiting, Opium suppository.

Wheezing, *Hep*. Ip. SQUILL. Tart e. TRIF P
—Pipes clogged with phlegm, Blatta or Ipe.
Squill. *Stan iod 3x. Stibi ars 3x*. Tart e.

Expectoration—Sputa Raised by Coughing:

—None during the night, Calc. Hep—None
during the day, Caust. Stap. Tart e—Only
in the morning, Pul. Nux v. Sep.

Blood, Aco. Cact Iod. Mer. Pho—(See Hæmoptysis)—Black blood, Cro. Nit a. Nux v.
Pul.

Bloody mucus, Arn. Ars. Chin. Ferr p. Iod.
Mer—after pneumonia, Acalyph.

Balls of mucus, Stan. Thuj.

Blue phlegm, Seneg.

Cold phlegm, Pho.

Cheesy particles, *Bar c*. Chin.

Frothy sputa, Ars. Kal p. Pho. *Silphium*.

Green slime, Carb v. Copai. KAL IOD. Kreo.
Nat s. PUL. *Sil*. Sul. *Stan*. STAN IOD. Thuj
—Green lumps, Sul. Stan iod.

Loosened phlegm, *but not raised*, CAUST. Ip.
Kal c. TART E. ZN.

Masses fly from the mouth, Bad. Kal c—on
falling break like batter, Pho.

Odor offensive, *Ars. Carb v*. Cal c. *Euca*. Pho.
Ph a. *Sang*. Sil. Sul—Like spoiled egg, Kal
iod. Sep.

Red sputa, Aco—Brick red, Bry—"Rusty,"
Bry. Pho. Lyc. Sang. *Rhus*. Tart e—"Prune
juice," Rhus. Tart e.—Reddish yellow, Bry.

Sticky, Alu. Stan iod 3x

Tough, hanging in ropes, Hydros. Kal bi—
Clear tough strings, Apis. Kal bi. Pho.

Transparent, clear slime, CHIN. Ferr. NAT M.
Sil—like starch, Arg m.

Taste musty, Led—Mouldy, Borax—Salty, Lyc

Pho. Sep. Stan. Mag c—Sour, Cal c. Pho—
Sweet, Cal c. Pho Sul. STAN. STAN IOD 3x.
Watery, Ars. Mer. SILPH. Squill—Enormous
   quantity of frothy liquid raised, SILPH.
Whole mouthfuls raised, as if the lungs were
   all dissolved, LYC.
Yellow sputa, Calc. Carb v. *Kal iod.* Lach.
   Mer. PUL. Sul. Stan. STAN IOD 3x. Verat a.
   —Yellow *purulent matter, Bacill* 200.
   Carb v. Hep. Iod. *Kal iod.* Kal s. *Sil 200.*
   Vaccin 200—Yellow lumps, Sil.

Hiccough :—Am m. Cyc. *Eup per. Glo 2x.*
Lyc. *Mag p.* Ice to the ear lobe. *Morsel of
sugar moistened with Vinegar, on the tongue—*
Induce sneezing by snuff or pepper—Desperate
case, Iodine tincture pure, 3 drops, ½ hour,
3 times, in a little water. QUINIA 10 grs.
(See Bandage. Dry cup.
In sleep, Cal c. Mer c.
During meals, Mer—After meals, Cyc. *Hyo.*
   Mer. Verat a.
Hysterical (globus), Asa. *Ig.* Mos 3x. NUX M
   θ. Verat v θ.
Vomiting, Tab. Verat v.
Drunkard, *Caps θ* 30 to 60 drops, in water.
   Nux v. Hot cayenne pepper tea.
Chronic, Ig. Hyo. *Sul a 1x.*

Whooping Cough : " Bromofom, 1 to 3 drops
according to age, in a little sweetened water,
6 times a day. Cure in 2 weeks." " Naphthalin ½ ounce, in a saucer, on live coals, daily
renewed. The patient to stay all the time in
the room where it is. Cure in 3 days." (See
Hydrogen. Turpentine.)
First stage, ACO.·*Ipe.* Spo.
Second stage—*Whooping,* BELL. CUP M.

Carbol a 2x. *Coral.* DROS. TRIF P *θ*, 5 to 10 drops, on sugar, or in water, 3 hours.

Blue face. Rigid, Ip. Laur.

Nose-bleed, *Arn.* Dros.

Spasm, Cup m. Laur. Pass *θ*, 15 drop dose.

Vomiting, Ip. Dros. Verat a.

Worse at night, Bell. Hyo. Mer.

Croup supervening, Hep. Pho.

Croup:—Mullein oil, drop doses. Vinegar dilute frequent sips (See Alum. Hot water. Hydrodrogen. *Iodine.* Kerosene. Onion.)

Dry stage, ACO and SPONG. Bell. *Iod.* Pho.

Loose, Blatta or. *Brom.* HEP. Ipe. TART E.

Throat full of tenacious mucus, Blatta or. KAL BI. Tart e.

Face blue, Kal bi. *Kal p. Lach.*

Cold sweat on the forehead, Verat a.

Worse on waking, *Lach.* Naj.

Crowing inspiration: Aco. Chlorine 1x. (See False Croup.)

Membranous Croup: Cal iod 1x. IOD 2x, 3 drops, ¼ hour. Kali m. KAL I. *Kaolin.* Tart e—Putrid, Ars—See Diphtheria—Croup.

False Croup: Spasm of the Glottis—Asthma of Millar:—*Aco.* Bell. CHLORINE 1x, 10 drops, ¼ hour. *Cup. m.* Iod. KALI BRO pure, 5 gr. doses. MOS. 2x. Sam. Spo.

— Dripping sweat, Sam.

By inhalation, Amyl. Hartshorn. MUSK.

Emphysema:—Am c. Arg n. Dig. *Pilo 1x.* *Kal p.* QUEBRACHO, pure, adult 10 drop doses, in water.

Hæmoptysis.—*Lung Hæmorrhage:* Am c. Bacill 30-100. *Cinnamon* oil or tincture, 1 or 2 drops on sugar or in water. "IODOFORM pills ¾ gr, 1 pill, 2 hours; rarely need more than 8 or 10 to cure any case." *Cocaine 2x.* Ice in cloth to genitals. Ice in mouth—Salt on tongue. ☞ See VINEGAR. See Turpentine. See BLEEDING.

Bright red blood, *Aco.* Dul. Ferr. *Mill.* Rhus—Dark, Ham—Frothy, Aco. Mill—Clotted, Arn. Pul.

Burning chest, Aco 1x. Tereb.

Red face, Aco. Ferr.

Vertigo, Aco. Bell. Dul.

Palpitation, Cact. Dig.

Tight chest, PHO.

Singing ears. Chin.

Gasping, Ipe.

Nausea, Ipe. Verat v *θ*.

From cold wind, Aco.

— Fall or blow, Arn. Hyper.

Sequel to pneumonia, Acalyph.

Vicarious, "Monthly," *Bry.* PHO. Puls. Senecio *θ*. USTIL 1x.

Hoarseness:—See Voice—Hoarse.

Hydrothorax:—

Idiopathic, Ars.

Involving the heart sac, Adon v *θ*. Cact 1x. Dig 1x.

Blue face—slow pulse, Dig. 1x.

With general dropsy, Ars. Apoc *θ*. Eup pur *θ*. See Heart—dropsy—See Dropsy.

Œdema of the lungs:—

Complication, Pho. Stab ars.

Blue face. Suffocation. Tart e.

Drowsiness, Ant c.

With general dropsy, Ars. Apo c. Tart e. See Dropsy.

Pleurisy:—Cact. Euca Ferr p. MELI. Kali m.

Hot and thirsty, Aco. Ars.

Very restless, *Aco.* Rhus.

Lying quiet, BRY—If Bry fails, try Asclep.

Extreme prostration, Ars. Pho.

Effusion, *Ars.* Apis Bry. Kali m—purulent, Mer. Sul. (See Bandage. Hot water. Iodoform)

Pleurodynia (False Pleurisy):—

Aco. Bry. Cimi. *Kan b*—especially left sides, Cimi—Near the heart, Ig. (See Iodoform.) See Chest-pains.

Pneumonia—Pleuro-Pneumonia :—

Ammon Caust pure, at the onset, 3 drop doses in water, Am c. *Cact. Ferr p.* Gel. Mer. *Sang.* Sul—Left lung, Chel.—"All through, even to hepatization, Ferr p." "Second stage, Kali m."—"Stand still" Lach.

"First three days, Aco and Bry; next three, Bry and Phos; next. Phos and Sulph."

Iodine treatment: Iodine, pure tincture, 15 drops in a glass of water. Of this, adult 1 teaspoonful, every ½ hour, until temperature under control, then occasional doses. (See Bandage. See CHLOROFORM, Hot water. Olive oil.) ·

Hot skin—Bounding pulse, Aco. Verat v *θ.*

Throbbing carotids, Bell. Gel.

Delirium, *Bell.* Bry. Rhus. Verat v *θ.*

Nostrils fanning, LYC—Wide open, flaring, Tart e.

Lying quiet, Bry—(If Bry fails, try Asclep).

Restlessness, *Aco. Ars.* Rhus. Tart e.

Sweat, Mer. Tart e.

Suffocation, Ipe. PHO. Sul. TART E.

Wanting to be fanned, Carb v.

"Rusty sputa," *Bry. Pho.* Rhus. Verat v.
Suppuration, Hep. Sang. Sul.
Typhoid type, Ars. Kal p. *Pho.* Rhus.
    See Fever—Typhoid.

Chronic Pneumonia:—Am br 2x. Am iod 2x.
Ferr iod. *Lyc. Sang.* Senega. *Squil.* Stan.
STAN IOD 2x. Stibi ars. 2x. See Cough.

Phthisis—Consumption:—Ars iod 3x. Arg n.
"*Acet a* 30 drops 6 hours." "Aurum mur 3x,
6 hours for 3 days; then wait 3 days, and give
again; and with it give Oleum j pure, 5 drops,
slightly salted, before meals." "BACILL 200
one dose a week, and Hydras 3x trit before
meals." "Baptisia controls the fever." "Cal p
6x is our best hope." CHINA ARS 2x
Drosera θ 10; 20 drops, 6 hours. Glycerine a
tablespoonful in sweet cream, 3 times a day, is
better than cod liver oil." Mutisia is a remedy of great promise. MYOSOTIS θ 5 drops
3 hours, cured a grave case in a few weeks.
Nat ars 3x. Petrol. is worthy of much confi-
dence. Stannum iod 3x and Stibium ars 3x,
if resulting from Pneumonia, or Chronic
Bronchial Catarrh. VACCIN 200, one dose a
week. *Ichthyol.*

From Suppressed Menses, Senecio θ 5 drops 6
hours. Ustil ix trit, 5 grs, 6 hours—See
Female.

Diet: Cream. Ice cream almost exclusive—
(See Diet. Climate. Iodine. Sulphur.
Turpentine. Vinegar.

Pains and Sensations in the Chest:—
Pain at top of right lung, Ars 30—Of left lung,
Nit a.
—At base of right lung, Lyc—Of left lung,
Kal c.

—Under collar bone, Rum c—Behind breast bone, Rum c.

—Under the nipple, Cimi. Ran b.

Burning in the Chest, Am c. Carb v. Pho— Like fire, Ars. Carb v. *Naj.*

Coldness, Cist. Lyc—In right lung, Sul—In left lung, Pet.

Pulsation, Spig—At night on waking, Sul— Morning on waking, Ran b.

Soreness, Apis. *Cal c. Pho.* Ran b. *ZN.*—As if raw inside, Arg n. Arum. Caust. Grap. *Kal iod.* Lyc.—From coughing, Spo. Sil. ZN.

Stitches, Aco. *Bry.* Borax. *Kal c.* Ran b. Squil.—On coughing, Bry. Rum c. Mer.— Tightness, Arg n. CACT. PHO. Stan. Verat a.—Sudden, Asa. (See Asthma).

Weakness, Carb v. Pho. Spo. Stan.—Especially on going up stairs, Iod.—On going down, Stan.

Respiration Difficult or Oppressed :—

As if every breath the last, Apis—As if chest too narrow, Arg n. *Bry.* Cact. Lach. Pho.— Painful, Ran b.

When ascending hill or stairs, Ars Cal c. Cact. Iod.

—Coughing, Sil—See Cough, *with.*

—Lying down, Ars.—On the back, Ars. Pho. SIL. Sul.

—Head low, Spo.—On left side, Pho, Spig.

—Stooping, Am c. Sil.

—Talking, *Caust.* Dros. Ph a. *Stan.*

—Walking, Aur., Ars. Jug r—In wind, Cham. Pho. ZN.

—Must sit erect, Ars. Apis. Bry. Sam. Tart e—

Lean back, Bell—Bend forward, *Kal c*—
Chin on the knees, Ars.
Every breath comes by double effort, Led.
Crowing, Cham. Lach.
Groaning, Bell
Hissing, Arg n.
Irregular—Unequal, Ail. Angus. BELL.
Cup m.
Panting, PHO.
Puffing, China.
Rattling, Cup m. Hep. Ipe. Lyc. Tart e.
Sighing, *Bry. Ig.* Ipe. Stram.
Slow, Bell.
Sobbing, Sec—In sleep, Aur.
Snoring, LEMNA. Nat m—*Stertorous*, Op.
Wheezing, Amb .Alu. Carb v. Chin. Nat m.
Sam. SQUIL.
Whistling, *China*. Kal c. Nit a—In sleep, Chel.

Voice altered :—

Failing or Lost: Am c. Bell. BROM. CAUST.
Gel. Mer. PHO. *Spo.* Sul. Stram—Sudden,
Alu. Bell. Gel. Glo—From being over heated,
Ant c—Fails when singing, or reading aloud,
Carb v. Caust. SPO. STAN. Piece of borax in
the mouth. Inhale Hartshorn.

Hoarse: Aco. Arg n. Bell. Cal c. *Ferr p.* Kali m.
PHO. SPO—Suddenly, Nux m θ. From long
speaking, reading aloud, or singing, ARUM.
Arn. PHO ix. Rhus—Walking against the
wind, Nux m. Pho—More in the evening, Alu.
Carb v—More in the morning, Carb v. *Caust.*
Cal c. Pho—With hawking, Pho —Chronic,
Caust. Carb v. Grap. Kal bi. *Kal iod.* Kali m.
Pho—(See Ham. Iodine).

Rough, bass: Arum. Bell. *Brom, Dros.* Kal bi.
Stan. Sul.

CHICKEN POX.

Squeaking: Stram.

CHICKEN POX:—TART E. Thuj.

Fever—Restlessness, Aco.

Headache—Sore throat, Bell.

Watery eyes, Pul.

CHILBLAIN:—AGAR 2x. Pet. Urti.

Burning—Spreading blisters, Ars. *Rhus.*

Bluish red—Itching, Abrotan. Pho. PUL.

Ulcerating, Hep. *Sil.* Sul. (See Euca. Glycer.
Lemon—See *Ointment.*)

CHILD-BED FEVER:—See Fever—Puerperal.

CHILD-BED MANIA:—See Female—Child-bed.

CHILDREN'S AILMENTS.—See Infant.

CHILL — CHILLINESS -- (See also *Coldness.*
See Ague). "Chill points to spleen."

Always Chilly, Arg n. Grap. Pul. Sep. Sil—
Cold and sleepless, Amb.

Ailments set in with a Chill, Aco.

Sudden Chill from exposure, Aco.

"Cold air goes right through," Calc.

Chilly from a drink of water, Ars. Caps. Cup m.

—From least motion, Nux v—Whenever she
walks, Am m.

Chills creep up the back, Gel. Sul—up and
down, Spo.

Chills at night, flushes of heat by day, Lach.

Chill and sweat alternationg, Pho.

Chill and heat mingling, Cham. Mer.

Nervous shivers, Cimi. Gel. Plat.

"Goose flesh," Gel—Indoors, Calc—Outdoors,
Sars.

Congestive Chill:—ACO 1x. CAMP. θ, adult 5
drops on sugar, 5 minutes; also rub chest,
back and abdomen with camphor spirits—
Quinia 10 grs, hypoderm. Hot spirituous drink.
See Bandages. See Lime SWEAT.

— Skin hot, Gel.

—Breath cold, Ars.

—Face blue, Verat v *0.*

CHLORAL—*Offensive foot sweat:*—"Lave with Chloral hydrate, 1 per cent solution in water; in two days, all offensive odor gone."

Unhealthy wound:—Dress with Chloral hydrate, 2 per cent solution.

CHLORINE—CHLORIDES—BROMO-CHLO-RALUM:—*Freckles:* If *yellow,* lave with Chlorine water night and morning: If *brown,* apply Chloride of Lime, weak solution in water, to suit sensation; brush it on every night, and wash it off in the morning, until the freckle is bleached out.

Diphtheria, Sore throat, Ulcerated Throat or Mouth, Foul breath, Scarlet fever, Small pox, Typhoid fever, Nasal catarrh, Ozæna: "Gargle with Bromo-Chloralum 10 per cent. solution in water, and swallow a little, every ½ hour in urgent cases, or at longer intervals as the case may require. *Inhale* the same also from a sponge to facilitate the cure. "There is no better remedy for *diphtheria;* in 6 hours the terrible odor will be gone, in 3 days, the cure effected. The same course, aided by *sponging the body* with a 10 per cent. solution in water and alcohol equal parts, once or twice a day, insures success in treatment of *Scarlet fever, Small pox,* and *Typhoid fever.*"

Local discharges offensive—Leucorrhœa fetid: "Inject a 10 per cent. solution of Bromo-Chloralum, two or three times a day. Directly every trace of foul odor will disappear, and the cure be promptly effected."

CHLOROFORM.

Antiseptic dressing for open Cancer—Putrid sore, Sloughing ulcer, Gangrenous wound, Purulent *Ophthalmia :* Bromo-Chloralum, 10 per cent. solution in water, lave the parts, and keep covered with cloths saturated with the same.

Disinfection : Saturate cloths with Bromo-Chloralum or Platt's Chlorides, and suspend them about the room. Sprinkle the bed and floors with the same. ☞ A splendid disinfectant—at cost of three cents a bucketful—suitable to pour down sinks and sewers, may be made thus: Dissolve ½ drachm of Nitrate of lead in a pint of boiling water ; then in a bucket of water dissolve 2 drachms of Common Salt; then pour the two solutions together, and allow the sediment to subside; now pour off the clear liquid; this is the disinfectant.

CHLOROFORM—*Retention of urine, strangury, spasm,* local or general: Chloroform by inhalation.

In Labor : Chloroform by inhalation, only during pain ; or equal parts of Chloroform and Sweet Oil, mix and apply to the abdomen from navel to pubes. Organic disease of the heart does not preclude the use of Chloroform by inhalation in labor, but rather calls for its careful use.

Myalgia, Neuralgia, Sciatica, Neuralgic headache or face ache : Chloroform, Ether, and Eau de Cologne, equal parts mixed, pour upon a handkerchief or cloth, *previously* dampened with cold water, and apply. Or anoint with Chloroform and Aconite tincture each 5 parts, with Lard 20 parts mixed; cover with light compress.

Pneumonia: Chloroform and Alcohol equal parts mix; saturate a roll of cotton, or small sponge with this, and cover it with a thin cloth; hold it within an inch of the mouth, a few minutes at a time every hour, or oftener if much pain. "No failure."

Pain-guard—Anti-pain spray, for minor operations: Chloroform 10 parts, Ether 10 parts, and Menthol 1 part mix; use in hand atomizer; after one minute Cut—no pain.

Bug in the ear: Wet cotton with Chloroform, and put in the bowl of a pipe, place the end of the stem in the ear, then with mouth over the bowl, blow the breath into it, thus forcing the vapor into the ear. The bug, insect or worm will roll out.

Earache: The same; or Chloroform 1 drachm, in olive oil 2 ounces mix; put 20 or 30 drops in the ear, and plug with cotton. Instant relief.

'Puerperal spasm: Dissolve 2 tablespoonfuls of brown sugar in a gill of lukewarm water, add a tablespoonful of Chloroform: draw it in and force it out the syringe a few times until well mixed, then inject the whole into the rectum, and cause it to be retained by napkin. No more spasms.

Sea-sickness, Vomiting of pregnancy, Acidity of the stomach: Chloroform, 1 drop on sugar.

Bleeding from operations in the mouth or throat, excessive bleeding of tonsils. Any surface bleeding: Spray the part with Chloroform, 2 per cent. solution in water. "This closes the mouths of all small bleeding vessels instantly."

Chloroform Narcosis: See Apparent death.

CHLOROSIS — GREEN SICKNESS: — Cal p. HELON. Pul. Sep.

73

CHOKING.

Bloodless, Chin. Cal c. Helon.
Bloated, Ars. Helon.
Crimson flush, Ferr.
Cold—Chilly, *Pul.* Sep.
Cold damp feet, Cal c.

CHOKING:—See Throat.

CHOLERA:—See Bowel.

CHOREA—ST. VITUS'S DANCE.—Ars. (FOW-
LER'S SOLUTION, 3 *drops after meals*). Avena.
Cic. *Cimi. Cocaine 2x.* Mag p. SCUT. Verat a.
ZN.

Leading remedies, ARG N. 3x. in water.
HYO. SCUT 3x.
All manner of antics, Tarant C.
Rapid movements, Stram.
Night *and* day, *Caust.*
Only when awake, Agar—"Agaricine 1x-1 gr."
Stammering, Stram.
Tottering, *Hyo.*
Blue hands and face, Coc. Cup m.
Boy, Nux v.
Girl, Bell. Pul.
From fright, *Ig.* Op.
—suppressed menses, Pul.
—second teething, Cal c. Cal p.
—worms, Cina, Ig.

CHORDEE:—See Gonorrhœa. See male-priapism.

CHOROIDITIS : — See Eye, Inflammation —
Choroid.

CHROMIUM:—*Cancer removed without the knife:*
" Apply Chloride of Chromium with a soft
swab, until the tumor is thoroughly saturated;
then apply Indian-meal poultice, made into
dough with glycerine; and keep it on until the
crust is detached; then apply the Chloride again,

and the poultice. So continue until the Cancer is entirely extirpated; then let it heal. If the poultice should render the patient restless mix it with some Stramonium leaf tea."

CHRONIC DISEASES:—In general, ARS. AUR. Bacill 200. CARBOL AC. *Hydroct.* SUL. Thuj.

"Persistent treatment with *Acon.* low and high."

"To set other remedies to work," Sul.

If Bacill will not work—Thuj. Then Bacill.

If Apis will not, give Acon. with it; or Nat. m.

If Nat s. will not, give Thuj.—then again Nat s.

If there is a *drug, dyscrasia,* see Cause—*Drug.*

CHYLURIA:—Berb. Ph a. Uva u.

CICATRICE-SCAR REMOVED: Cut it cleanly off, and dress it daily with Perchloride of iron 1 drachm, and Collodion 2 drachms mixed. A barely perceptible line will be the result.

CIRRHOSIS:—Aco. Ars. Pho.

CLAIRVOYANCE:—Aco. Cann i. Pho.

CLAVUS:—Coff. *Ig. Nux v.* Pul. Mag. p.

CLAY—FULLER'S EARTH—"MINERAL EARTH:"—*Black pores in the skin of the face.* "*Black-heads*": Make a paste of Potter's Clay 4 parts; Glycerine 3 parts; and Vinegar 2 parts, and cover the face daily with this for an hour; then wash off with sand soap, or pumice stone soap. In a few days this will remove them.

Sprain, Swelling, Gathering, Throbbing Tumor, Painful Enlargement of the Scrotum, Gathered Breast, Swollen Diseased joint, Wounds foul, unhealthy: Clay paste, made with water, Cosmoline, Vaseline, or other base apply thick coat, and cover with compress, two or three times a day, washing the part each time before renewing the paste.

75

CLERGYMAN'S SORE THROAT.

Bed Sore, Raw Surface, Chafing, Foul ulcer, Gengrene: Keep the part well coated or filled with Clay dust; and cover with Carbolized absorbent cotton. There will be no fetor after 12 hours.

CLERGYMAN'S SORE THROAT:—See Throat.

CLIMACTERIC AILMENTS:—See Female—change of life.

CLIMATE CURE FOR CONSUMPTION:—
Texas is regarded as the "Italy of America." Western North Carolina, centre at Asheville, is called "The Home for Consumptives." As likewise California, Colton as a centre. And the Cumberland plateau Tennessee. Dwelling on HIGH, DRY SOIL is a requisite for recovery.

CLUB FOOT, AND OTHER DEFORMITY, PREVENTIVE: Phos. during gestation.

COCAINE:—*Facial Neuralgia:* Cocaine 1 per cent. solution, by camel-hair brush; or dropped in the ear of *that* side. Same for *Earache.* Instant relief.

Diphtheria: "Cocaine 2 per cent. solution, *local;* relieves the pain and dissolves the patch."

In labor: "Cocaine oleate, (4 : 100) to cervix in first stages, and to vulva and perineum during expulsion; subdues the pain."

Surgical operation upon the Eye. Mote in the Eye: Cocaine 2 per cent., a drop or two at intervals of 5 minutes, for three times; renders the eye insensible to pain.

Local anæsthesia—(for ear, nose, throat, vagina, os uteri, urethra): Cocaine 4 per cent. ex. *Vaginismus. Pruritis. Pain* of *ingrowing nail:* The same.

Fistula in Ano—Anal fissure or ulcer. Stricture of Anus. Painful piles: Coca butter suppository, containing 10 to 15 grains of Iodoform. "Unrivalled."

To remove Cancer without pain or use of knife; especially open Cancer: "Paint the growth with a 10 or 20 per cent. Cocaine solution, then apply an escharotic, with which some Cocaine may be incorporated. The process may be completed at one sitting, or several, until the growth is removed. A cancerous growth of the os and cervix uteri was destroyed without pain, by means of a 10 per cent. solution of Cocaine, and stick of Potassa fusa." See Solar Cautery.

Gastralgia, Gastritis, with excessive vomiting: Cocaine 4 grains; Lime water 1 ounce; Cinnamon water 1 ounce; mix; Adult take a teaspoonful every ½ hour. Sure relief.

COFFEE: — *Delirium Tremens. Brain Fag. Nervous Sick-headache. Headache in general. Weak heart. Palpitation of the heart from slight excitement, Fainting from sudden emotion, Nervousness, Sleeplessness, Spasmodic Asthma:* Caffein, adult 1 grain, every ½ hour in urgent cases; or at longer intervals as the case may require.

Delirium Tremens, Colic, Vomiting. Typhus of Children. Cholera Infantum — Moaning Stupor. Hernia. Opium poisoning. Ague, before or during Chill: Inject coffee into the bowel, strong decoction; freely; and give to drink repeated draughts of hot coffee.

Disinfection: Ground coffee, sprinkled upon live coals, in a shovel or pan, and carried around in a room will in a few minutes, clear

COLDS, RECENT.

the atmosphere of all impurities, especially of animal effluvia.

COLDS, RECENT—AMMON CAUST pure, drop doses in water. CAMP *θ*, drop doses. *Cep 1x* drop doses. Ferr p. NAT M 2x trit. *Acon and Nux v.* Gel *θ.* In the Throat, Bar c. Fl ac. Guai *θ.*

COLDNESS:—(See Chill. Chilliness).

Want of vital heat, Arg n. Alu. Ferr, Led. Pul. Sec. Sep. Sil

When in pain, Led. Pul. Verat a.

Cold but averse to covering, Camp. Sec.

" Horrid Coldness "—paralytic, Helo h 200.

Cold and blue, Helo h 200.

Cold and clammy, *Cuprum ars.* Mer. *Pic a.* Helo h 200.

Cold veins, Aco. Verat a.

Cold spots, Sul—as if touched by icicle, Agar.

Internal coldness, *Am. Ars.* Cist. Lith c. Kal bro—with external heat, Ars.

Local coldness. See the part of body, or limb.

COLD WATER:—*Delirium Tremens :* " Stream of cold water from a height, upon the back of the head and neck, until pulse rate falls to forty. Sleep then ensues, and recovery."

Lightning Stroke :—Dash Cold water upon the the naked chest and back, turn about, as rapidly as the patient can conveniently be rolled back and forth on the left side. If not successful after half an hour, wrap the patient in woolen blankets, and in a half sitting position, cover with fresh earth, except the face, and administer *Nux v.* or perhaps Amyl.

Nose-bleed : Ice cold water or ice, to root of nose, or back of neck.

Hydrocele.—Congenital: Cold water, a small stream from a height upon the scrotum for several minutes daily.

Erysipelas from an injury: Cold water on cloths. Keep constantly wet.

Hernia: Make bare the abdomen and chest—patient lying on the back, Knees drawn up—Cover the face with a towel, and without the knowledge of the patient suddenly dash a cup of cold water on the stomach. The sudden shock causes retraction of the bowel, and reduces the rupture.

In Dropsy: Water should not be withheld; it encourages the kidney to action.

In Scarlet fever, Measles—and other eruptive diseases: Water may be freely taken. With this precaution, that small quantities be taken at a time. It is the sudden chill from a *large* cold drink that does harm, not the water itself.

Infantile ailments, Colic, Diarrhœa, Fever, Restlessness: Give the baby cool water, a teaspoonful every hour or two. This alone may prove curative.

When baby cries: Offer it water, it may be thirsty. Washing the baby's mouth daily with cold water prevents *sore mouth*.

COLIC: See Abdomen.

COLLAPSE:—Ars. *Cocaine 1x.* Glo 2x. KAL P 3x. in hot water. Pho. Opium hypoderm—See Musk —See HYDROGEN.

COLLODION (Flexile):—*Birth Mark, Pimple— Sore Nipple. Wen:*—Repeated Coatings of collodion, with camel-hair brush.

Sprain: Paint on a Coat of Flexile Collodion, and when dry, which will be in a few minutes, another coat, until six in all. No further treatment needed.

Cholera: "With camel-hair brush paint with collodion the abdomen (previously shaved if hairy). This arrests all symptoms. Try the same in Cholera Morbus. The effect of this treatment is immediate stoppage of discharges and vomiting, restoration of warmth to the whole body, and resumption of perspiration, even profuse, which is indispensable to success."

Eruption in the face from shaving. Pimples. Sore Nipples: Collodion ½ drachm; Glycerine 1 drachm; Rose water 2½ drachms; Mix; Use as a wash.

COLORING FOR TINCTURES AND POWDERS:—Scorch *Sugar of Milk*, until dark brown, in a porcelain Mortar, or Common Saucer upon a stove; add to this sufficient distilled water to form a syrup, stirring until all the sugar is dissolved, when it will be ready for use. A few drops of this syrup, added to an alcoholic solution, will give a light or dark brown color, according to quantity used. *Coloring Powder* is made by using the scorched Milk Sugar pulverized, and mixed with common sugar, or unscorched sugar of milk, to any shade required.

COMA—STUPOR:—Aco. *Hyo. Op.* VINEGAR.

Of infant with jaundice, Pod.

When menses fail to appear, Ham.

Sleep day and night, continuous, Verat a. See cause.

COMEDONE:—"Black heads." Grap. Nit a. Sul. See Clay. See Face.

COMPOUND FRACTURE:—See Wound—See Pain—fracture.

CONCUSSION. Aco. *Arn.* Bell. CIC. *Glo 2x.*
Hyper. See Cause—injury.

CONDYLOMA.—Nit a. Phyt. THUJ in. and ex.

CONFINEMENT.—See Female—Child bed.

CONGESTION ACUTE:—In general, ACO. Ferr
p. GEL *0.* MELI *0.* See Bandage.
Setting in with a chill, Aco.
Threatening spasms, Verat v *0.*
Livid, Kal p. Ustil. See Chill—*Congestive.*

CONJUNCTIVITIS:—See Eye-lids, *inflamma-tion.*

CONSCIOUSNESS LOST:—See Apparent Death
—See Mind.

CONSTIPATION:—See Bowel.

CONSUMPTION:—See Chest—*Phthisis.*

CONTAGION AND INFECTION GUARD:—
Keep in the sick room Bromine Water in a dish,
or Bromine in a bottle uncorked; or sliced onion
in a dish, renewed daily; or burn a thimbleful of
gun-powder in the room daily. Smoke or chew
tobacco. Keep myrrh in the mouth. See "*Air
indoors kept pure.*" See disinfectants.
Against Diphtheria :—Apis 2x. Lach. See Salt.
Against Scarlet Fever:—*Atrop 2x.* Bell. ZN 3x.
Exclusive milk diet. "Sweet spirits of Nitre is
a mild and safe prophylactic of scarlet fever."
"Quinia prevents the spread of scarlet fever. In
no case will it attack a child, when taking, according to age, 2 to 3 grains, 3 times a day.
After 5 days, lessen the dose, but keep up the
use of it for 3 weeks." See Lard.
Against Small-pox :—THUJ. VINEGAR, adult
2 tablespoonfuls twice a day. Cyanide of
potash strong solution, *sprinkle* about the

CONVALESCENCE.

floors and stairways—Vaccininum 30. " Ma-
landrinum, 30-200, even after exposure to infection."

Against Malaria: ARS IOD 2x. Euca θ. G1 θ.
NAT M. Gun powder burned in bed-room or
tent daily. Put on flannel jacket, in the early
evening. A fire, kindled in the evening, and
continued through the night, in apartments
occupied, is indispensable for the preservation
of health in malarial regions.

Against Yellow Fever: Salicyl ac, adult 5 to 10
grains, daily for two weeks.

Against Whooping Cough : Pul.

Against Rabies: See Hydrophobia.

CONVALESCENCE:—See Diet. R—See Tonic.

CONVULSION:—See Spasm.

CORNEA:—See Eye-balls.

CORNS:—See Limb—leg, *foot.*

CORPULENCE:—See Obesity—See Person.

CORYZA:—See Nose.

COUGH:—See Chest.

COURSES:—See Female—*menses.*

CRACKING IN JOINTS:—See Limb.
Jaw, when chewing, Grap. Sep.

CRACK—FISSURE:—See Skin.

CRAMP:—CUP M. Mag p. *Meli. Pass.* Verat a—
At night in the legs, VIB OP θ. See part affected.
See Sulphur.

CRAVING:—See Stomach.

CROOKED BY RHEUMATISM:—See Limb—
drawn *crooked.*

CROUP:—See Chest.

CRUSTA LACTA—MILK CRUST:—See Head
—*scalp.*

82

CUT:—See Cause—injury.

CYANOSIS:—Dig. Cup m. LAUR 30 Op. Verat a. Have baby lie on its *right* side, head high.

CYNANCHE CELLULARIS.—Anthracinum 30-200. See Throat.

CYSTITIS:—See Urinary organs.

DANDRUFF:—See Head—Scalp.

DEAFNESS:—See Ear—*hearing.*

DEATH SIGNS:—See Apparent Death.

DEBILITY:—In general,CHINA 2x. *Ferr.Helon.* Hydrogen. Kal p. KOLA NUT, 5 to 10 grain doses. Stan. ZN p. Oleum j; 5 drops after meals.
Rapid prostration, *Ars.* Ph a. Verat a.—As soon as pain sets in, Cham.
Alternate weakness and strength, China.
In hot weather, *Bry.* Hyo. Nux v.
Old age, Con. See Cause. See Tonic. See Diet T.

DEFORMITY IN UTERO - PREVENTIVE: Pho, during gestation.

DELIRIUM:—See Mind.

DELIRIUM TREMENS:—See Mind—Delirium. (See Cold water, Coffee, Musk.—See Mind—Mania).

DENGUE; —"BREAK-BONE FEVER": Ars. *Bry. Cimi.* EUP PER. Gel. *Rhus.*

DENTITION.—See Mouth—Teething.

DESQUAMATION.—See Skin.

DEVELOPMENT ARRESTED.—Barc c. Thuj. See Person.

DIABETES — GLYCOSURIA. — See Urinary Organs.

DIAPHRAGM.

DIAPHRAGM.—
Inflammation, *Aco. Bry.* Ferr p. Lyc.
Myalgia, Bry. Cimi.
Spasm, *Arg n.* Cact. Cic. Mag p.

DIARRHŒA.—See Bowel.

DIET.

A. *Prostration. Faintness from overtaxation of body and mind:* Yolk of egg beaten up with brandy. Egg nogg. *Sore throat of public speakers:* Yolk of egg, raw.

B. *Cough from Cold :* To the white of an egg, beaten up with a teaspoonful of sugar, add a teacupful of hot water, stirring the white; take on going to bed.

C. *Nausea. Sick-stomach:* Stir a little of the white of a fresh egg in cold water—ice water if preferred—and beat the remainder of the white to a froth, and put it on top of the water, drink freely whenever thirsty.

D. *Cholera Infantum.— Nothing stays on the stomach:* Put the white of an egg, well beaten, into half a glass of water, season it with a very little salt and sugar, and give 2 teaspoonfuls, every 2 hours. When the stomach becomes settled, try pure milk, warm from the cow, every 2 hours, for a few days; then perhaps sweet cream, and hot water mixed to consistency of milk.

E. *Diarrhœa of Infant at breast* (Mother's milk not good): Give in the course of 24 hours, the white of one egg, stirred well into 5 or 6 ounces of water, previously boiled, and add condensed milk 3 or 4 drachms. The quantity can be gradually increased to two or three times this amount.

F. *Atrophy, Marasmus:* Boil an egg "stone hard," crumble the yolk, and feed it to the child. This is good for baby at any time.

G. *When milk disagrees:* Treat it thus: Into one pint put a glass of water, a tablespoonful of sugar, and half teaspoonful of salt; and if necessary beside, a tablespoonful of lime water.

H. *When milk sours on the stomach of infants, reared by bottle:* Add a little chalk to the milk when boiling it.

I. *Exhaustion of body and mind:* A glass of hot milk. This is more invigorating than alcholic stimulants.

J. *Consumption:* Hot milk, adult, 4 to 8 glasses daily. This increases the weight and strength of the patient, and lessens cough and diarrhœa.

K. *Diarrhœa—Dysentery:* Hot milk.

L. *Night Sweat:* Skim-milk, a wine glass full on retiring to bed. "A pinch of German Chamomile flowers, stirred in a cup of boiling water, and taken at bed time, will cure night sweat in a week. It never leaves you in the lurch."

M. *Dropsy of old people:* Skim-milk, freely taken.

N. *Diabetes:* Skim-milk, 8 to 10 pints daily, *no other food.* In two weeks the sugar will have disappeared from the urine. In seven weeks the cure be effected. *Lactic acid,* 10 per cent. solution in alcohol, 5 drops, morning and evening, cured a case of Diabetes Mellitus of six months' duration.

O. *Bright's Disease:* Skim-milk diet exclusive. Persevere for two or three months. Reported cures.

DIET.

P. *Epilepsy:* Milk diet exclusive. Cure in three months.

Q. *Incrustations of the valves of the heart. Ossification of the arteries. Cystitis. "Kidney complaints." Consumption:* Butter milk, to the heart's content.

R. *Disease of the Throat. Consumption Nervous exhaustion. Exhaustion from surgical operations. Convalescence from fevers. Nervousness. Dyspepsy. Hip and Spine disease. Debility from chronic discharges. Typhoid fever. Scarlet fever. Diphtheria:* "Koumis. Made thus:—Into a quart of new milk, put half pint of fresh butter milk, or a teaspoonful of yeast, and three lumps of loaf sugar (inch cubes). Mix well, and see that the sugar becomes dissolved; put it into a warm room, to stand ten hours, when it will be thick; now pour it from one vessel to another until it becomes smooth and uniform in consistency; then bottle it; and keep it in a warm place, twenty-four hours, it may require thirty-six hours in winter. The bottles should be *tightly* corked, and corks *tied* down. Shake well *five* minutes before decanting it from the bottle."

S. *Nervousness.* Suitable for nervous persons, subject to *neuralgia*, and *mental depression:* Rich juicy meats, cream toast, sweet bread and butter; also fish and cracked wheat to supply phosphorus "Fish diet for brain work."

T. *Dyspepsia. Indigestion. Defective appetite. Debility*, especially *with red* tongue: Baked flour in beef tea. Beef peptonoids. Malt extracts and pepsin, "Beef tea alone, stimulates but does not nourish." "Malt extract is

86

the best food for weak digestion, even for baby."

U. *Diabetes:* In this disease the storage of grape sugar in the liver is disturbed, too much passes off by the kidney, the urine is milky, contains sugar—we have *Glycosuria or Diabetes:* Abstain from food containing starch and sugar. Partake only of meats, green vegetables and skim-milk. Reported cures by eating nothing but meat and fish, and taking at each meal *Lactic acid* three or four scruples, in six ounces of water. Two complete cures by taking two teaspoonfuls of Lactic acid in a goblet of water once a day, with exclusive meat and egg diet.

V. *Gravel, Gout, Bright's Disease:* In these affections the liver fails to change the meat waste into soluble urea, and leaves the consequent insoluble urates and lithates in the system to be deposited in the joints (Gout); in the urine (Gravel); or else to break down the Kidney (Bright's Disease). The food from which this trouble comes — the nitrogenized—must be withheld:—Partake of no meat, eggs, or new milk. Let the diet be mainly farinaceous— Bread, cakes, green vegetables, skim-milk.

W. *Scrofula, Phthisis, Tubercular Meningitis, chronic Hydrocephalus;* In these affections *fuel food*—Hydrocarbon—is defective. The system calls for fat in natural emulsion,—Rich Milk, Cream, Milk puddings, suet puddings. Artificial fat emulsions are better borne, and prove more useful when taken one and a half hours *after* meals.

X. *Emaciation:* In order to get fat eat all manner of sweets, nothing sour. "Two ounces of loaf sugar, and two pounds of sweet grapes,

DIET.

three times a day will fatten a skeleton, and Cure Consumption.''

Y. *Obesity:* In order to get thin, eat all things sour, nothing sweet. "Abstain from bread, butter, milk, sugar, potatoes, salmon, pork, soups and beer; eat and drink anything else, and you will lose a pound a week.''

Z-1. *Baby's Best Food:* SUGAR OF MILK 1 ounce, in water ½ pint, boil 15 minutes, then add ½ pint of fresh milk, and boil again. Give from the bottle moderately warm. Obstinate cases of *Dysentery* have been cured by this food.

Z-2. When the baby is *losing flesh*, *vomits food*, and has *sour stool*. A grain or two of MILK SUGAR, placed dry upon the tongue several times a day, may correct the trouble.

Z-3. With children brought up by hand, the subtitution of MILK SUGAR, for loaf sugar, will frequently obviate *sour vomiting*, and acid stools.

Z-4. For the sake of change, if the *bowels are loose*, crack a teaspoonful of BARLEY in a coffee mill, boil it 15 minutes in ½ pint of water, with a little salt, skim it; and for a young child, add half as much cow's milk as there is barley water, sweeten and give warm from the bottle. If the *bowels are bound*, use oatmeal instead of barley.

Z-5. CREAM skimmed off two hours after milking in the morning, diluted one-half, or three-quarters with boiling water, very slightly sweetened with loaf sugar, often agrees with a child, and stays on the stomach when milk does not.

88

Z–6. To a quart of milk just boiling, add a heaping tablespoouful of CORN STARCH, and as
much white sugar; continue the boiling until
it thickens, *no longer*, and feed warm.
"This will make the baby fat."

Z–7. Pure unfermented GRAPE JUICE—pre-
served without boiling, and without chemicals
—is the food *par excellence*, for sick children,
as well as for adults. They will take it when
all other nourishment is rejected. Just the
thing in scarlet fever.

Z–8. Squeeze the JUICE FROM RAW LEAN
MEAT, with lemon squeezers, salt it slightly,
and dilute it a little with warm water, put it
into the nursing bottle, and give four times a
day as much as seems well tolerated by the
stomach. This cures "*Summer Complaints.*"

Z–9. Instead of the expressed juice, the PULP
OF RAW MEAT, especially the soft, inside
part of dried beef pounded to a jelly, may be
freely given. This has cured wasting *Summer
Diarrhœa* of infants.

Z–10. Permitting the baby to suck a RAW
OYSTER, or the raw soft part of DRIED
BEEF, held in nurse's fingers, often proves
curative in cases of *Bowel Complaint.* Beef
peptonoids are good.

Z–11. RICE carefully cleansed, and *browned* in
an oven, a tablespoonful in a pint of water,
allowed to stand, and simmer on the stove for
an hour or more, then the watery portion
draiued oft, and cooled to blood heat, and
slightly sweetened (colored if you wish with
a teaspoonful of milk), will agree with the
most delicate stomach, and is almost as
nourishing as milk.

89

DIPHTHERIA.

Z-12. Take two tablespoonfuls of UNBOLTED WHEAT FLOUR, and wet it with cold water, to thickness of cream, then add this to two quarts of boiling water, and boil thirty minutes, strain, and serve. This agrees with children raised upon the bottle, sometimes, when milk does not. It arrests *Cholera Infantum.*

If baby's *stools are bloody,* boil a piece of MUTTON SUET with the milk, and season with a little salt.

DIPHTHERIA.—See Throat.

DIPLOPIA.—See Eye—Sight.

DISCOLORATION FROM A BRUISE. PREVENTIVE.—Apply Arnica oil. Calendula oil. Hamamelis *Raw beef. Raw Oysters.* "Cigar wrapper moistened." See Starch.

DISEASE, PREVENTIVE. — See Contagion guard.

DISINFECTANTS. See *Chlorine.* Potash. Salt. *Sulphur.* See under Contagion, mention of Bromine, Coffee, Gun powder, Onion, Tobacco, etc.

"To disinfect clothing, *bake them.* This is effectual.

DISLOCATION.—See Sprain.

DISSECTING KNIFE CUT.—Ars. LACH. See Alcohol. Ichthyol.—See Cause—*blood poison.*

DIURESIS.—See Urinary organs. Urine—flow copious.

DOSE.—The dose should be of a strength no greater than is simply sufficient to induce the needful reaction of the organism; all in excess of this, remains as an obstruction in the system, and delays recuperative action; hence minute doses frequently repeated, are more efficacious than large ones given at longer intervals.

It has been asserted that drugs administered in hot water, are much more sure and speedy in their action, than when given in cold water, and that half the usual dose will produce the desired effect.

If a medicine taken in minute doses, according to homœopathic indications, should aggravate existing symptoms, be not too readily discouraged; it may be a good omen; wait a little while, until the exacerbation has passed off; when perhaps improvement will set in. If it does, let it progress undisturbed, by further medication to the complete cure.

Omitting medicine. Every third week is a good plan in treatment of chronic ailments.

If the *adult* dose be stated, then for a child one year old, give one-twentieth of that dose, and for each year older one-twentieth more.

A SYSTEM OF OFFICINAL DOSAGE.
(G. A. W., M. D.)

1. The dose of all INFUSIONS, is 1 to 2 ounces, except infusion of digitalis, which is 2 to 4 drachms.

2. Dose of all poisonous TINCTURES, is 5 to 20 minims, except tincture of aconite, which is 2 to 5 minims.

3. Dose of WINES, is from ½ to 1 fluid drachm, except wine of opium, which is 5 to 15 minims.

4. Of all poisonous SOLID EXTRACTS, you can give ½ grain, except extract of Calabar bean, which is $\frac{1}{18}$ to $\frac{1}{4}$ grain.

DREAD.

5. Dose of all DILUTE ACIDS, is from 5 to 20 minims, except dilute hydrocyanic acid, which is 2 to 8 minims.
6. Dose of all AQUÆ is from 1 to 2 ounces, except aqua lauroceracus, and aqua ammonia, which are from 10 to 30 minims.
7. Of all SYRUPS, you can give 1 drachm.
8. Dose of all MIXTURES, is from ½ to 1 fluid ounce.
9. Dose of all SPIRITS, is from ½ to 1 fluid drachm.
10. Dose of ESSENTIAL OILS, is from 1 to 5 minims.

DREAD.—ACON.

When alone, Ars. Lyc.

In the dark, Camp. Stram. See Mind—Fear.

DRINKING GREEDILY. — Hell. Hep. See Nerve.

DROOPING SHOULDERS — STOOPING GAIT.—Pho. Sul. See Person.

DROPSY.—(See Diet M—See cold water).

"Feet bloated only, the *heart* in fault; abdomen only, the *liver;* all over bloated, the *kidney.*" *Apis.* APO C θ. *Ars.* EUP PUR θ. Nat s. PILO. Urti. Tab 1x. Oxyden θ, 1 drop before meals, increase 1 drop daily.

Region.—

Abdomen, Apo c. Ars. Chin.

Brain. Acute, APIS. Bry. HELL—Chronic, Bacill 200. Cal p. Kal iod. (See Head.)

Chest, Ars. Bry. Dig. (See Chest.)

Heart, Cact. *Dig* θ. Spig. (See Heart.)

Ovary, *Apis.* Bell. Lach. (See Ovary.)

Scrotum, Chel. Iod. RHOD. (See Scrotum.)

Joint, Aco. Bry. Pul—Knee, Bry. *Dig*—Ankle, Bry. Ferr.

Origin :—
    Ague, Elat. Ferr. Hell.
    Rheumatism, Bry. Colch.
    Scarlet fever, *Apis.* APOC θ. Hell. *Tereb.*
    Typhoid fever, *Apo c.* Ars. Chin.
    Amenorrhœa, Helon. Senecio θ 20 drop doses.
    Suppressed Eruption, Sul.

Symptomatic Indications :—
    Acute, febrile, Aco. *Apis.* Bry.
    Lips blue, Dig—Dry cracked, Bry.
    Thirst burning, Aco. *Ars.*—Constant sipping,
      Ars. Chin—Absent, Apis.
    Skin waxy pale, Apis. Ars—Greenish, Ars—
      Livid, Ars—Blue spots, Ferr. Sul.
    Pain Burning, Ars—Stinging, Apis—Stitch-
      ing, Bry.
    Urine thick yellow, Apo c θ—Pale copious,
      Senecio θ—Coffee-ground sediment, Hell—
      Red sand sed., Lyc.
    Strangury, *Apis.* Tereb. Urti.

DROWNING.—See Apparent death.

DROWSINESS.—See Sleep.

DRUNKENNESS. See Alcoholism.

DRY CUPS. *Carbuncle:* "Upon the appearance
of one or more of the little ulcers on the carbuncle apply a dry cup, saturating the paper
used with turpentine before lighting it. In a
moment the section of the cup will open the
cells, and there will exude into it a teaspoonful
of thin pus. Follow this with poultice to keep
up the discharge, and in a *few days* the carbuncle will vanish. In this way we obviate from
three to six weeks' suffering."

Strangulated Inguinal Hernia: Cured after
    collapse had set in, by using a jar, as a dry
    cup, applied upon the abdomen.

DUODENUM.

Obstruction of the bowel, with stercoraceous vomiting: Cured by the same. A very large bowl, capable of covering the abdomen below the navel was applied as a dry cup. In 15 minutes there was relief, then rumbling was heard, and in 20 minutes after, by aid of copious injections of hot water, there were several free stools of undigested food.

Dangerous flooding: Cured by the same.

Hiccough: After all usual remedies had failed, was arrested at once by the same.

DUODENUM.—See enteritis.

Inflammation, Ars. Pod. Kali m.

Ulceration, Ars. Cal iod. Cal p. Uran n.

DYSCRASIA.—See Cause.

DYSMENORRHŒA. — See Female — Menses, *painful.*

DYSPEPSIA.—See Stomach—Derangement.

DYSPNŒA.—See Chest—Respiration, *difficult.*

DYSURIA.—See Urinary Organs—Urine flow, *painful.*

EAR.—

Earache—otalgia—otitis :—

From a cold, Acon. Cham. Pul.

In cold damp weather, Dul.

Pains shooting, Mer. Pul—Stinging, Apis. Mer—Stitching, Cham. Mer. Spig. Throbbing, *Bell.* Mer. Nat m.

With one red cheek, Cham—Headache, Bell.

Worse in the evening, Pul—At night, Mer.

(See *Aconite.* Chlorof. Cocaine. Hot water. MULLEIN OIL. *Olive Oil.* Onion. VERATRUM).

Deafness: (See Arnica. Glycer. *Mullein.* Tan. *Veratrum*). CAL C. Led. Pul. Sul. Vis a.

As from stoppage, Calc. *Pul.* Mer—Coming and
going, Mag c. Nit a. Spig.

From Ague, Chin. Mer—Catarrh, ARS IOD.
Bellis p LED. Nit a. Pet—Enlarged tonsils,
Ars iod. Cal p. Kali m.

With oozing discharge, Hep—Moisture, Cal c.
Lyc. *Sil*—Cracking in the ears, CAL C. SUL
—Dryness, Grap. Thuj.

Better when riding in car or carriage, Grap—removing wax. Con—Can hear the human voice
better than other sounds, Ig—The reverse,
Pho.

Worse in the fall, Sil—in winter, Sul 30.

Otorrhœa—Suppurative otitis: Aur 3x. *Aurum mur and oleum* j. Lyc. Nat p. *Sil. Sul. Skook, in. and ex.*—Mullein oil in the ear.

Bloody, Grap. Mer. MER D 3X. Pet.

Excoriating, Ars. *Ars iod. Sul.* TELL.

Fetid, *Ars iod.* Bovis. *Pso.* Sil. TELL. THUJ.

Green, Mer. *Pul.* Kal s.

Yellow, HEP. Kal s. Kal bi. Nat m. PUL.

Watery, thin, Ars Elaps. Sil. TELL.

From catarrh, Ars iod. Aurum mur—Measles,
Pul—Scarlet fever, Grap. Hep—Vaccine, *Sil.*
THUJ—(See ACETAN. Alum. BORAX. *Car-
bola.* EUCA. Hydrogen. Tann).

Outer ear:—

Burning, Hyper. Kreo. Sang—As if frost bitten,
Agar—One ear burns Ig.

Numbness, Plat.

Redness, Aco. Sul—Bluish red, Tell—with
burning, *Agar*—with swelling, Apis. Grap.

Eczema, Bacill 200. *Skook* 3x.

Herpes, Cist. Sep—moist, Grap. Kreo. Ol.

Behind the Ear:—

Dampness, Cal c. GRAP. Lyc. Ol. Pet—Oozing row, Grap. Ol—Offensive, Grap. Ol.

Scurf, Cic. Grap. Hep.

Swelling, Caps, *Carb a*—Of the bone, Carb v.

Ulcer, Aur. Nit a. Sil.

Under the Ear:—

Glands swollen BAR C. Cal c. MER PROT. Sil. Sul—and dark red, *Rhus*—Gathering, Cist. Cal p. Hep. Sil.

In the Ear:—

Bug or grub; Dislodge with Tobacco smoke, see Chloroform.

Foreign body in the ear; insert a horse-hair loop, as far as it will go, give it a turn, and draw it out, the patient the while lying down with *that* ear up. A few trials will insure success. Instillation of oil brings about spontaneous expulsion; after introducing the oil a cotton plug is to be inserted, and patient directed to lie as much as possible on *that* side.

Boil in the ear, Mer. Pic ac. Sil.

Polypus, Cal c. CAL P. Hep. Sang. TEUCR. Thuj 30.

Gathering, Hep. Mer. Sil. See Onion.

Swelling, tenderness, *Bell.* Hep. *Mer.* Pul. Sil.

Sensations in the Ear:—

Coldness, Lach. Mer. Verat a.

Fulness, Cann I—As if stuffed with air, Aur.

Pulsation, Rhus—Preventing sleep, Cact.

Pressing out, Con. Kal c. PUL. Sil.

Stoppage, Ana. Con. Lyc. PUL. Spig. Sil. Mer—with every step the ear seems to open and shut, Graph.

96

Throbbing, Bell. Mer. Nit a.

Tingling, *Aco.* Bell.—From quinine, Bell.

Wabbling as of water, Sul —as of a worm, Rhod.

Sounds in the Ear:—(See Borax.)

Buzzing, Caust. Iod. Sabin. Mer.

Banging, Grap. Sil.

Cracking, Bar c. Sil. Nit a—Cracking when chewing, Grap. Kal c. Pet.

Fluttering, Agar. Sil. *Spig.* Tart e.

Hissing, Grap. Sul.

Humming, Bell. Con. Cro. Sul.

Re-echoing of the voice, CAUST.

Ringing, Cann I. CHIN. FERR. *Ferr p.* Nux v. Sil. Sul—As of bells, Alu. Cann I. Pet.—At " Change of Life," Con.

Roaring, ACO. Mer. Nit a. Nux v. Ph a.

Rushing, Pet.

Whizzing, *Chin.* Pho. Sul.

All noise intolerable, *Aco.* BELL *Nux v.* Sil. THERID.

Ear wax:—

Black, Elaps. Pul.

Red, Con.

White, Con. Lach. Sep.

Hard, Con. Lach.

Moist, Hep. Sil.

Thin, Con. Mer. Sil.

ECLAMPSIA.—See Spasm.

ECTHYMA.—See Skin.

ECZEMA.—See Skin.

EFFUSION.—Apis. Ars. Bry. Kali m. See Œdema.

ELBOW.—See Limb—Arn.

D   97

ELM.

ELM.—*Constipation:*—Take at night on going to bed, or in the morning before breakfast, a heaping tablespoonful of *powdered* slippery elm bark in a convenient quantity of water. Continue the daily dose until the bowels become regular. Chronic cases may require several weeks.

Acidity of the Stomach—Milk curdling in the Stomach:—Slippery elm bark finely pulverized, added to cow's milk, boiled or unboiled, will prevent it. A teaspoonful will serve for a pint of milk, but it may not be best to mix so much at one time.

Punctured wound.—When you do not want a wound to close, insert into it a tent, made of a smooth piece of elm bark; it will not cause pain to introduce it; and it expands gradually, thus enlarging the opening. The same to keep open an incision into an abscess if desired.

EMACIATION.—See Atrophy. Person. Infant. Charcoal. Diet x. z.

EMETIC.—Alum 120 grains in water. Ipecac 20 to 30 grains in water. Sulphate of zinc 15 to 20 grains in a little water. Apomorph $\frac{1}{8}$ grain in solution *hypoderm* (in any case of poisoning except that of opium, or morphine); repeat the dose if necessary. Salt, an ounce, in luke warm water. A pinch of snuff on the tongue. Injection of tobacco smoke or tea. Copious draughts of tepid water. Titillation of fauces with feather, etc.

EMISSIONS, SEMINAL.—See Male—Spermatorrhœa.

EMPHYSEMA.—See Chest.

EMPYEMA.—*Ars. Carbol ac.* Chin. Kal p. PYROGEN in water, 2 hours. *Sil.*

98

ENCEPHALITIS.—See Head—Brain.

ENCHONDROMA —Arg m. Sil.   See Bone.

ENDOCARDITIS.—See Heart.

ENDOMETRITIS.—See Female—Uterus.

ENTERITIS.—See Abdomen.

EPILEPSY.—Seek for cause, examine eyes, teeth, urethra, etc. (See spasm.)

In general, *Aurum bro 3x. Atrop 2x and Strych 2x.* Arg n. Avena. *Bufo. Borax* 5 to 20 gráins. Cal c. Cic. Coc. Hyo. INDIGO 2x. Kal p. Laur. MELI *θ. Œnanth θ* 5 drops Pæon. PASS *θ.* 60 drops. *Pothos f θ* 10 drops. Sil. *Solan c* 10 drops, 6 hours. Stram. MER and LACH. (See Amyl. See Bandage.) (See Diet, P.   )

Infants at the breast, Arn. and Hep. *Hell. Eer.* Mer. and *Lach.*

EPISTAXIS.—See Nose-bleed.

EPITHELIOMA.—See Lactic acid. Resorcin. Thuj.

EROTOMANIA.—*Canth. Lach. Pic-ac.* Dul. Pho. Plat. *Hyo.* Stram. " Mono-bromide of Camphor, 10 gr. doses."

ERUCTATIONS.—See Stomach—Derangement.

ERUPTIONS.—See Skin.

ERYSIPELAS.—(See *Alcohol.* Bism. Cold water. Ichthy. *Lead.* Log wood. Starch). PILO 1x. *Urti.* "No remedy acts better than Passiflora *θ,* adult 30 to 60 drops as occasion requires. It even controls the delirium." "Cantharis *θ,* 1 drachm in water 1 pint, bathe 3 times a day, cure in 3 days." "Bathe with Aqua Ammo. and let it evaporate. Three applications cures." "Apply raw cranberry pulp." "Paint with Iodine."

99

ERYTHEMA.

Blackish, Am c. Ars. Crotal.

Erratic, Bell. Pul.

In the joints, Bry.

Moist, Grap.

Œdematous, Apis.

Smooth, Apis, Bell.

Vesicular, CANTH. Carbol ac 30. Euphorb.
RHUS.

Ulcerative, Grap. Hep. Sul.

Chronic erysipelas: Grap. LAPPA. Sul. Bathe
it daily with alcohol. See Ichthyol.

After amputation: Cinchona. (See Calend Logwood).

From mechanical injury, Arn. *Rhus.* See
Cold water.

ERYTHEMA.—See Skin.

ETHER.—*Local external pain, rheumatic, myal-
gic, neuralgic:* Pour on ether, or apply by spray.
until the parts become numb. Guard the eyes.
Internally for *pain,* adult 1 drachm in ice cold
water.

Spinal Irritation. Nervous affections. Chorea:—
Ether spray to the spine.

Hernia, strangulated: Place absorbent cotton on
the rupture and saturate it with ether. It will
reduce itself.

Extraction of tooth without pain, local anæthesia:
Into ½ ounce of ether, put 3 drachms of pulv.
Camphor; soak cotton in this and apply it for
5 minutes around the tooth (and *in it if* hollow)
or until the gum becomes white, then operate

Lockjaw: Inhale ether until the jaw relaxes, and
from time to time afterwards, to keep up the
relaxation. To render relaxation more prompt,
safe, and pleasant, and recovery quicker, shut

off the circulation in the extremities, upper
and lower by tight bandage.

To disinfect a *musty room*—"ratty parlor":—
"Fill a small single wick lamp with chloric
ether, and burn it in the room, for a short
time."

EUCALYPTUS.—*Ulcerative Ophthalmia:* "Eucalyp. fl. ex. 1 drachm, in distilled water 1
ounce, mix; shake well together, and drop a
little into the suffering eye several times a day.
Quick relief and speedy cure."

Otorrhœa:—Fl. Ex. Eucalyp. 1 ounce, and water
1 ounce, mix; inject this into the ear, two or
three times a day, after cleansing each time
with tepid water. "Cure in 3 weeks."

Diphtheritic Croup:—Fill an atomizer with oil
of Eucalyptus, and oil of Turpentine, equal
parts mixed, and spray the throat every ½
hour. "Relief in an hour, cure in a day."

*Gastric Ulcer. Stomach Pains. Old stomach
troubles:* Fl. Ex. Eucalyp , adult, teaspoonful
doses in milk before meals. "Works won-
ders."

Diabetes: Fl. Ex. Eucalyp. adult, 20 drops, 4
times a day.

Ague: "Not failed once in a hundred cases,
Eucalyp. fl. ex. adult, 60 drops, 3 times a day."

Traumatic Fever: Eucalyp. fl. ex. adult 5 drops
every hour. "Superior to all other remedies."

Wound:—*To prevent suppuration--Stump dressing.* Oil of Eucalyp, 10 per cent. solution in
Olive oil. "The best thing ever yet tried."

Chitblains: Oil of Eucalyp. apply with Camel-
hair brush, "prompt relief, and speedy cure."

Typhoid Fever: (all stages and types):—"Eucalyp
2x, controls the high temperature, better than

EXCITEMENT, MENTAL, NERVOUS.

any other remedy, and conducts the case safely through from beginning to end. In case of *tympanitis*, or hæmorrhage from the bowels, aid internal treatment by enema of Eucalyptol. To 1 drachm of the oil, beaten up with the yolk of an egg, add a mixture of 1 pint each, of milk and water, and throw it well up into the bowel."

EXCITEMENT. MENTAL. NERVOUS—See Mind—Nerve.

EXCORIATION.—See Skin.

EXCRESCENCE.—See Tumor. Wart—See Skin.

EXHAUSTION.—See Diet. A. I. R.—See Cause.

EXOSTOSIS.—See Bone.

EXPECTORATION.—See Chest—Cough.

EXUDATION.—See Effusion.

EYE.—

Inflammation. Ophthalmia :—ACO. Ars. *Aur.* BELL. EUPH. Grap. Pul. SUL. Lave with carbonated water. (See * Alum. Bell. Borax. Chlorine. Eucalyp. Hama. Hydrast —Hydrogen. Mullein oil, Salt. SILVER. Soda Zinc. *Purulent Ophthalmia.* See especially Hama. SILVER.

Of the Lids—Blepharitis:—ACO. ARS. BELL. Calc. Clem. Euph. Ferrp. GRAP. Hep. Kali m. *Kal bi and Mer bin.* MER. NAT M. Pul. Sil. Sul. Stap—(See * especially Hydrast. Soda.)

Of the Conjunctiva—Conjunctivitis:—Simplex, *Aco.* Ars *Bell.* EUPH. Grap. Pul. Sul—Purulent, Aco. ARG N. Apis. Calc. Cal p. *Hep. Mer.* PAL. Sul—Neonatorum, *Arg n.* Apis. Hep. *Kals.* Mer. *Nat. p.* Pul (See * especially *Acetan* Bell. Borax. Ham. Silver.)

Of the Choroid Coat. Choroiditis:—Bry. Gel.
Ig. Mer. *Santo.* Thuj.—Worse at night, Mer.
Of the Iris—Iritis: Bell. Bry. Clem. Euph.
Gel. Ferr p. KAL IOD. Kali m. MER. RHUS.
Thuj—Worse at night, Mer—Suppurative, Hep.
Mer. Sil. Sul—Syphilitic Asa. *Aur.* KAL IOD.
MER C. Nit a. Hot dry applications. (See
* especially Bella.)
Of the Eye Ball—Keratitis: Apis. ARS. *Aur.*
BAR IOD. Cal c. Euph. GRAP. Hep. Mer. Sul.
—Suppurative—Ulcerative, Ars. Cal p. HEP.
Mer. Sul. Dry hot applications every hour,
10 minutes at a time. (See * especially Bell.
Euca. Hydras.)
Of the Retina. Retinitis: Bell. Ferr p. *Gel.* Kali m.
PIC AC. Lach. *Santo*—Worse at night, Mer—
Of the Sclerotic coat. Sclerotitis: Ferr p. Kali m.
Thuj.

Symptomatic Indications of Eye Remedies;—

Burning, Aco. ARS. Cal c. Carb v. Euph.
GRAP—Sul. ZN—Like fire shooting out,
Dul—More in the evening, Pul. ZN—Burn-
ing and itching, Ars. Canth. Pho. Pul. *Sul*
—Burning after reading, *Ruta.*

Coldness, *Alu.* CON. Pho. Plat—As if cold air
under the lids, Fl ac—As of cold air flowing
out, Thuj.

Dryness, *Bell. Grap.* Mer. Nux m. SUL.
Verat a. *ZN.*

—More in the morning, Sul. ZN.

Heat, Bell. *Cham.* Carb v. Ran b.

Itching, Pul. Rhus. Sep. Sul—More in the
evening, Pul. Sul—More in the morning,
Sul.

Smarting, Iod. Lyc. Sul—As from Salt, Nux v—

As from sand, Alu. CAUST. Euph. *Grap.*
Pho. Rhus. *Sep.* SUL. THUJ. ZN—More in
the morning, NAT M.

Sensitiveness to cold air, must have the eyes
covered up warm, Hep. *Sil.* THUJ—Lids
sensitive, easily reddened, GRAP.

Pains in the Eyes. CIMIC in. and ex. EUPH.
Onos. *Pic ac.* Prun s. SPIG.

(See Euca. Hama. Opi. Zinc).

From eye strain, *Agar.* Carb v. Chin. *Nat m.*
RUTA.

Pain in the eye better by:—

Cold applications, Arg n. Apis. Alu. Nit a.
Pul.

Being in cold air, Asa.

Gentle touching, Bry. Caust.

Rubbing, Caust. Cina.

Pain in the eye worse by:—

Cold water bathing, Sul.

Looking down, Lyc.

Stooping, Con. Ferr p.

Moving the eyeballs, BRY. Kalmi. Ph a. PB.
SPIG.

Touching the eye, Aur. Asa.

Eye suffering caused by:—

Bruise, Arni. Con. Tight shoes, Sec.

Cold in the eye, *Cal iod.* Jac. Sang—Red and
watery, EUPH. NAT M 2x. Pul. Kali iod.
" *Rhus and Lach.* "

Close application to books writing, or fine
work, *Agar.* Carb v. China. Lith c. *Nat m.*
RUTA. SYMPH.

Use of improper glasses, Cro. Fl ac.

Dreg of Diphtheria, Gel. NUX V. Kal p.

Eruption suppressed, Ars. Bacill 200. Cal c.
SUL. Viol t.

Foot sweat checked, Sil.

Gonorrhœa suppressed, Mer. Pul.

Gout, Colch. Pul.

Rheumatism, Aco. *Bry.* COLCH. Kalmi Pul. RHUS.

Scrofula, ARS IOD. *Cal c. Cal p.* CIST. Grap. Hep. Lyc. Mer. SUL.

Syphilis, Asa. *Aur.* KAL IOD. MERC. *Nit a.*

Vaccine, Ars. Bacill 200. SIL. THUJ. "Thuj 30 then Nit a 6."

Flow of tears—Lachrymation: *Cep. Euph.* NAT M. Pilo. Pul. Thuj—(See Hama).

Acrid corroding, making lids and cheeks sore, *Ars.* Euph. Mer. NAT M.

Burning, *Cep.* Mer. Nat m.

From reading or writing, Ferr. Ip. Ol—with every attempt to use the eyes, Ipe.

When out in open air, *Cal c.* Sil. Sul—In the wind, *Pho.* Pul. Sul.

Tear duct closed, the tears flow out over the cheek, Cal fl. Fl ac. Sil. Thuj.

Phlegm in the eyes—"Blear-Eye": Arg n. Euph. Gel. Lyc. Pul—Forming a film, Apis—Yellow, Kal s.

Constant need to wipe the eyes, Arg n. Cro. *Euph*—or wink, Cro. *Euph.*

Dread of Light—Photophobia: (See Iodine).

Carbonated water lavement. *Aco. Ars.* BELL. Caust. CON. Euph. Gel 30. GRAP. RHUS. Sul—More in the morning, Nux v. *Pet.* Rhus—More at night, Bell. *Glo.* Hep. MER. Pho. THUJ—Without inflammation, Con. Ig.

Light causes blinking, Caust. Spig, or aching of the balls, Hep; or darting pain, Grap. or Stitches, Sul.

Desire for Light—Photomania: Aco. Am m. GEL. *Stront*—Light and company, Stram.

Lids :—

Agglutinated, BAR IOD. Carb v. GRAP. KAL C. Lyc. Mer. *Pul.* Sil. Thuj. ZN. *Mullein oil lavement.* (See Borax. Salt).

Blue, DIG. Dros. Plat—edges, Verat a.

Bloated, Apis. Ars. *Ars iod.* Dig. Kal iod—like bladders, Apis. Rhus—Under the brow, KAL C.

Bulging conjunctiva, between the closed lids, Ars. Rhus. Sul.

Closed lids, tight, and if forced open, hot tears gush out, Aur. *Con. Rhus*, or blood, Bell. Nux v; or Matter, Arg n. Hep. Lyc. Cracked and bleeding, *Grap.*

Dryness, *Grap. Sul.* Verat a—Dry mucus on the lashes, *Grap*—Lashes turn in, Grap.

Drooping Lids—Ptosis: Arg n. CAUST. Con. Euph. GEL. Kal iod. PB. *Rhus. Sep.* Verat a. ZN.

Granulated Lids—Trachoma: ACO. ARS. Bell. EUPH. *Mer iod.* Py ht. Sang 6x. *Sul* 30-200.

Apply Apis. cerate, Lactic acid 50 per cent. solution by swab daily. Mullein oil daily: (See *Alum.* Hydrast. Hydrogen. QUINIA. Salt Silver.)

Hard swollen, *Aco.* Nit a. Thuj—Hard and scaly, Thuj.

Heavy, Gel. *Grap.* Nat m. *Rhus.* Sep. Sul.

Inverted, Apis. Mer.

Itching, Pul. Rhus. Sep. Sul—Edges, Sul. Stap.

Pustules inside, Kal bi. Mer. Nit a.

Quivering, Alu. Plat—Upper lids, Arum. Cal c.

Redness intense, *Aco.* Bell. Mer. NAT M. *Sul*

—Dark red, Ars—Shining red. ACO. Apis.
BELL. Ferr p. Hep—Red when in open air,
THUJ—Redness and pain from the least use,
Kal c—Redness from the least irritation.
Grap 3x.

Raw lids, Bacill 200. NAT M—Calendula oil ex.

Smarting, Arg m. *Clem.* Lyc. *Nux v.* Sul.

Scurfy, scaly. GRAP. *Mer.* Sep. *Thuj.*

Stiff, Kalmi. Rhus. Spig.

Stye—Hordeolum: Hep. *Grap.* Mer. PUL. *Sil.*
Sul. STAP. Thuj. URAN N—Ailments from
suppressed styes, URAN N. (See *Iodine*).

Tightness, as if they did not cover the balls:
Sep—As if glued to the balls, Mer.

Twitching—Blepharo, Spasm: Agar. Cic. PLAT.
Mag p. Ruta. Pho. PHYSOS.

Ulcerated, Euph. *Kal iod.* Lyc. *Mer.*

Warty, Caust. Thuj.

Wild hairs, Grap. Lashes turn in. Grap. Tell.

Corners.—Sore, Bacill. Grap. Kal c. ZN.

Inner corner, blue, Sars—Itching, Alu. Ruta—
Red, Z N—"One red mass," Arg n—Smarting
Con. Stap—Skin from the corner spreading
over the ball—*Pterygion*—("Bat wing"):—
Thuj. ZN.

Outer corner. Sore, Aut c—sore, cracked and
bleeding, Grap.

Balls :—

" Bloodshot," Aco. Bell. *Nux v*—"One gore,"
CRO. Thuj.

Bulging, Bell. Como. Guai. Stram. ZN—
Staphyloma, Thuj.

Drawn toward each other—Convergent Squint:
Alu. Bell. *Cyc. Mag p.* Mer—In brain affec-

tions, Apis Bell. Hell—In new born babe, Arn. Hep.

Drawn apart. Divergent Squint:—Alu. Con. Cyc. Mag p. *Ruta.*

Enlarged feeling, Lach. Nat m. Spig.

Gyrating sensation, Cro.

Glazed, as in death, Lyc. Ph ac.

Glistening, Bell. Stram.

Jerking, Agar. Cic. Mag. p.

Oscillating, Physos.

Rolling, Hyo. Physos. Stram.

Rolled up, Hell. Naj. Verat a.

Sparkling, Bell. Stram.

Staring, Cic. Hyo. Stram—In stupor, Op. ZN— As of terror, *Aco.* Sec. Stram.

Specked. See Cornea.

Cornea :—

Blue, Spig.

Gray, Apis.

"Ground glass," Sul.

Opaque, Apis. Arg n. Aur. Cal c. Cann s. Cal fl. Fl ac. Teucr.

Specked with blisters, Mer. Nat m. Sang— Pimples, Arg n. Kal bi. Mer. (See Resorcin)

Ulcerated, Aur. CAL C. Cal fl. CIMI θ dilute in. and ex. Euph. *Fl ac. Hep.* MER. Sul— With adhesion, Mer. Sul. See reference under Ophthalmia especially, EUCA. *Resorcin.* Lactic acid.)

Yellow color, Chel. Crotal. Lach. PB. Sep— Dirty yellow, Chel. Iod. *Kal bi.* Kal c. Pod. See Jaundice.

Pupils :—

Too large—Dilated, BELL. *Cal c. Cina. Gel. Hyo.* Nit a. OP. *Stram.* Verat a.—In concussion of the brain, Arn. Cic.—Dilated and insensible, Bell. Cic. Op.

Too small—Contracted, Bell. *Camp.* Mur a. Pilo. *Sep.* Tab. Verat a. ZN—In spasm, Cic. Hyo. Physos.

Green Color—Glaucoma:—ARS. *Arg n 200.* AUR. Bell. Bry. COLO. GEL. Mag p. Pho. SPIG. "Eserine sulph; 2 grs to the ounce of water; a drop in the eye, every 2 or 3 hours, to contract the pupil.

Sight—Vision—Defective :—

Amaurosis—Amblyopia. See indications subjoined.

Astigmatism, Lil t. Physos.

Cataract, Caust. Con. CAL FL. Colch. FL AC. Kal s. Pho. Sec. SIL. CINERARIA, 2 drops in the eye, 3 times a day. It does not produce inflammation, only a slight burning for a few minutes. Shows signs of improvement in a few days. "Cure in 3 months."

Hemeralopia—night blindness: Con. *Nux v.* 6. "Evening or night blindness, may be cured in a few days by placing a slice of calf's liver on live coalts, and holding the face over it, so as to receive the fumes upon the eyes, 10 minutes at a time twice a day."

Sudden total loss of sight, ACO 3x 2 hours.

Blur, Euph. Gel—From falling of the womb, Sep.

Dazzle, Con. Ph. ac. SIL.

Dimness, Pilo—"Massage of the ball and Apis"—On waking, Cyc. Pul—Going into a warm room, Pul—As if looking through gauze, Ars. Caust. Pho. Sul—Yellow gauze, Kal bi—Through mist, Cal c. Caust. Grap.

Mer. Pet—Veil, Sul—Smoke, Gel—Edges of objects dim, Bell.

Momentary loss of sight—vanishing vision: Mer. *Pho.* SIL. Sul. Stram—*With* vertigo, Aco. Bell—*When* blowing the nose, Caust—Stooping, Ferr p. Grap. Nat m—Rising up, Hep—Looking down, Nat m.

Weak sight, CAL FL. *Con.* Sil. Sul—After Diphtheria, Kal p. *Nux v 2x.* Sil—Seek cause.

Can see only one-half of an object (Hemiopia): Aur. Lith c. Nat m. Sep—The left half, Lith c. Lyc.—Upper or lower half, Bovis. Caust. Lyc. Nat m.—Can see an object only when looking sideways, Chin 200.

Cannot see well after 4 p. m., Lyc—After sun set. Bell—Can see better in twilight, Pho.

When reading, the letters seem to move, Agar, Aur. Cann I. Nux v—Quiver, Bell—Run together, Arg n. *Cann I.* Grap. NAT M—Also look pale, Chin. Sil, or Red, Pho; or double, Grap.

Objects Appear:—

Black, Pho—also double, Cic.

Blue, Lach.

Double—*Diplopia:* AUR. Bell. Cic. LYC. Dig. *Gel. Hyo.* Nit a. Sil. Verat a—Mixed, Aur. Nat m—Inverted, Bell—Oblique, Stram—Out of place, Sul.

Green, Ars. Dig—Green halo, Pho Sep. Sul 200.

Red, Bell. Con. Hep. Pho—Letters look red. Pho—Red halo, Bell. Lach.

Yellow, Alo. Canth. Cin. Dig. SANTO—As through yellow gauze, Kal bi.

Too large, *Æth.* Hep. HYO. *Laur.* NUX M. Too small, Hyo. *Plat.* Stram.

Too near, Agar. Bovis. Cic—To each other, Nux m.

Too remote, Ana. Nux m. Pho. Stan.

Appearances in vision, of:—

Black points, motes, spots, Bell China. Hyo. Mer. Nit a. Pho. Sep. Sil. Sul—Floating, dancing motes, Agar. Con. Pho.

Cobweb, Bell.

Colors various, Con. Pho. Mag p.

Dark stripes, Sul.

Distortions—Grimaces, Bell, Hyo. Stram.

Flashes, Bell. Mag p. Nux v. Spig.

Flickering, CYC. Lach Sul. Thuj—More in the morning, Lyc.

Feathers, Lyc.

Fiery points, Nat m—Rays about the light, Bell. Lach.

Fog, Caust. Mer. Pet. Pho. Pul. Sul.

"Golden shower," ZN.

Green halo, Pho. Sep. Sul 200.

Red halo, Bell. Verat v.

Rays of light broken, Bell.

Shadows, Cal c. Senecio.

Serpent like forms, Arg n. Physos.

Smoke, Bell. Cyc. Gel. Pho. PB.

Sparks, Bell. Chin. Lyc. Mag p—Flashing, Glo.

Stars, *Cyc.* Mag p—White, Kal c.

Yellow spots, Am m. Ph ac. Santo.

Yellow rings, Alo.

Zigzags, Ig. Nat m.

FACE.—

Pain in the Face. Faceache. See Pain. See Neuralgia. See Cocaine. Glo 3x. SPIG 2x. ZN v 2x—Periodical, Ars. Chin. *Spig*—One side,

Colo. Kalmi. Pul. Spig—Left, Colo. Lach.
Stap—Right, Con--Extending from cheek
bone to ear, Lach—Involving the ear, Hep.
Pul—Starting from, or involving the eye,
Cimi. Pho. *Ruta. Spig.* Strap—Neath the eye,
Arg n—Eyebrow, Sil—Root of the nose, Nux
v. Pul—Extending into the head, Thuj.
Burning pain, Ars. Rhus.
Crampy, Mez. *Plat.* Thuj.
Tearing, Pho. Vis a.
Worse in the evening, Con. Pho. *Pul*—Night,
Con. Led. *Mer.* Sil—Eating, talking, Pho—
Touch or motion, Colo. *Spig*—Draft of air,
Verb 200—Cold damp weather, Dul.

Condition of the Face :—

Barber's Itch: Carbol ac 2x—Remove the crust
with flaxseed poultice, cut off all the beard
possible, apply for half hour hot water, by
sponge or cloth. Then with camel hair brush
apply lotion of water 100 drops, alcohol 100
drops, and Kreosote 1 drop, every other day.
In a week double the Kreosote. Moisten the
parts with spittle, and rub on ashes of cigar 3
times a day.
Beard falling out, Cal c. Grap. Nat m.
Mustache falls out, Kal c. *PB.*
Beard on Lady's face removed: " Mix Barium
Sulphide 1 drachm, Quick lime 1 drachm,
Starch powder 2 drachms; and make of this
mixture a paste, with alcohol, sufficient for
use each time, and apply; allow it to remain
on until some pain is felt, and then remove it· '
Continue from day to day, until the hair roots
are destroyed." See HYDROGEN. " Yellow Sulphate of Arsenic, and Quick lime equal
parts, make into a paste with hot water, apply

the paste, and allow it to remain and *dry* on
the face. No hair will show *there* for two or
three weeks. May be never." "Sulphide of
Calcium paste is the least irritating, and at the
same time most effective. The hair falls out
readily, after the paste has been allowed to remain some hours upon the bearded parts.

Black pores. "*Black heads*" *Comedones:* Grap.
Nit a. Sul.

   (See Clay. Sali acid. Vinegar.)

Blisters around the mouth—Herpes Labialis—
Hep. Mer. NAT M. *Rhus.*

Bloat—Œdema: Pho.—Glossy, Aur—Over the
eye, KAL C—Between the eyes, Lyc—Under
the eyes, Apis, Ars. Pho—Puffy face, Apo c θ.
Apis. Aur—Red, soft puff, *Bry.* Sul.

Chapped skin, Arum.

Enlarged feeling in the face, Aco

Eruptions around the eyes, Ars. *Euph.* Hep.
 Mer. In the eye brows, Caust. Kal c. Stap
 —Around the mouth, *Arum.* Bry. NAT M.
 Rhus. Kreo—At corners of the mouth, Mer.
 Nit a—On the lips, Mer. *Nat m.* Sil. (See
 Benzo, Collod).

Feeling like Cobweb on the face, Alu. Bar c.
 Borax. Grap; or white of egg dried on, Alu.
 Kal iod.

Formication, Plat.

Freckles. Pho. Lave with milk-whey; or white
 of egg stirred in water—(See Benzo, Chlorine,
 Hydrogen and Lactic acid).

Greasy skin, Nat m. PB. Thuj. Lave with
 weak lye.

Grin—Lips drawn back showing the teeth,
 Angus. Nux v.

Lumpy jaw, Hec. 1. Kal iod.

 D*   113

Lupus: Ars. Bacill 200. Canth. Carbol ac. 2x.
HYDROCT 6: 12 in and ex. Nat p. Oleum j.
THUJ in. and ex. Dip a camel-hair brush into
Kreosote, then into Calomel powder dry, and
apply daily.

—Non exedens, Bacill 200. Kal bi.

(See Glycer. Ichthy. Lact acid. Ointment).

Mentagra. Chin eruption: Cic. Kali m. Thuj—
Raw chin, Arum. *Bry.*

Moth Patches: Caul. (See Hydro. Lact a.)

Netted veins, Plat. Thuj 30.

Numbness, Asa. *Plat*—Of the skin, Ol—Paralytic, Caust. Coc. Nux v.

Paralysis, Bell. *Caust. Coc.* Nux v.

Pimples—Acne: Ars bro. *Ars iod 2x.* FL AC.
Gel. LED. NIT A 1x, 3 drop, 12 hours, in
water, in and ex. *Psor.* Sul. From masturba-
tion, Bellis p—vaccine, Thuj—Blue pimples,
Lach. Mer—Mattery, Ant c. Grap. Thuj—
(See Alo. *Borax.* Collod. Glycer. Icthy. Lime
Sulph. Sali ac.)

Pustules, Ant c. Grap. Hep. Mez. *Tart e.* THUJ.

Spots, " Mottled skin," *Carb a.* Laur. Rhus.
Sil—Wine colored patches, see Solar Cautery.

Scabs, Cic. Rhus. SARS 2X—with sore nose,
ANT C—*Crusta lacta,* Lyc. Mer. *Rhus.*
Stap—Sycotic Scab, Thuj.

Scurf around the mouth, Pet. Sep—On the
chin, white, Cic.

Sore raw spots, bleeding by picking, *Arum*—
Sore raw chin, Arum. Bry—Sore mouth corners, Ant c. Mer. Rhus—Sore cracked mouth
corners, Ant c. Arum. *Condu.*

Stiff jaw, from a cold, Dul. Gel. Kreo—Tightness, can hardly open the mouth, Caust. Nux v
--Sweat around the mouth, Aco. Rheub--On the

nose, Ruta—Cold sweat, Hell. Tart e. verat a.

Tan: (See Hydro. Lact a.)

Tetter, around the mouth, Kreo. Nat m—on the lips, Sep.

Twitching, Agar. Bell. Cic. Ig.

Wrinkled, old look, *Arg n.* Cal c. Fl ac. LYC. SARS Sep—In brain trouble, Hell—In old age, rub them out with Lanolin—See Person.

Lips:—

Black, Ars. Chin. Mer c. verat a—"Sooty coating," Pho.

Burning, Am m. Ars. Mur ac.

Cracked (See Glycerine), *Grap 30.* Sil 30. Nat m—Lower lip cracked in the middle, Am c, Dro. NAT M—Mouth corners, *Ant c.* Arum, Condu. *Grap.*

Crimson, Sul.

Dry parched, ARS. BRY. Con. *Nat m.* Grap. Sil.

Drawn back showing the teeth, Angus. *Nux v.*

Pale, bloodless, Caust. Cal c. *Ferr. Helon. Pic ac,* Kal p—Whole upper lip death white, angular, ÆTH.

Slimy, ZN—Gummed together, Cann I. Fl ac. Kal iod. *Mer bin.*

Swollen upper lip, Nat m. Sul—More in the morning, Bovis. Cal c.

Trembling lower lip, Arn.

Color of face:—

Blue, Camp. Con. CUP M. DIG. Hyo. Ipe. *Kal p.* LACH. *Verat a.* ZN—Around the Eyes, Ars. Bell. *Chin.* CINA. Cic. *Cimi.* Hyo. Ipe. *Lyc.* Ol. Pho. Rhus. Sec—Around the mouth, Ars iod. *Cina.* Cap m. Ph ac.

FAINTING.

Brown, Iod. Nit a. Sep. Sul—Brown patches, Sep.

Changing color, pale and red, Bell. *Ig*. Pho. *Plat*—red to pale on rising in bed, Aco. Bry —on leaving bed, Verat a.

Greenish, *Ars. Carb v.* Ferr iod. Verat a.

Pale and bloated, Aur. Cina—" Like polished ivory," Pho—"Waxy white," Apis—Pale and sunken, Ars. Carb v. Tart e. Sec—With red or blue spots, Ferr—Death white, Am m. CANTH. Carb v. Cro. DIG. Ferr. Ph ac. PB. Sec. Verat a,

Red flushed, Aco. Bell. Bry—On emotion, Ig. *Ferr*—with wild stare, Hyo—Red *hot* face, Aco. *Bell*—Dark red, Ail. *Bap. Bry.* Gel— Fiery red, Amyl. FERR. *Meli* — Cheeks flushed and eyes dull in low fever, Bry. *Mur ac*—One red cheek, Aco. CHAM. Mos. (left, Nat m). Sang—One side of the face red, burning, Bell. Ig—Red hot flush and faintness, Sep. Sul. ZN—Flushes at the Change of Life, Lach. Sep. Sul—Flushes from the least excitement, *Ferr*—Redness and heat of the face with cold ears and nose, *Arn.*

Yellow, Arg n. Chel. *Card* (see jaundice)—Pale yellow, *Lyc.* Mer—Brownish yellow, Ars iod. Iod—Yellow around the eyes, Nit a. Sep— Around the mouth, Nux v. Sep—On the temples, Caust—Yellow patches, Sep.

FAINTING:—

Habit: Amb. Alet *0.* AM C. Asa. Crotal. Ig. Laur. MOS. NUX M *0.* Verat a—From the least motion, Verat a.

Long faints, rigid, Laur.

Speechless spell, Sep.

From pain, *Aco.* Cham. Coc. *Hep.* Verat a.

—Loss of blood, Chin. Ip. Glo.

—Fright, Aco. Op.

—Any emotion, Ig.

Guard; Hydrogen 1 vol. 10 drops in water— Alcohol dilute, hot—Caffein 1 gr. Cinnamon tea. *Nutmeg tea.* "Smelling Salts." See Heart—See Cause.

FAINTNESS.—See Debility.

FALL—CONCUSSION.—See Cause—Injury.

FALLING FIT—PETIT MAL.—*Kal bro.* pure 5 to 10 gr doses. *Kal p.* PHO. Opi—See Epilepsy.

FALLING OF THE WOMB OR BOWEL.—See Female, or See Bowel

FALSE LABOR PAINS, OR FALSE PRESENTATION.—See Female—Labor.

FATIGUE.—See exhaustion.

FATTENING DIET.—See Diet X—See Charcoal.

FATTY DEGENERATION, Ars. PHO. Phyt.— See Person.

FAVUS.—See Head—Scalp, *scab.*

FEAR.—See Mind.

FEET.—See Limb—Leg, *foot.*

FELON.—See Limb—Arm. *hand.*

FEMALE ORGANS, AND AILMENTS—.

Breasts:—

Dimple—Look out for cancer.

To prepare the breasts in advance of Labor; Lave with Arnica oil, or Culendula oil. (See Tannin).

To harden the nipples before confinement: Lave daily with lemon juice, or alcohol dilute. Nipple retracted; Sars—See Dry cup.

Sore Nipples: Arnica oil, Calendula oil. Pulv. Gum Arabic ex—Blistered, Grap—Cracked, Grap. Hydras. dilute in. and ex. Sul—Ulcerated *Sil*—(See Bism.Benzo. Calend. Colloid. Glycer. Hydras. Tannin. *Ointment*).

" *Broken Breast*," (Suppuration)—Hep. Phos. Mer. PHYTO θ dilute in. and ex.—Deep opening, Pho. *Sil.*

(See Clay—*Ointment.* Poultice).

"*Caked Breast.*"—Inflammation, threatening abscess, PHYTO θ dilute in. and ex.—See Bella · don—Burning stinging,Apis—Hard and heavy, Bry.

—Glossy red, Bell—Red in streaks, Bell—Red in spots, Pho—(Baby's breasts, swollen, tender, Arnica oil ex.)

Hard Lump. Tumor. Mammary Growth: Cal fl. CON. Fl ac. Grap. Iod. Sil. *Hydras and Phyto alt.* each low, cured—Movable tumor, nipple retracted, Bell 1x cured—See cancer.

Pain when milk flows in, *Phyto* 1x—When child suckles, Croton. Phel—Stitching pains, Borax. Cham. Con.

Scars, itching burning, *Grap.* Sul.

Scurfy nipples, Lyc. Pet.

Shrunken   breasts—Atrophy.   Dwindling; Chimap. *Con.* IOD. *Kal iod.* Sabal ser 1x. (See Ice.)

Tender Breasts, Con. Iod. LII, T. Mer. ZN.

Milk, quantity and quality :—

Fails to come, PHO.

Scanty, Agn. Caust. Ferr p. Pho. *Pilo 1x* 5 gr. Pul. STICT θ 5 drops, 6 hours. Ustil 2x. "Jaboran fl. ex. 20 drops, 6 hours." Urtica 1x.

Too much, Calc. Pho. Rhus—with exhaustion,
Chin.

Depraved, the babe refuses the breast, and
vomits soon after nursing, Lach. Sil.

Blue thin, Lach. Pul.

Bloody, Apis.

Red, Ipe. Sul.

Thready, Sul.

Weaning—See Belladon. Hama. See Diet Z.
(1:12.)

Ovary :—

Abscess, Hep. Lach. Mer. Sil.

Enlargement, Apis. Con. *Ham.* Iod. Lach.
Spo. Thuj—"Like a bag of water," Apis—
Dropsical, Apis. Cann I. Iod. Nat s—Left
enlarged, Lach. Ustil—Right, Apis.

Inflammation. Ovaritis: (See Aconite.) APIS.
Bell. Canth. Con. Ferr p. *Ham. Hot Ham. 0
fomentations.* Kali m. LACH. LIL T. PUL.
Induration, Aur. Con. Grap. Iod. Kali m. Spo—
Induration and enlargement, Con. Spo.

Pains, Neuralgia: Fell., *Cann I* 1x trit 3 gr. 3
hours. "Hemp extract ¼ to ½ gr. 12 hours."
Cimi. Colo. GEL. LIL T. Plat. *Pod. Sabal scr
3x.* Sec. Sep—Left, Grap. Lach. Ustil. ZN—
Right, *Apis. Bett.* Pod. Ustil—Bent double with
pains, *Colo.* Cimi.

—Boring pain, ZN.

Burning, Plat. Ustil. Thuj.

Cutting and tearing, Ham. Vis a.

Stitching, Bell. *Bry* Cimi. *Colo.* Canth—Extending down the thighs, Cimi. Lil t.

Better, by menstrual flow, Lach. ZN—Pressures,
Lil t.—Lying down, Thuj.

Worse from the least jar, Bell—Walking or riding, Thuj—Inability to lie on the left side be-

cause of a painful sensation of something
within rolling over to that side, Lach.
Tumor, APIS. Plat. Thuj—See enlargement.

Uterus:—

Inflammation. Metritis: (See Hot water. See
suppository.) ACO. Apis. Ars. *Bell.* Carbol ac.
Ferr p. Kali m. Mer. NUX V. Op. *Verat v.*

Pain: Sabal ser 3x. with great nervous excitement, Aco. Tarent 200.

—Aching, *Cal c.* Con. Ig. *Mang. Sabin.*

—Bearing down, Agar. *Bell.* Caul. *Cham.*
Cimi. LAPPA. LIL T. Nit a. *Pul SEP.*
Plat. Nat m. NUX V. Sec.

—Bruise-like, Apis. *Arn.* Bar m. *Ham.*

—Cramp-like, Caul. CHAM. COC. Gel. IG.
Thuj.

—Drawing, Pul. Sabin.

—Stitching, Coc. Ig. *Kal c. Sep.*

Bloat: Lyc. Ph. Ph a—Flatus escapes, Brom.
Lyc. Sang.

Cancer: Ars. Iod. Ergot. Kreo. Ova t. Thuj.
Bleeding, Carbol ac. Kreo. Ova t—Burning like
fire, Ars. Kreo. Alcohol lavement daily.
Thuja fl. ex. on tampon of borated cotton.
(See Iodoform. See Suppository.)

Gangrene: Sec.

Hæmorrhage. Metrorrhagia: (See Ice. Suppos-
itory) APO C θ 2 drops, ½ hour, in water.
"Apocy. fl. ex. 4 drops, every hour or two."
"Hydrast. fl. ex. 20 drops, 4 times a day."
Mill. Trill. USTIL 1x. See Menorrhagia—
See Flooding.—Constant bleeding, *Ham.* Iod.
Sec. Ustil. (See Suppository.)

—Renewed by slightest cause, *Amb. Cal c.*
Sec. Sep.

—Stopping and starting, *Kreo. Nux v.* Sul.

—Blood bright red, Sabin. Trill—Black and stringy, Cro—Clotted, Cham—Dark, Ham. Sec.—Nausea, *Ipc.* Verat v.

—Menses too early and too profuse, *Cal c.* Nux v. *Trill.*

—Preventive, Cal c. and Sul.

Induration:—Carb a. Con. Sep. (See Suppository.)

Polypus: Cal c. Nit a. *Stap.* Thuj in and ex. (See Suppository.)

Prolapsus—Displacement — version: — Alston c. Alet *θ* ("cordial.") Bell. HELON. LAPPA. *Pod.* Pul. Sep. LIL T. Nat m. Nux v. (Cal c. Ferr. Hydroct. Onos. *Vib op*). (See Alum. Hot water. Ice. Suppository.)

—Aching in the vagina, *Cal c.* Con. Sabin ; or burning, Sul.

—Backache, Nux v—As if it would break, Bell —Spine tender, Agar. Nux v.

—Bearing down, Alet *θ.* ("Cordial.") *Bell.* LIL T. Sep. Plat. LAPPA—Dragging down from the shoulder, Alston c. *Lil t*—Must sit to dress in the morning, Nat m—Must cross the legs for support, Sep—Must support the womb with the hand, Lil t.

—Breasts indurated, Con.

Constipation the cause, Collin.

—Head hot, on top, Sul—Vertigo on turning in bed, Con.

—Faint spells, Sep. Sul.

—Frequent vain calls, or urging to stool, Lil t. Nux v.

—Intolerance of pressure upon the womb, Apis. Cal c. LACH. Nux v.

—Feet cold and damp, Cal c—Soles hot, Sul.

—Flooding, Trill.

—Morning sickness, Lil t.

—Menses too early and too profuse, Bell. CAL C. *Nux v.* TRILL.

Rigid os: Bell. *Gel.* Cimi. Belladon Ointment.

Spasm: Coc. Cic. *Ig.* Nux v.

Tumor—Fibroid: CAL IOD 1x. Sec 2x. Ergot. Nit a. *Thuj.* USTIL 2x—Cauliflower, Thuj. in. and ex.—Warty growths, Thuj. in. and ex. See Suppository.

Ulceration: Arg n. AURUM MUR. Con. HYDRAS θ dilute in. and ex. HYDROCT. *Nit a.* Thuj. ZN. Alcohol lavement daily— (See Chlorine. Hydras. Hot water. Iodo. Potash. Suppository.)

Vagina:—

Abrasion, excoriation: HYDRAS θ dilute in and ex. Grap. *Helon.* Sep—See Suppository.

Aching, Cal c. Canth.

Burning, Amb. BERB. *Cauth.* Con. KREO. Lyc. SUL. *Thuj.*

Dryness and heat, ACO. *Bell.* Lyc Sang. *Sep.*

Prolapsus: Cal p. Mer. Sang n. Senicio θ. Thuj— Raw, Mer.

Soreness, tenderness: *Aco.* BERB. HYDROCT. Kal bi. KREO. Lil t. Sep—(See Suppository.)

Smarting, HYDRAS θ. dilute in. and ex. Sep.

Stinging, Ars. Apis. Con. *Mur a. Nit a.*

Swelling, Kal bi. Mer.

Ulceration, Arg n. *Aurum mur.* HYDRAS θ. in. and ex. *Hydroct.* Nit a. Thuj. (See Suppository).

Vaginismus: Cup m. Ham. PB.

Vulva—Pudenda:—

Abrasion—Excoriation: HYDRAS θ. dilute in. and ex. Grap. Sep.

Aphthæ—Erosion: Carb v. Thuj θ. in. and ex.

  Burning, Amb. *Berb.* Canth. *Hydroct. Kreo.* Lyc. SUL.

  Dryness and heat, ACO. *Bell.* Lyc—with tenderness, Aco. Sep.

Eczema: Aur. HYDROCT. Plat 30. *Skook.* Thuj in. and ex.

Itching—Pruritus: Amb. Canth. Caust. Con. Grap. HYDRAS θ dilute in. and ex. *Hydroct* in. and ex. *Kreo. Sep. Sul.* Tarent 200.

  —Itching and burning, *Carb v.* Cal c. Kal c. *Nat m.*

  —Itching pimples, CROTON. *Hydroct.* Mer. Sep. *Sul.*

  —Voluptuous itching and tingling, Coff. HYDRAS θ dilute in. and ex. *Plat. Sul. Apply* Alcohol dilute. Menthol 5 grains, in water 1 ounce. Calomel 1 drachm, in vaseline 1 ounce. Linseed oil. *Peppermint water.* (See Acetan. Glycer. *Ichthy.* Naph. Soda. Thuj.)

  Induration, Con Iod. Plat.

  Œdema, Apis.

  Soreness. Tenderness, Apis. Berb. *Hydroct.* KREO. Lil t. Sep—Painful to touch, *Aco.* Coff. PLAT. Sabin. *Sep.*

  Smarting, HYDRAS θ dilute in. and ex Kal c. Sep.

  Weight and Pressure in pubis constant, Bar c.

During Pregnancy:—

  Bleeding—Coca, 1x, 3 drop doses (see flow).

  Bruise-like soreness, *Arn. Cypr.* Lil t. LAPPA.

  Child's motion painful, Pul. *Thuj.*

  Pain in bladder and urging to urinate, Thuj.

  Pain and distress in the womb, Alet θ ("Cordial."). *Cypr.* Gel. θ. Pass θ.

123

Dropsy, Helon.

Exhaustion, See Celery.

Flatulence, CAL FL. Nux m.

Hysteria, Caul. *Gel.* NUX M. Pass. Sabin.
See Celery.

Insomnia, CYPR.

"*Morning Sickness.*" *Amygdal* θ 5 drops.
Ferr p. Mag c. "Pepo θ 10 drops, before
meals." SYMPHORICARP 200. *Tab 2x.*
With salivation Mer. "Ingluvin 5 to 10
grains"—"Oxalate of Cerium, 4 to 5 grains
once a day." "Insert end of index finger,
three-quarters of an inch, within the neck of
the womb, thus dilate the *external os*, but not
the internal. This arrests the nausea or vomiting at once." "Vesicate over the 4th and 5th
dorsal vertebrae. This not only arrests
"morning sickness," but also *pruritus*, and
Toothache of pregnancy." "Lie with hips
higher than shoulders." *Inject a pint of
salted milk into the vagina daily.* Malted
milk diet. (See Chloroform. See GLY-
CERIN.)

"*Evening sickness.*" KREO. Pul. Tab 2x.

Miscarriage—Abortion—Threatening: Alet. θ
"Aletris Cordia.l" *Camp. θ.* Caul. Cimi. GEL θ
1 drop, ½ hour. *Lil l.* VIBURN OP θ 3 drops,
½ hour. "Viburn pru. fl. ex. 1 drachm, 1
hour, until pain abates, then as a guard ½
drachm once or twice a day." "Opium and
rest." "Inject per rectum, Tincture of
opium, 15 drops in 2 tablespoonfuls of lukewarm water, every hour, the patient lying perfectly still in bed. No danger inside, six
doses." Opium Suppository. Morphia hypoderm. See Glycerine.

From a fall or hurt, Arn.
—Grief, Ig.
—Fright, Aco.
With great fear and anxiety, Aco.
   —Chilliness, coldness, Camp. Pul.
   —Drowsiness, Gel.
   —Goneness of stomach pit, Ustil.
   —Nausea, Ipe.
   —Urinary tenesmus, Canth.
   —Urging to stool with every pain, Nux v.
   —Pains irregular, spasmodic, Caul. Cimi.
   —Dragging down, Lil t.
   —Drawing from back to pubes, Sabin.
   —Flow black, *Sec*—Clots, Cham. CRO. Sabin
     —Dark oozing, *Sec.* Ustil—Bright red, Arn.
Bell. *Ipe.* Sabin—Worse from slightest motion, Cro. Sabin Sec.
—*Habit of abortion*, Caul. Cimi. *Mer. Thuj*—
Early, SABIN—Third month, Cro. Sabin—
Later months, *Sec.* Mer. Thuj.

Labor :—

To *insure early and quick labor:* Begin several weeks in advance, and take twice a day. either *Cal fl.* Caul 1x. or *Cimi* 1x. or vib op θ 5 drops.

To *induce strong vigorous pains, and quick safe labor:* Take at the onset, QUINIA 9 grains, or Jamaica Dogwood, fl. ex. ½ drachm, doses. "No ill effects." "Sugar 1 oz. in water." See Chloroform.

Fetus in false position, Pul.

Placenta prœva: "Pass the index finger around between the womb and the placenta, and thus thoroughly detach the placenta, two inches from the os, in every direction. This at once arrests the hæmorrhage."

Rigid os, Bell. *Camp θ.* Cimi 1x. GEL θ. Nux v.
Belladon Ointment. Hot Sitz bath.

Cramps, Camp θ. Mag p in hot water.

Fainting, Pul.

Feeble Pains: CAMP θ 1 drop, ¼ hour on sugar.
Gel 1 drop, ¼ hour. Kal p. NUX 2x. *Ustil*
1x. Thuj. "Borax may be used as a substi-
tute for ergot, 2 scruples in water, repeat in
20 minutes if needful." "*Sugar,* 1 ounce in a
little water, repeat in ½ hour if necessary."
"Ipeca. pure 2 grains, better than ergot."
"Ustil fl ex. ½ drachm, ½ hour." HOT
MUSH POULTICE TO FUNDUS OF THE
WOMB, renew several times if needful. See
Poultice.

Flooding: Grasp the womb with the hand upon
the abdomen, and hold it firmly until it remains contracted. If clots in the womb, remove them, bandage abdomen tightly, apply
cordage to limbs at groin and axilla. Give
vinegar, dilute, a wine glass full, repeat the
dose if necessary. Inject dilute vinegar or
lemon juice, or saturate sponge or cloth with
the same and introduce it in the hand into the
womb, and hold it against the walls, for a
minute, and then withdraw it. In death door
conditions, apply hot sand bags to the back of
the head, and keep up tight cordages. Give
Cocaine 2x, or Hydrogen perox 1 vol. 10 drop
doses; or put a teaspoonful of chloroform into
two teaspoonfuls of sweet cream, and administer half, and in 15 minutes the rest
—Emergency remedies, ERIGERON C 1x
trit, dry on the tongue, CINNAMON θ 30 to
60 drops, ¼ hour. Strong Cinnamon tea.
Canu I 1x. 5 drops, ¼ hour. Cro 1x. IPE 1x.

5 minutes. *Ustil i.x.* MELI 2x. Mill. Till.
(See Alum. *Dry Cup.,* Hot water. Vinegar.)

Hysteria: Ig. Gel.

Loud outcries, Cham. Coff.

Palpitation of the heart, Pul.

Restless excitement, Aco. Coff. Nux v. Pass θ.

Spasms: ACO. Bell. GLON. Hyo. Mag p. *Meli θ.*
Stram. PASS θ.

—with every pain a spasm, Bell.

—Foaming, Bell. Hyo. Stram.

—Screaming, Ig.

—Trembling, Op. Verat v.

—Stupor, Op.

See Amyl. CHLOROFORM. Ether.

Child-bed:—

Good recovery insured, Arn. Lil t.

Hæmmorrhage when nursing, Sil.

After pains: ANTIPYRIN 3 to 5 gr. *Camp θ.*
GEL. θ. Vib op. Xanthox. "*Paregoric 60
drops.*"

—Bruised feeling all over, Arn.

—Abdomen very tender, Bell.

—Call to stool with every pain, Nux v.

—No cessation of pain, Cro. Sec.

—Drawing from back to pubes, Sabin.

—Cramps, Cup m.

—Frightened feeling, Aco. Xanthox.

—Sleeplessness, Coff.

—Nervous excitement, *Cham.* Caul. *Cimi.*

—Sighing, Ig.

—Urine retained, Aco. Arn.

Fever puerperal.   Peritonitis: ACO. Carbol a.
Verat v θ. dilute "*Opium Suppository.*"

—Restless and thirsty, Aco. Ars.

—Lying quiet, Bry.

Lochia "cleansing:"

—Scanty or suppressed, Bry. Cimi. FERR P.
3x. Pul. PHYT ιX. Sec. Stram.

—Prolonged, Aco. Calc. *Ferr p.* Phyt. Rhus.

—Offensive, BAP. HEP 3x. *Kreo.* Nux v. Phyt.
Sec—See Potash.

—Steaming hot, Bell.

—Back bad, Bell. Nux v.

—Vomiting, Verat a. Verat v.

—Sinking, Ars. Verat a.

—Cold, Ars. *Sec.* Verat a.

—Urine retained, Aco. Arn. Ars.

—Womb inflamed, Aco. Bell. NUX V.

—Typhoid type, Ars. Rhus.

Mania: Bell. CANN I ix. 5 gr, 6 hours. " *Hemp
extract* ¼ to ½ gr pill, 12 hours." Verat a.

—Deep gloom, CIMI. Hyo. STRAM.

—Face blue, bloated, Verat a. *Ustil ix.*

—Furious rage, Bell. *Stram.*

—Wild shrieks, Stram. Verat a.

—Erotic furor, *Coca* ix. 3 drops. Kal bro. pure
5 to 10 gr. HYO. *Plat.* Stram—See Mind.

Milk Fever: ACO. *Bell.* Cal c. Pul—See indications under Fever Puerperal.

Milk Leg—Phlegmasia Dolens: "*First Aco. then
Pul.*" HAM *Θ.* dilute in and ex,—See Ham.

—Heat all over—Violent pain, *Aco* Bell.

—Dread of the least jar, or knock, Arn. Bell.

—Dare not move the limb, Bry.

—Red streaks, *Bell.* Rhus.

—Veins knotted, Pul.

Menses Suppressed—Amenorrhœa: (See Suppository.) Alet *Θ.* ("Aletris Cordial.") Bacill
30-200. *Cimi.* HELON. Kal p 30. PULS *Θ.* Sep.
Senecio *Θ.* USTIL ix. XANTHOX ix—Delay
of first flow, Caust. Ferr. *Pul* Xanth.

From sudden chill, Aco.

—Damp feet, *Dul.* Pod. *Pul.*

—Fright, *Aco*—Long standing, *Lyc.* Ustil.

With bleeding, vicarious, Senecio *0.* USTIL 1x.

— —from the nose, *Bry.* Bell. Pul. Ustil.

— —from the lung, *Pho.* Ustil.

—Chilliness—Despondency, Pul.

—Colic, Cham. Coc. *Colo.* Pul.

—Cold feet, Grap – Cold and damp, Cal c.

—Cold vertex, Sep. *Verat a.*

—Goneness at the stomach pit, Sep. Ustil.

—Heat flushes, Sep. Sul.

—Heat on top of the head, Sul.

—Hysteria, Cimi. *Plat.* Pul.—Globus, Sep.

—Œdema, *Apis.* Ars. *Ferr. Helon.*

—Weight in the anus, Sep—In the back, Grap.

Instead of menses; stupor, Ham—headache, ZN—
Leucorrhœa, Ceanoth. Coc. Hyper. Sil—Vicarious bleeding, *Ham.* Ustil.

Menses scanty: (See Ice.) Alu. BAR C. Bacill.
Con. HELON. Kal c. Kal p PUL 30. Sul.
USTIL 2x.

—Short and scanty, *Lach*—Pale, *Grap.* Sil—
Putrid, Ig.

—Only by night, *Bovis.* Helon. Kreo. ZN.

—Only by day, Caust. Ham—When on foot,
Cact. Caust. Lil t.

—Only in the morning, Sep. Mag c.

—Less when walking about, Sabin. Mag c.

—Less and less every month, *Nat m.*

(See Hot water.)

Menses Irregular: Caul. Cimi. *Helon. Nux v.*

—Too early, CAL C. Carb a. Coc. NUX V.
Sabin.

—Too late, Con. Grap. Nat m. Pul 30.

Menstrual flow excessive, Menorrhagia:
Atrop 2x. Bell. CAL C. Cro. *Ferr.* HELON.

NUX V. *Plat. Sabin.* Sec. TRILL. *Ustil 1x.*
See Lemon.

See Uterus—*Hæmorrhages.*

Menstruation painful. Dysmenorrhœa :—

In general, ANTIPYRIN 5 gr, ½ hour. Chloroform 10 drops on sugar. Codeia ½ gr. 6 hours. HELON 1x. "Hemp extract ¼ to ½ gr pill, 12 hours." Passif *0* 60 drops in hot water. "Paregoric 60 drops in hot water, ½ hour." XANTHOX 1X. *Vib op Vis a 0.* (See Amyl. Celery. Hot water. Suppository.)

Pains insupportable, *Cham.* Coff. Stram—Writhing in agony, *Aco* Cimi. Nux v. *Pul.*

—Bearing down, Agar. *Bell.* Borax. *Cham.* Cimi. Caul. *Plat.* Pul. Sabin. Sep.

—Spasmodic, *Caul. Cimi.* Coc.

—Squeezing, Gel. Plat—Crushing, Cimi. Coc.

—Tearing, Cham. Grap. *Vis a.*

Ailments during menses :—

Abdomen, tender, Apis. Bell. China. Coc—Distended with gas, Chin. Coc. Crotal—Rumbling, Lyc—Life-like motion in it, Cro—Tearing pains, Cham. Grap. Vis a—Violent Colic, *Coc.* Pul. Plat. Pass *0.*

Back, severe pain every few minutes, Ustil—Aching in the small of the back, Cimi. Kal c. Pul—As if it would break, Bell. Borax. Nux m—Drawing pain from back to pubes, Sabin—Lame back can hardly turn in bed, Nux v.

Breasts, painful, Grap—Enlarged or tender, Cal c. *Con.* Helon. *Mer*—Pain under the breasts, Cimi. Ustil—Ulcerative pain in the breasts, Mer—Darting in left nipple, Sil.

Chilliness, Cal c. Cimi. Hep. KREO. Mag c. MOS. Nux v PUL. Sep—Icy cold spells, Sil —Shuddering, Cimi. Sep.

Constipation obstinate, Grap. *Lyc.* Nux v. SIL —Debility profound—Extreme prostration, CARB A. Iod. Mer a. Sul a. Sep. Sabin— —Back and limbs enfeebled, Coc.

Eyes watery, Nat m. *Phyt.* Pul—Sight dim, Cimi. Cro. Pul. Trill—Double vision, Cyc. Mag p—Flickering sight, Cyc. Mag p.

Face fiery red, *Ferr.* Meli—Flashes, Sep. Sul— Puffy, Ferr. Helon—Swollen, Sep—One cheek red, Cham—Pain in molar bones, Stan.

Fainting fits, Nuv v. Lach. Mag m—Tendency to faint, *Mos.* Nat m. *Sep.* Sul—Faintness, Nux v. Pul—Feet puffy, Ferr. Helon—Cold and swollen, Grap—Cold and damp, Cal c— Numb, Ig—Fetid sweat, Sil.

Headache, Cimi. *Ferr p.* Gel. *Nat m.* Sep. ZN —Throbbing pain, Glo—Vertigo, Aco—Sick headache, Sang—Morning headache on wak- ing, Nat m—Involving the eyes, Onos. Sep. —Heat on top of the head. Sul. Lach—Cold vertex, Sep. *Verat a*—Cold sweat on the fore- head, Verat a—Heat flushes, Sang. *Sep.* Sul. Ustil. Uran m.

Legs painful, Bry. Spo—Pain in the thighs, Cham. Cimi—Crampy, Nux v—Weariness of legs and twisting at the knee, ZN.

Liver pain, Ph a.

Mind, anxiety and fear, Aco. Ars. Sec—Sad- ness, gloom, Cimi. *Ig. Nat m.* Plat. Stan— Tearfulness, Pul. Sep—Suicidal gloom, Aur —Wanting to die, Lil t—Irritability, Cham. Nux v—Hilarity, Cro—Loquacity, Stram—

Mania, Bell. Hyo. Stram—Erotic fervor, Plat. ZN.

Mouth dry on waking, Nux m—Gums sore, Mer—Toothache, Cal c—Teeth "on edge," Mer—Tongue red, Mer—Salivation, Mer. Phyt—Salty taste, Mer.

Nervous excitation, Cimi. Coc. Stram. Tarent —Hysteria, Caul. *Ig.* Ph a. *Plat.* Sabin. Tarent—Spasm, Cimi. *Mag p.* Plat. Sul.

Ovary, hard swelling, Apis. Con—Pain, Ham. Lil t. Ustil—Tenderness, Cimi—Left ovary very sore, Ustil—Left burning, Thuj.

Sexual excitement, *Pho.* PLAT. Kal bro. low. MOS. Thuj. ZN—Even to masturbation in sleep, Thuj—Voluptuous tingling, Plat.

Skin eruption, *Dul.* Grap. Kal c—also excoriation, Kal c.

Sense of Weight about the pubes, Bar c—In the anus, Sep—in the pelves, Alo.

Sleeplessness, Cimi. Lach. Mag m—Night mare, Sul a.

Stomach fluttering, Cact. Xanth—Sinking, gone feeling, Apo c Sep. Ustil—Pain from stomach through to the back, Borax—*Vomiting,* Carb v—Also *purging,* AM C. Verat a —Morning sickness, Grap. Mer. Nux v. Pul.

Throat sore, Mag c—Globus. Lach. Sep.

Vulva pain violent, Rhus—Itching, Croton.

Womb pain severe, Cimi. Ustil—Tenderness, Apis.

Wind escapes from the womb, Lyc.

Condition of the Menses:—

Acrid, excoriating, Kal c. Sil. Sul.

Black, *Cact. Coc.* Ig. Pul. SEC. Mag c. Nux v. Sul—Thick black, Nux m. Plat—Black and putrid, Ig—Black clots, Cham. Cro. Lyc.

Brown, *Bry*. Carb v. Con.

Dark and thick, Plat. Pul. Nux m—Dark liquid, Sec.

Clotted, CHAM. Cimi. CRO. PLAT. Pul. Rhus. Sabin. TRILL. Ustil—Clotted and fetid, Trill—Lumps drop, ZN.

Gushing, Bell. Pul—Fits and starts, *Kreo*. Pul. *Nux v.* Sul.

Hot, Bell. Borax.

Increased by the least motion, Cro. Helon. Sec.

Membrancous, BORAX. Cal c. Ustil. VIB OP. See Iodoform.

Odor offensive, BELL. Bry. *Carb a. Cro*. Sec —Putrid, Ig—Pungent, Kal c. Kreo.

Pale, watery, *Ferr*. Grap. Pul. Sil. Ustil.

Stringy—Tenacious, Cro. Pul.

Thick. Bell. Pul. *Nux v.* Plat. SUL.

Leucorrhœa. See Suppository.

(See Alum. Carbol a. Chlorine. Hama. Hydras. Hydrogen—Hot water. Ice. Eucalyp. Potash.)

In general, Ars. *Canth*. HELON. HYDRAS *θ* dilute in. and ex. HYDROCT. KREO. *Nat m* 2x. OVA T 2x. *Kal bi*. Jac. Kal s

Acrid, *Alu*. CARB A. Carb v. *Kal bi*. MER. Nat m. Pho. *Thuj*—Corroding, *Alu*. Ars. Carb v. EUCA in and ex. IOD. KREO. Kal iod. Mer.

Albuminous, Am m. BORAX. Bovis. Pul. Sang n—Only by day, Plat.

Black, Chin. Cro. Kreo

Blue, Amb.

Bloody, Amb. *Chin Coc*. Ham. Kreo.

Burning, Alu. AM C CAL C. *Carb a*. Mer. *Pul*.

Excoriating, ARS. Con. Grap. KREO. *Lil t*. *Nat m*.

133

Gushing, Coc. Grap.

Green, Asa. CARB A. Lach. Mer. *Nat m.* Pul. Thuj.

Hot, Borax.

Itching, CAL C. Chin.KREO. Mer. *Mez*—More at night, *Mer.*

Offensive odor, CARB A. EUCA in and ex. Hep. KREO. *Ova l* Sec. *Sep* Ustil—Stopping and starting, Kreo. Sec.

Streaming, Arg n. ALU. Carb v.

Stringy—ropy, HYDRAS. KAL BI.

White, BORAX. CAL C. Con. *Pul* Lyc. Sep. SIL.

Watery, AM C. Coc. GRAP. Lil t. Pul—Fetid liquid, CARB A.

Yellow, *Alu.* Ars. HYDRAS *θ.* dilute in. and ex. KAL BI. *Kreo* Lil t. *Nux v.* SEP. Stan.

Occurring—Before the menses, Bar c. Cal c. *Carb v.* Chin. *Grap*—During or instead of menses, *Coc.* Hyper. IOD. Sil—After menses, Alu. Amb. Coc. Grap Pul.

Leucorrhœa of little girls: Cina. Ham. Hyper. Teucr.

Change of Life:—

In general, Alo. *Glo* 3x. LACH. *Sep.* Sang.

Headache a great deal, Cimi—On top, Cact.

Rush of blood to the head, FERR P. GLO. Plat. Sul.

Burning vertex, Gel. Lach. Sul—Cold vertex, Sep. Verat a.

Fiery red face, Amyl. Cardu. FERR. MELI.

Flashes of heat, Amyl. *Cardu.* Euca. *Gel.* LACH. *Sep.* Sul—With sweat, Sep. Sul.

Flooding, *Arg n.* Trill. USTIL 1x.

134

FEVER:—

"Attendant's hand on patient's forehead, twenty minutes induces sweat, and reduces temperature."

"Anointing the body all over with Lard, or Olive oil, several times a day, may be the means of conducting almost any inflammatory, or eruptive fever safely to the end."

In fever of infants, water alone given systematically, by the teaspoonful, may prove curative.

Water may be freely given in all eruptive fevers, with this precaution, that small quantities be given at a time.

Our two greatest antipyretics are, I suppose, *Antifebrin* 2 to 5 gr. doses, and *Antipyrin* 2 to 5 gr. doses. Some one however has had the temerity to say that "Sepia corresponds precisely to Antifebrin, and Chelidonia to Antipyrin."

"The first remedy in all congestive and inflammatory fevers, before effusion takes place, and while the parts affected are tender, and painful to pressure, and pains worse from motion, is *Ferr p* 6x. (Aco).

"The second remedy, answering to the stage of effusion, exudation, infiltration, *patch*, is *Kali m* 6x. (Bry).

"The third remedy, answering to the stage of suppuration, ulceration or induration, is Calcium s—(Hep. Sil)."

Bilious Fever—Remittent Fever: *Euca*. Euony. *Eup per*. Homar 3x. Pod. "*Quinia* 5 to 10 gr. hypoderm."

Chilliness dominant, Bell. GEL. *Pul*—With flushed face, Gel—Pain in head, back and limbs, Gel—Vomiting, retching, Bell. Ipe. Pul.

Fever high, especially at night, Ars. *Bell.* Mer.
Nausea persistent, Ipe.

Tongue white, Carbol a. Ipe. Pul—Dry brown,
Ars. Bry. Rhus—Yellow, *Bry.* Ipe. MER.
Nat s.

Taste bitter, Bry. Pul. Mer. Nat s.

Liver pains severe, Aco. Bell Bry. Mer—Shooting, ACO. Bell. *Bry*—Involving the shoulders, Bell. Chel. Mer—Obstructing respiration,
Aco. *Bry.* Bell—Cannot lie on the right side,
Mer.

Thirst intense, Ars. Mer—*Absent,* Pul.

Great *muscular* weakness, *Gel.* Rhus.

Prostration extreme, Ars. *China* with humming in the ears, China.

Constipation, Bry. Nux v.

Diarrhœa, Ars. Mer. Pod—More at night,
Chin. Pul.

Brain Fever—Congestion or Inflammation of the Brain, or Meninges.—See Spotted fever.

Anxious fear, Aco.

Rapid speech, Mer. Stram.

Restlessness—Thirst, Aco. Bell. Hell.

Quietude.—Faint on rising, Bry.

Delirium, Agar. Bell. Hyo. Stram—Eyes open,
Op—Eyes closed, Hyo—Attempts to leap
from bed, escape and "go home," Bell. Bry
—Chewing, Bry. Hell—Gnashing, Apis.
Stram.

Headache violent, throbbing, Bell. Glo—As if
bursting, Aco. Bell. Bry—Vertigo on rising
up, Aco. Bry.

Face red, bloated, Aco. Bell—White, Apis. ZN.

Eyes distorted, Bell. Hyo. Stram—Glistening, sparkling, wild, Bell. Stram—Pupils dilated, Bell. *Cic.* Hyo.

Starting in sleep, *Bell.* Bry. Hyo—Screaming, Apis. Bell.

Stupor, Bell. *Op.* ZN.

Twitching, *Cic.* Hyo. Op—Head jerking up, Stram.

Spasms, *Bell.* CIC. Cup m. *Hyo.* Op. *Stram.* See Hydrocephalus acute.

Catarrhal Fever.—See Chest—Bronchitis *acute.*

Child-bed Fever.—See Female—Child-bed.

Gastric Fever.—Continuous Fever :—

"The First remedy," BAP.

Violent headache and sick stomach, *Bap.* Bry —Throbbing carotids, Bell— Hot head, sweat, Cham.

Intense heat—Thirst, ACO. ARS. Bell. *Mer.*

Restlessness—Tossing, ACO. *Ars.* Bell.

Quietude—Faint on rising, Bry.

Irritability, *Bry.* Cham. Nux v.

Chillness, Bap. *Pul. Mer.*

Cold sweat, *Ars. Mer.* Tart e. VERAT A.

Nausea, vomiting, Ars. ANT C. Bell. Bap. *Bry.* IPE. *Tart e.* VERAT A—Bloody vomit, Pho—Sour, Ars. IRIS V. Mer. *Nux v—* Water rejected immediately—Ars; or as soon as warm in the stomach, Pho.

Lips blue, Verat a—Parched, Ars. *Bry.*

Tongue white, ANT C. *Bap.* Carbol a. Pul— Dry brown, Ars. Bap—Yellow, *Bap. Bry.* Kal s. MER.

Taste bitter, Bry. Nat s. Pul—Rancid, Pul.

Stomach tender, Bap. Bry. Mer—Burning pains in the stomach, *Aco.* ARS. Canth. IRIS V.

Constipation, Ant c. BRY. Nux v.

Diarrhœa, Ars. Ant c. IRIS V. Mer. *Verat a.*

Hectic Fever: *Aco.* BAP. Carbol a. CHAM *0.*
Hep. *Iod.* SANG. SENECIO, *Sil.* Sul. USTIL.

Inflammatory Fever: See Inflammation, and
parts affected.

Intermittent Fever: See Ague.

Lung Fever : See Chest—*Pneumonia.*

Milk Fever: See Female—Child-bed, *fever.*

Remittent Fever: See Bilious Fever.

Rheumatic Fever: See Rheumatism, acute.

Scarlet Fever—Scarlatina:

(See *Alcohol.* Carbol a. *Chlorine.* Lard. Soda
Onset—Nervous excitement, Aco.

Smooth, Apis. *Bell.*

Rough—Vesicular, Am c. Rhus.

Raw spots in the face, Arum—Raw chin,
Arum. Bry.

Malignant, AIL. Am c. Ars. *Bap. Crotal.*
LACH. Mur a. Phyt.

Eruptions receding, Bry. Ip—Body Cold, Ars.
Camp. Cup m—Spasms threatening, Bell.
CAP M. Mos. *Verat v.* ZN.

Dropsy preventive, Hell *0.* See Soda.

Dregs: Desquamation tardy, Ars. *Kal s.* Sul.

—Dropsy, *Apo c 0. Apis.* Ars. Hell *0.* Tereb.

—Nasal flux, Ars. Aur. Mur a.

—Otorrhœa, Grap. *Hep.* Mur a. *Sil.*

—Mattery eyes, Sul.

—Swollen glands, Lach. MER IOD. *Rhus.*

—Slow convalescence, Cal c. See Tonic.

Guard—See Contagion.

Diet—Grape juice. Milk. "Malted Milk."
Koumis. Broth. Gruel. Toast.

Spotted Fever—Cerebro-Spinal Meningitis:
" Alcohol, ½ ounce, put in twelve teaspoon‑

fuls of water, and give of this, one, two, or
three, teaspoonfuls according to age, every
½ hour, until there is decided amendment,
then lengthen intervals. Free warm sweat
is very favorable. Alcohol thus administered
in the early stage subdues the disease."
See Lime—*Sweat.*

" First," GEL.

Bruised feeling all over, Arn. *Cimi*—Powerless
to move, Gel.

Drowsiness, Bell *Gel.*

Deafness, *Cic.*

Diplopia, Bell *.Gel.* Hyo.

Dilated pupils, Bell. *Cic.* Verat v θ.

Jerking eye balls, Cic—Rolling, Verat v θ.

Headache violent, Bell. Verat v.

Moaning, Bell. Laur.

Stiff neck, Bell. Bry. *Gel.*

Numb spine, Aco.

Opisthotonos, Bell. CIC. Op. Verat v.

Face red, Bell—Pale, Cic—Purple, Laur.

Jaw fallen, stupor, Lyc. Op.

Vomiting persistent, Gel. IPE. Verta v.

Spasm as a *dreg*, *Cimi.* Hyo. Lach. and Mer.

Sweating Fever—Sweating Rheumatism :
Bry. Eup per. TART E. *Pilo* ix. Hep. MER—
Rapid cure of a desperate case with Nitrous
Ether and Buchu fl. ex. each ½ drachm mixed.
Relief in half an hour. (See Lemon.)

Traumatic Fever: *Acon.* Arn. EUCA θ 3 drops,
1 hour.

Urethral Fever : ACO. Arn. Euca

Worm Fever : ACO. Bell. *Mer.* Sul.
Boring at the nose, CINA. Chin.

Blue circles around the eyes, Cina. Cal c. Lyc.

Fear, timidity, Aco.

Restless sleep, Aco. Mer—Coughing, Cina—
Starting, Bell.

Typhoid Fever—Enteric Fever: (See Carbol
a.) ECHIN. EUCALYP. "*First stage*--hyper-
æmia--Ferrum *phos. Second stage*—infiltration—Potassium Chlori, *Third stage*—Ulceration—Calcium Sulph. Thus we lay hold directly
upon the process of the disease, control and
cure it." .

" Pyrogen 6, three tablets dissolved in water,
and given every 2 hours, keeps temperature
down and conducts the case safely through."

" Oil of Turpentine, Gum Arabic and Sugar, 2
drachms of each. Mix; and while triturating
them in the mortar, slowly add 4 ounces of
cinnamon water; of this to adult, give one
teaspoonful every four hours. This the only
treatment needed in all cases."

" Pure Cider Vinegar, adult, 5 drops on sugar,
every hour or two, all that is needed. The
same for Typhus."

" Typhoid Fever should be treated with Quinia
5 to 10 grains in solution, combined, with
minute doses of Morphia. Three injections,
(hypodermic) a day. This treatment brings
about convalescence generally at the end of
the second week."

Sponge patient with tepid water, containing a
little alcohol, morning and evening. If temperature as high as 104°, give Antifeb. 5 gr.
doses and 'use simply cold water, sponging
every half hour or hour until temperature
falls.

Bathe the back daily with alcohol dilute to
prevent bed sores.

" Rhus and Bryonia in alternative, every 2 or

3 hours, *with good coffee as the main article of diet*, all that is needed in most cases."

" First Remedy," BAP.—" Forlorn hope," Upas 30.

Mind anxious, fear, Ars.

—Fear of death, Ars.

—Fear of being alone, Ars. Lyc. Stram.

—Irritability, Bry.

—Indifference, Arn. Ph a.

—Slow answering, Mer. Ph a—Falls asleep answering, Bap.

—Moaning, Bell. Bry.

Delirium—Furious, *Bell*. Hyo. Stram.

—Loquacious, Hyo. Lach. Stram.

—Muttering, Apis. Lach. Mer. *Rhus*.

—Picking at bed-clothes, Ars. Hyo. Mur a. Op. Stram.

—Speechless, Bell. Hyo. Stram.

—Wanting to leap from bed and " go home," Bell. Bry.

—Tossing about " to get pieces of head or body together," Bap.

—Stupor profound, Bell. *Lyc. Op.* ZN.

Head—Burning on top, Lach.

—" Bursting," Bell. Bry.

—Throbbing, Bell.

—Vertigo on rising up, Bry.

Face—Blue, Op.

—Bloated, Ars.

—Blisters around the mouth, Rhus.

—Red, Bell—Dark red, Bap. Bry—Red and swollen, Bry.

—Pale, sunken, Ars. Pho.

Eyes—Distorted, Bell. Stram—Squinting, Bell.

—Glistening, sparkling, *Bell*. Stram.

—Glazed, Rhus. Lyc.

—Red, Bell. Bry.

Nose—Liquid flow, Ars. Mer.

—Epistaxis, *Ars.* PHO. *Ph a.* Rhus.

—Fanning nostrils, LYC.

Mouth—Foul breath, *Bap.* ECHIN.Mer—With Salivation, Mer.

—Open mouth—"Jaw down," *Ars.* Lach. *Lyc.* Mur a. *Op.*

—Gums bleeding, Mer. Ph a—Sputa bloody, Ars. Rhus.

—Teeth covered with sordes, Ars. *Bap.* Rhus.

—*Lips* dry, cracked, Bry—Black, Ars. Pho.

Tongue—Burning, Ars.

—Black, Ars.

—Brown, Bap. Rhus.

—Red, Ars. Bell. Tereb—Shining, Lach. Tereb—Red tip, Ars. *Rhus.*

—Yellow, Bap. Bry. Mer—Moist and yellow, Mer.

Taste—Bitter, Bry. Mer.

—Putrid, Mer.

Throat—Dry and sore, Bell.

—Tender to pressure, Bell. Lach.

Stomach—Tender, Bry. Mer.

—Nausea on rising up, Bry.

—Vomiting up food, Bry—Water as soon as swallowed, Ars—As soon as warm in the stomach, Pho.

Abdomen—Bloated, *Tympanitis*, Ars. Lyc. Pho. Ph a. *Rhus.* TEREB—Rumbling, Lyc. Pho. Ph a—With diarrhœa, Ph a. Stram.

—Tenderness, Mer. Nit a.

—Weak empty feeling, PHO.

Liver—Burning, Bry.

—Stitching, Bry.

—Stinging, Mer.

—Soreness, Mer.

—Tenderness, Bell. Bry. *Mer.*

Stools—Bloody, Am c. Ars. *Pho.* Tereb—Like charred straw, Lach.

—Black fetid, *Ars.* Op. Stram.

—Involuntary, Arn. *Ars.* Hyo. *Op. Rhus.* Mur a.

—Hæmorrhage, Am c. *Alu.* Carb v. Mur a. *Nil a. Sec* 200.

Urine—Hot, scanty, Canth.

—Red as if bloody, Mer—Smoky red, Tereb— Red Sand sediment, Lyc.

—Involuntary, Hyo. (See Stool Invol.)

—Suppressed, Arn. Ars. Canth.

Chest—Constant desire to take a deep breath, Bry. Lach.

—Soreness in the lungs, Pho.

—Tightness across the chest, Pho.

—Weakness in the chest, Pho.

—Pneumo-Typhus, Pho. Tart e.

Skin—Burning hot to the hand, BELL— Steaming hot, Bell.

—Sweat profuse, Bry. PH A. Tart e—Cold clammy, Mer.

General symptoms—Bed feels as "*hot* as an oven," Op; or "*hard* as a board," Arn. Bap.

—Faintness on rising up in bed, Bry.

—Jerking, twitching, *Hyo.* Lyc. Op. Ph a. *Stram*—Head jerks up from the pillow, Stram.

—Sudden starting in sleep, *Bell.* Bry. Hyo.

Restlessness, *Ars.* Rhus.

Rapid speech, Mer. Stram.

Trembling, Bap. Op. Rhus.

Prostration extreme, ARS. Carb v. Mur a. *Rhus*—Must be fanned, Bap. CARB V.

143

FIBROID TUMOR.

Pulse—Intermittent, Mur a. Nit a—Very slow, Op. Diet:—*Exclusive milk diet best.* No solid food until stools normal.

Typhus Fever:—See Remedies indicated under Typhoid.

Leading remedies, Bap. ARS. Pho. PH A.
(See Coffee. Vinegar.)

Yellow Fever—Icteric Fever:—(See Carbol a.)

Cold stage, CAMP *θ*, 2 drops, ¼ hour—See Camphor. GEL *θ*. 5 drops.

Hot and thirsty, Aco.

Delirium furious, Bell.

Headache, "bursting," Bell. *Bry.*

Vertex. burning, *Lach.* Sul.

Carotids throbbing, *Bell.*

Face death-like, Ars. *Verat a.*

Tongue black, Ars—Trembling, Lach.

Nausea persistent, IPE. Tart e. Verat a—Black vomit, *Ars.* CROTAL. Sul. *Verat a*—Bloody, Ars. *Arg n. Crotal. Pho—Violent* vomiting, Mer. *Verat a*—Water rejected immediately, Ars—As soon as warm in the stomach, Pho.

Stools bloody, CROTAL. Carb v. Canth. Mer—Involuntary, Ars.

Skin cold, Ars—Cold sweat, Tart e. *Verat a.*

FIBROID TUMOR.—See Female—Uterus.

FIDGETS.—ZN. Val.

Of the feet, Apis. ZN.

Attendant upon Locomotor Ataxia, *Atrop.* hypoderm.

FINGER.—See Limb—Arn, *hand.*

FISSURE.—See Anus—Skin—or part affected.

FISTULA: Cal fl. FL A. Pæon in. and ex. Pho. SIL 200—With cough, Berb. "Inject Aqua

Silica and give Sil 30-200." "Inject essence of Turpentine. In seven cases of *Anal fistula*, five were cured: In six cases of *Caries* of the petrous bone all were cured; in eight cases of *Dental fistula* no failure: In fifteen cases of *Fistula Steno's duct*, only one failure. It may be injected pure or diluted with olive oil, or almond oil. But it does better undiluted. With timid people it maybe mixed with a solution of Chloride of Morphia."

FIT.—See Spasm.

FLATULENCE.—Arg n. *Cal fl.* Carb v. *Collin.* Colch. *Lyc. Nux m*—Fetid, Am. Carb v. Sul— Odor of garlic, Agar—As of spoiled egg, Sul— Hot, Alo—Sour, Rheum.

FLIES AWAY.—"Oil of Bay—A few drops in a saucer; or in paint the slightest trace."

FLOATING SENSATION.—In the lower limbs STICT—See Nerve.

FLOODING.—See Female — Labor. Also see Uterus—*hæmorrhage.*

FLUSHES.—See Heat—See Face.

FLUTTERING.—At the heart, Cact. Lil t. Laur Rhus—See Heart. At the stomach pit, Cact. Xanthox—See stomach.

FOMENTATIONS.—See Hot Water.

FONTANEL, OPEN.—Cal c. Cal p. Sil.

FOOD.—See Diet.

Food by injection: First empty and wash the rectum by injection of clean warm water. When thus prepared, slowly force the nourishment up into the bowel, as far as possible, every 2 hours; half teacupful at a time, temperature 98° to 100° F.

E* 145

FOREBODING OF DEATH.

Sweet milk or cream, slightly salted, or egg and cream beaten together, are suitable for nourishment. Always a little pepsin should be added to insure digestion.

FOREBODING OF DEATH.—ACO. Cal c. Grap.

FOOT.—See Limb—Leg, *foot*.

—Foot sweat offensive, Bar c Cal c. Pul. Sil. (See BISM. Borax. From Potash.)

FRACTURE.—See Arnica. Calendula Lead.

Slow uniting, *Cal p*. Ruta Kali m. *Symp*.

" Glacial Acetic acid, inject between fracture ends."

Pain of fracture, HYPER. *Symp*. ZN p.

FRECKLES.—See Face.

FRIGHT.—ACO. *Ig. Op*. Kal p. Stram.

Frightened feeling, Aco Xanthox.

FROZEN.—Treat same as a burn—See Soda.

Insensible, see Apparent Death.

FUNGUS.—Ars. Ant c. Lach. Sang. root pulv. THUJ. in. and ex. (See Lactic a.)

Bleeding, Ars. Carb a. Lach. PHO. Sil.

GAGGING.—*Ant c.* Cup m. Ipec. *Kreo* Lob i.

From teething, Pod. Kreo.

From worms, Cina.

GALL STONE.—See Liver.

GANGLION.—See Benzo. See Seaton.

GANGRENE.—*Ars.* Carbol a. Crotal. ECHIN. HYDROCT. Kal p. Lach. PB. *Sec.* THUJ. in and ex. (See Calend. Chlorine. *Charcoal. Clay*. EUCALYP. Hydrogen. *Logwood*. Potash. Turpen. Yeast.)

In mouth or throat, Thuja. See Potash.

In lungs, Caps. Sali ac. Kal p.

In Bowels, Ars. Carb v. Kal p. Tereb—See Yeast.

In stump, Cinchona. HYDROCT. See Logwood.

Humid, Cinchona. Hell. Kal p.

Senile, Ant c. Kal p. *Sec.* THUJ in. and ex. See Thuj.

GAPING SPASMODIC.—Ant c. Cinnamon *0*. IG.

GASTRALGIA.—See Stomach.

GASTRIC CATARRH.—See Stomach.

GASTRIC FEVER.—See Fever—*gastric.*

GASTRIC ULCER.—See Stomach.

GASTRITIS.—See Stomach.

GENITALS.—See Male or Female.

GIDDINESS.—See Head—vertigo.

GLANDS.—*Enlarged: Bar c.* Bell. CIST. Cal c. Carb a. Con. KAL IOD. Kali m. Lyc. Mer. MER PROT. *Nat p.* Nat a. Pho. *Pilo.* RHUS. Sil. Sul —(See Iodine.)

Especially the salivary glands, Pilo. Mer.

Induration. Especially, Ars bro. Bell. CARB A. Clem. CON. Nit a. Rhus. SIL.—Bony hard, Cal fl.

Inflammation—Adenitis—Hot swellings: Bar c. BELL. Mer. MER PROT. Pho. RHUS. Thuj.

Suppuration—Ulceration—especially: Ars. Bacill 30–200. CIST. HEP. Mer. Nat p. Nit a. Pho. Phyt. SIL. See Clay. Iodine.

Syphilitic engorgement, KAL IOD. *Mer.* Nit a. *Pod.* PHYT.

GLAUCOMA.—See Eye.

GLEET.—See Gonorrhœa.

GLOSSITIS.—See Mouth—tongue, *inflamed.*

GLOTTIS ŒDEMA.—APIS. Nat s.

— spasm: See Chest—Croup, *false.*

GLYCERINE.

GLYCERINE:—*Impetigo, Prurigo, Encrusted Lupus, Herpes exedens, Syphilitic and Strumous Eruptions, tending to fetid discharges and hard crusts, Fetid Ulcers, Skin Scurf, Dandruff, Chilblains, Chapped Skin, Acne, Eczema—Scabby stage of Small pox to prevent scars and pitting, Cracked nipples, Cracked lips, Burns and scalds, Erysipelas. Wounds:—*Pure Glycerine, in the proportion of a dessert spoonful to a tumbler of water, apply as a *lotion;* and also *take,* adult, one, or two tablespoonfuls before meals.

Local Itching: ("Frantic")—Glycerine 5 ounces, with Bism. submit 1 ounce, mix; and apply as often as needful: Or Pure Glycerine 1 ounce, Tannic acid 1 drachm, and Morph. sulph. 10 grains, mix, and apply, 3 times a day; especially for *anus* or *vulva.*

Medication by Inunction : This is well effected by mixing the medicine with Unguentum Glycerine—or with *Lanolin* or *Agnine.* The medicine comes into effect in two or three minutes.

During Fever to Subdue Thirst :—Pour a little Glycerine upon the tongue, from time to time.

Deafness :—A drop of Glycerine in the ear occasionally. In old people, a pledget of raw cotton alone, pressed well back is helpful.

Vomiting in Pregnancy, Miscarriage Threatening :—"Take a little wad of cotton, or small sponge, tie a piece of tape to it, and saturate it with Glycerine, and push it up to the mouth of the womb, and in a short time moisture will flow, and the sickness will cease. Then draw it out by the tape."

148

GLYCOSURIA.

GLYCOSURIA.—Ars. Pho. Ph a. Ura.
Diet, N. and U.—See Urinary organs.

GOITRE.—Cal fl. IOD.Ova t. *Fl ac.* FUCUS VES*θ*.
Nat p *Spo.* (See Iodine. Iodoform.)
Exophthalmic, Apis. Fucus ves. Amyl. gently,
inhale 5 minutes, daily. Naj. Thuj.

GOOSE FLESH.—Gel. Cal c—when outdoors,
Sars.

GONORRHŒA.—See Borax *Hydrogen.* Potash.
Vinegar.
Of Females. See Borax. Salicyl.
In General, Canth 2x. Cann s 2x. Cann I 2x.
Gel *θ. Hydroct.* Hydras. Jacaran. Kreo. Mer.
Nat s. Sabal s. Thuj. Vesicar.
From the Beginning and Through to the End.
Cure in from 5 to 15 days. Cann I 1x, 10
drops, 4 hours, day and night: As improvement advances diminish strength to 2 or 3x.
Gelsem *θ* 10 drops, 3 hours, day and night,
until *vision dim*, then stop; no harm to the
sight, but the cure is complete. Hydroct 3d
to 6th, 5 drops 3 hours, day and night, rapid
cures. Jacarand *θ* 5 drops, 3 hours, day and
night, persevere and cure. Nat s 3d to 6th,
from the first, but if it fails to take hold at
once, change to Thuj 30 one dose, then after
6 hours, begin again with Nat s, a dose every
3 hours, and cure without fail. Piper m *θ*, 20
drops, 4 hours, in tumbler of water, cure in
two or three weeks. No danger. Sabal ser *θ*
5 drops 3 hours, day and night and conquer.
Vesicaria *θ* 5 to 10 drops, every 3 or 4 hours.
Sure victory—Kreosote low, a good record.
Burning urine, Canth 2x. Cann s 1x. Vesicar—
Thread stream, *Mer.* Sul.

149

GOUT.

Chordee—Priapism; Canth. CANN S. Mer.
Pic a. " Antikamnia 10 gr."

Bloody discharge, *Canth.*

Green, Kal iod. Mer. Nat m. Nat s. Thuj.

Yellow, Copai. Hydras. Hydroc. Kali iod.
Mer. Sul—Muco-purulent, *Hep*, Sil.

Watery, thin, Cann s. Thuj. See Gleet.

Gleet, Agn. Copai. Hydroc. Nat s. Sabal s.
Stigm. THUJ fl ex 10 drops—With enlarged
prostate, Sabal s. Thuj. Stigm. *Pass θ.*

GOUT—ARTHRITIS. — See Limb-joint. See Joint.

In general, Bacill 30-200. BENZ A. Lith bro
1x, 5 grs. LITH LAC 2x. URTICA URENS *θ.*
Vis a.

Red hot shining, ACO. Ars. BELL. Rhus—
White spot from pressure, Bell. *Colch.*

Preference for the *wrist, Abrotan. Caul.* Pho.
Rhus. *Ruta. Sabin — Fingers,* ANT C.
BENZ A. *Colch. Led.* Pho. Rhus—*Ankle,*
Arn. LED. RUTA. Sabin—*Toes,* ARN. *Ben a.*
Led. *Sabi*—Throat, Benz a.

Pains Burning, *Aco.* ARS. Pul—Cold, LED—
Sprain-like, ARN. Pho. *Ruta.* RHUS—
Throbbing, Bell—Shifting, Caul. Pul.

Better in a warm room, Ars—By quiet rest, Bry—
Gentle motion, Aco. RHUS—Firm pressure,
Nux v.

Worse by rest, RHUS—Motion, BRY—First
motion, Rhus—Least knock, ARN—In a warm
room, Pul—Evening, Pul—Night desperate,
ACO. Ars. *Colch.*

Nodosities, Concretions, BEN A. in. and ex. Bry.
CAL C. *Cal p.* Grap. *Nat m.* Nux v. PHO.

" Drink a tumblerful of tepid water, every 20
minutes for 3 hours, after breakfast daily for

3 days. This will cure the gout."

To prevent the gout: Cal p. POD ix. Take a tumbler of hot water every morning.

(See *Ichthyol.* Kerosene. Lime *Sweat.* Vinegar. See Diet V.

GRANULAR EYELIDS.—See Eye-*lids.*

GRATING, GNASHING THE TEETH.—Bell. Pod. Stram.

GRAVEL.—See Urinary Organs.

GREEN SICKNESS.—See Chlorosis.

GRIEF.—Ig. Ph a. See Cause—Emotion.

"GRIP."—See La Grippe.

GROIN.—See Abdomen—groin region.

GROWTH STUNTED.—*Bar c.* Cal p. THUJ. See Person.

Too rapid, Ph a.

GUM ARABIC.—*Acidity of the Stomach:* Pulverized Gum Arabic, adult one teaspoonful taken after meals. Half teaspoonful of the same, put into a child's nursing bottle, once a day, when filling it with milk, obviates *sour stools*, and *vomiting of sour curds.*

Sore nipples: Gum Arabic pulv. apply as often as convenient

GUMS.—See Mouth.

GUM-BOIL.—See Mouth—*gums.*

GUMMATA.—Mer. *Kal iod.*

HÆMORRHAGE.—See Bleeding. See the Affection, or part affected.

HAIR.—See Head.

HAMAMELIS.—*Aneurism—Varicose Veins:* Inject Ham. θ dilute, 20 drops, behind the vein.

Throat affections—Hoarseness of public speak-

ers:—Ham. θ in glycerine (1:2), lave, gargle, spray.

Eye affections — Purulent Ophthalmia — Excessive Lachrymation :—Distilled extract of Hamamel. dilute, pour warm into the eye.

To " Dry up the Milk :"—Rub the breast with Ham. unguent several times a day.

Milk-leg :—Place patient in horizontal position, bathe the part with Ham. θ and hot liquor, equal parts mixed, every 3 hours, and wrap in cotton. Administer Ham. ix. After the acute stage passed, bandage from toes to hip until swelling all subsides. If pus forms let it out.

Boil—Carbuncle:—Ham. extract or tincture, 20 drops in ½ teacupful of water; apply on cloths.

Anal affections—Fissure, Ulcer, Tender Piles:—Ham. ungent. See Ointment.

Leucorrhœa:—Ham. extract or tincture, a tablespoonful in a teacupful of warm water; inject this three times a day into the vagina.

HAND.—See Limb—*Arm—hand.*

HANKERING.—See Stomach—Craving.

HARDENING OF TISSUES.— Kali m. Sil. Of glands—See Gland.

HAWKING.—See Throat.

HAY FEVER — ROSE COLD.— See Nose — Catarrh.

HEAD, BRAIN, MENINGES.—

Anæmia of the brain—*Failing brain power—" Brain fag:"*—Apis. Avena θ 10 drops in water at bed time. KALI PHOS PHO. Sil. ZN. ZN P. See Diet, S. W.

Hyperæmia of the brain—*Congestion :*—From injury, Arn.

—Sudden chill, Aco.

Violent Headache, Bell. Gel. Glo.

Throbbing carotids, Bell. Glo. Verat v.

Hæmorrhage of the brain:—Arn. Apis. Op. Phos.

— From injury, Am. See Apoplexy.

**Hydrocephalus — "Water on the brain,"
Acute** :—Bacill 200. "Bell. and Stram."

—Automatic motion, Apo c θ. Hell θ. ZN—Left leg, Bry.

— Head hot, Bell. Cup.—Boring into the pillow, Apis. Bell. Hell θ.—Rolling, Hell θ.

— Frantic screams, APIS. Bell. Hell θ.

— Face dark red, Bry.—Cold sweat on forehead, Hell θ.

— Eyes red, protruding, Bell.—Rolled up, Hell θ.—Squinting, Apis. Bell. Hell θ.

— Jaw in motion, chewing, Bell. *Bry.* Hell θ—Relaxed, Hell θ.

— Tongue dry, brown, Bry—Moving in and out, Hell θ. Pulse slow, Dig.

— Drowsiness, Bry.—Sopor, Cup. Dig. Heil θ—Hands cold, fingers blue, Cup. ZN.

— Vomiting, BELL.

— Twitching, Cup.—Spasm, Dig. Cup.

Hydrocephalus, Chronic :—(See Diet W.)

In general, Ars iod. Bacill 200. "*Cal c. and Sul.*" Cal p KAL IOD. Kali m. Mer. Sil.

— Incipient stage, Iod.

— Automatic motion, Apo c θ. Bry. Hell. ZN·

— Cold head sweat, CAL C. Sil.

— Hot vertex, Sul.

— Blindness, Kal iod.

— Precocity, Bell. Mer.

Hydrocephaloid (Brain exhaustion from Diarhœa), PHO. Mag p. Pod. ZN.

153

Meningitis. See remedies indicated under Hydrocephalus.

Initial stage, Aco.

"Boiling" heat in the brain, Aco.

From injury, Arn.

— sudden chill, Aco.

Head hot, Bell. Cap—Boring into the pillow, Apis. Bell. Hell—Rolling, Hell—Hot vertex, Sul.

Carotids throbbing, *Bell.* Glo. Hyo.

Frantic screams, APIS. *Bell.* Bry. *Hell θ*

Face red, bloated, Aco. Bell—Dark, livid Bry—Pale, Hell—Cold sweat on forehead, Hell.

Eyes red sparkling. Bell—Rolled up, Hell—Half open, ZN—Pupils dilated, Apis. Bell.

Jaw in motion, chewing, Bell. *Bry.* Hell θ.

Limbs in motion, automatic, Bry. Hell. ZN.

Teeth grating, gnashing, Apis. Bell. Stram.

Sopor, Apis. Hell θ. Op θ. ZN—Hands cold and blue, Cap. ZN.

vomiting, BELL.

Syphilitic cachexia, Kal iod. Mer.

Chronic Meningitis:—PB.

—Deep seated brain disturbance, Ox a 2x. Pic a 2x.

Headache constant for days, months, years, HEMP extract. ¼-½ gr, 12 hours

Softening of the Brain: PHO. Kal p. ZN p. See Diet S.

Headache. Congestive:—*Antipyrin* 5 gr, 10 minutes. "Antikamnia 10 gr, 10 minutes." *Atrop.* 2x, 2 gr. *Aco.* Bell. Bry. FERR P. GLO 3x. Gel MELI θ—Sul. (See Chloroform. Coffee. Mustard.)

Daily headache constant, China. *Cann I* 1x. 5 gr. 12 hours. Kalmia 3x.

For relief of headache, Hot mustard water foot bath. Hot solution of soda in water by compress. Scent of the Oil of Rosemary; or extract of sweet Clover. Induce nose bleed, by inserting a small roll of mustard paper into the nose, and leaving it *in situ* for a few minutes.

Headache Neuralgic Nervous:—*Antifebrin*,
5 gr, *Atrop* 2x, 2 gr. Ars bro 3x. "Caffein 1 gr." Glo. Ig. *Mag m.* MELI. PASS *θ*. *Pho.* SPIG. Thuj. ZN P. 2x, 2 gr. ZN V. 2x, 2 g.

Headache Rheumatic: Bry. *Cimi.* GEL. Phyt.
SPIG—Nightly, *Mer.* Phyt.

Sick-Headache. Bilious:—*Antifebrin* 5 gr. ¼
hour. Charcoal powder, 2 teaspoonfuls, in ½ tumbler of water, at the onset. Chionanth Vir 1x. *Epiph.* Vir 3x. *Glo 3x.* Geranium 2x. Hydras. IRIS V. NUX V *θ* 5. drops. ¼ hour, in hot water. Phyto—SANG. Sul. Verat. a.

Deathly nausea, Ipe.

Sour vomit, IRIS V.

Cold sweat, Verat a.

Weak sight, Gel. ZN.

From a "flurry," EPIPH.

—Riding in car or carriage, Coc. "Place a sheet of paper next to the skin, over the stomach." Begins in the morning in the occiput and extends up over the head, and settles in or above the right eye, Sang.

Prevention of Sick Headache: Give the selected remedy—perhaps in preference,—Chionanth. Iris v or Sang. before meals for several weeks.

Headache occurring:—
After meals, Bism. NUX M *θ*. 5 drops, before eating. Nux v.

In the evening, Pul—From 4 to 8 p. m., Lyc.

At night, Merc. Thuj—Throbbing, Sul—
With sick stomach, Sil.

In the morning on waking, Bry. Cal c.
Carb v. NAT M. NUX V—With foul taste,
Nux v—Lasts all day, Nat m. Spig.

"Monthly," Bovis. Cimi. *Cyc.*, *Ferr p.*
Nat m. Sul. ZN—Over the eyes, Iris v.

Headache From :—

Catarrh, Kal bi. *Nux v.*

Constipation, Alu. Lyc. Nux v.

Indigestion, Hydras. *Nux v.* Sang.

Intemperance, Carb v. *Cimi. Nux v.*

Excitement—"Flurry," EPIPH VIR.

"Ironing", Bry.

"Washing," Pho.

Reading, studying, Cal p., CIMI. *Nux v*
Viola od.—School girls, Cal p. Nat m—Eye
strain, Gel. Onos Vir.

Riding in car or carriage, Arn. COC. Kal c.
Nux v.

Sea Bathing, Nat m.

Smoking, *Bell.* Glo. Ig.

Strong light (electric), Glo.

Sun's heat, Ant c. Bry. GLO 3x—Coming and
going with the sun, Kalmi. Nat m. Spig.

Malaria, Nat m.

Headache with :—

Coldness About the head, Cal c. Sep. Sil. Val
—In the vertex, Cal c. Sep. Verat a.

Delirium, Agar. Bell. Stram. Verat a. *Meli.*

Dim vision, *Cyc. Gel.* Mag p—Begins with a
blur, *Gel. Iris v.* Kal bi. Nat m. Pod—Eyes
"bloo -shot," Bell. MELI. Nux v.

Drowsiness, Gel., Nux v. *ZN.*

Heat on top of the head, Lach. Kal c. *Sul*—
Heat in the head and face, body cool, Arn.

Hunger, Pso.

Noise in the ears, Aco. CAIN. Coc.

Pressure here or there, *ZN*—Like a board
against the forehead, Coc. Rhus.

Red face, Gel. *Ferr.* Ferr p. MELI.

Sore throat, Bell. Homar 3x.

Throbbing Carotids, Bell. Glo.

Vomiting—See Sick-headache.

Pains in the head located or extending into :—

Base of brain, Crotal. Avena. Gel.

Top of the head, CACT. Ferr p. Sul—As if the
top would fly off, Cimi—Opening and shutting, Cann I.

In the temples, Bell. Chin. Nit a. Spig—Left
temple and eye, Onos Vir.

Through the temples as if screwed together,
Lyc—Bolted together, Ham.

From ear to ear, Pul.

Root of nose, Ars. Stict.

Involving the eye, Cimi. Coc. Ig. *Onos.* Pul.
Spig—As if the eyes would be torn out, Coc—
Over one eye, Gel. Kal bi. Nux v. Onos—
Over the left eye, Ars. Nux v. Sep. *Spig.*
Plant—Over the right eye, Chel. Gel. Kalmi.
Spig. Sang.

In the back of the head, Coc. Con. Ig. Kal p.
LIL T. *Sil.* THUJ—Rising from the back of
the head or nape of neck, Cimi. Fl. ac. GEL,
KAL C. Lil t. *Sang.* SIL—Extending from
head down the spines, *Cimi.*

Pains in the head relieved by :—

Eating, Ana. Sep—Eating breakfast, Bovis.

Flow of menses, Lach. ZN.

Tight bandage, ARG N. *Apis.* Bell. Chin.
Cal c. Gel. *Glo.* Pul. Sep.

Warm wrapping, Pho. SIL. Thuj.

Uncovering the head, Glo. Led. Sul—Removing the hat, Carb v. Nit a. Mez.

Thinkiug of the pain, Camp. Cic.

Touching the place of pain, Asa, Colo.

Urinating, GEL. IG. Scutt. Sil.

Sensation in the head as of:—

A ball rising into it, Aco. PB—Ball seated firmly in the forehead, Stap—Ball lodged in the brain, Con.

Beating like little hammers, Ferr. Phos. NAT M. *Lach.* Psor.

Boiling, ACO. Alu.

Boring, *Arg n.* Mer.

Bubbling, Sul.

Bursting, splitting, *Aco.* Bell. BRY. Mer. MELI. *Nux v.* Verat v.

Burning, Aco. ARG N. *Canth.* Hyper. Pho.— On top, Canth. Lach. Kal c. SUL—Burning spot on top, Grap. Kal c.

Coldness, Arg n. Sep. Sil. Val—On top, Cal c. Verat a—On one side, Calc—In the back part, Chel. Pho—As if cold air blowing through it, Aur. Nat m—Cold water dropping on it, Cann s—As if touched by icicles, Agar.

Diminution, sense of, Aco.

Enlargement, sense of, ARG N. Bovis. Cann I. Glo. NUX M. NUX V—Face also, Æth. Alo—the hands, Bap. Diad.

Elongation, sense of, Hyper.

Emptiness, Hollowness, COC. *Ig.* Sep

Fullness, as of too much blood, Chin. Con. Glo. Sul.

Heaviness, LACH. Mos—As of a weight on top, CACT. Cann s. Sul—At base of brain, Laur.

Lightness, *Coc.* Val. ZN.

Looseness of the brain, Am c. *Cro.* Nux m. Rhus—Rocking, Chin—At every step the brain seems to rise and fall, Bell.

Nail driven in—"Clavus"—Coff. IG. Mag p. NUX V. Pul. Thuj—In the back part, Mos. Thuj—On top, Nux v—Through the bone, Hep.

Numbness, *Coc.* Grap. Plat. *Tart e.*

Opening and shutting, *Coc.* Cann I—Feeling as if the top would fly off, Cimi; or fly to pieces, Coff.

Pressure here or there, Bell. ZN—Pressing out at the forehead, ACO. Asa. *Bry*—On top, *Cact.* Sul.

Pulsation. Throbbing, Amyl. *Bell.* Chin. *Glo.*

Soreness deep in the brain, Phyt.

Tired feeling in the brain, APIS. *Pho.* Ph a. *ZN P.*

Wild feeling as if going crazy—Cimi. Lil t.

Vertigo :—

In general, CAMP. *Ferr p. Gel.* Glo. *Mur a. Nit a.* Pet—In the occiput, Sil. ZN—Of old people Cal p. Con—As if intoxicated, Gel. Grap. Nux v. Sil

After eating, *Nat m.* Nux v. PUL. Sul.

—Sleeping, Carb v. *Hep.* Lach.

—Smoking, Borax. Sil. ZN.

When ascending a hill or stair-way, Borax. *Cal c.* Con. *Sul—Descending*, Ferr.

—Closing the eyes, *Ars.* Chel. Hep. LACH. Pet. Thuj—*Opening* the eyes, Aco. Pul. Sang.

—Eating, Am c. Aur. Sil.

—Entering a room, Pho.

—Looking up, Lach. *Sil*—Down, Spig. Ol—
Around, Con.

—Lying down, Cham. Con. Ferr. Grap. Lach.
Ptel. Sang. Thuj—On the back, *Mer*. Nux v
—Preventing sleep, Coc. Merc.

—Reading, Am c. Aug. Arn.

—Reaching up, Lach.

—Rising from a seat, Pul. Bry. Rhus.

—Rising up in bed, *Aco*. Coc. *Bry*. Pet—In
the morning, BOVIS. *Dul. Lyc*. Nux v.
Rhus—Turning in bed, Con—Morning in
bed, Kalmia.

— Standing, Cann I. Caust. Cyc. Ol.

— Stooping, Bar c. *Bry*. Bell. *Cham*. Nux v.
Pul. SUL.

— Talking, Cham. Borax. Thuj.

— Thinking, Agar. Agn. Pul. Nux v.

— Walking, ARN. Con. Ferr. Nat m. Nux m.
Pho. Pul. Spig. *Sul*—In open air, Aur. Cal
c. Lyc. Sep. SUL—In the dark, Arg n.
Stram.

With appearance of objects moving, Mos. Sep.
Thuj—In a circle, *Bell. Con. Cyc*. Mur a. Rhus.
Sil—Around each other, Sabad—Seat seems
moving, ZN —Rising up, Pho.

—Blindness, Aco. Bell. Kalmi. Nux v.—
Diplopia, Cyc. Gel.

—Buzzing in the ears, *Arg n*. Chin. Nux v.
Pul.—Ringing, Ferr. Sang.

—Fainting, *Bry*. Coc. Glo Lach. MOS. NUX
V. *Pho*. ZN.

— Falling, Agar. CON. Pho. Physos. Pul.
Rhus. SIL.—Forward, *Agar. Alu*. FERR P.
Nat m. *Sil*.—Backward, *Chin*. Kal c. Led.
Pho. Rhus—Sideways, Cann I. *Con*. Sul.—
Swaying to and fro, Pet.

— Nose bleed, MELI. Pho. Sal.

— Palpitation, *Ferr*. Plat. Sal.

— Sick stomach, Coc. Mos. Sul.; or gagging, Sil.

— Trembling, Carb v. Dig. Dul. Zinc v.

Motion of the Head:—

Boring into the pillow, Apis. Bell. Hell.

Falling back, Æth, Agar. Dig.

Falling front, Cup. Nux m—As if pushed, *Fer p.*

Jerking, Agar. Alu. Cic. Verat v—Back and forth, Bell. Sec. Sep—Up from the pillow, Stram.

Rolling of the head on the pillow, Bell. Hell. Pod.

Trembling, Asa. Bell. *Coc.* Mer. *Tart e.* Verat a.

Position of the Head:—

Drawn back, Alu. Gel. Lyc—In spasm, Bell. *Cic.* Op. Verat a.   See Neck—stiff.

Scalp:—

Baldness.—See Hair.

Dandruff: Alu. ARS. Carbol a. *Canlh.* Lyc. OL. Pho. GRAP—Yellow, Kal s. (See BORAX. Glycerine. Resorcin. Tannin.)

Eruptions on the head :—

— Burning, Cic. Mer. Ol.

— Itching, *Mer.* Mez. Ol. RHUS. *Sul.* STAP— At night especially, *Cal c.* Ol. RHUS. Sul— After scratching burning, Ars. Hep. Sul— Moist, Ol.

Favus. Porrigo. Scald-head : See *Scab* and *Scale.*

— In general, Dul. *Iris v.* VIOL T. Pet.

— Bleeding easily, Sul.

— Dry, Cal c. Sul.

—Humid, Clem. Graph. Hep. RHUS. *Sil.*

Skook—Oozing, Graph. Ol. Skook—Extending back of the ears, *Grap.* Ol. Pet. *Sep*— Eating away the hair, Mer. *Rhus.*

—Invading the eyes, CLEM. HEP. *Graph.* Mez. Sul.

—Itching intensely, Cal c. *Rhus.* Sul.

—Suppurating, Hep. Rhus. Sil.

Clip hair short. Use Skookum Soap. "Calomel ointment." (See Acetan. Glycerine. Ichthyol. Soda. Vinegar. Ointment.)

Lump. Node: See Tumor.

Scab. Crust: Grap. Hep. IRIS V. *Mer. Mez.* RHUS. Sil Sul Stap VIOL T—"One mass," Cal c—"Leathery," Mez—"Stinking," Stap—Green, Mer—Eating away the hair, Mer. *Rhus.* Skook.

Scale. Scurf: Alu. ARS. *Bar c.* Cal c. KAL C. Kal s. Nat m. Skook.

Sweat:—See Hair—*Wet.*

Tenderness, *China.* Pet. *Spig.* Sil. Sul.

Tetter: Alu. BOVIS. Pet—"Ring-worm", Bacill 200. Bar c. Dul. Sep.

Tumor—Node: Aur. Cal c. *Cal fl.* KAL IOD. *Sil*—Blood tumor at birth, Fl ac. Sil.

Ulcer: Ars Mer. Nit a. Ol—Invading the bone (caries), Aur. Fl ac. Ph a. Stap.

Hair :—

Baldness, Arnica oil. (See Carbol a. Onion.) Aas. *Bar c.* CAL FL. Euca. Kal c. Lyc. NAT M. PILO in. and ex. Thuj—Syphilitic, *Kal iod.* Thuj.

—From ring worm, Bacill 200. See Tetter.

—Off in patches, *Alo.* FL AC Pho—On top, Bar c.

—Spots smooth, Grap 30.

—Wooly spots, Vinc min.

Hair feels as if " on end ", ACO. Spo.

Hair growth arrested, Thuj; or very slow, Thuj; or too abundant, Thuj; or in tufts, out of place, Thuj.

Brittle, *Cal fl.* Fl ac. Kal bi.

Dry, harsh, Alu. Cal c. CAL FL. Kal c.

Split, Thuj.

Tangled, Bovis. Lyc. Pso—At the ends, Bovis. Fl ac—" Kink ", Lyc.

Greasy, Bry. Ph a. PB.

Wet with sweat, RHEUM. Sil—Hot Sweat, Cham—Cold, Cal c. *Mer.* Sil—Pillow wet with sweat during sleep, CAL C. Sil. Mer.

HEARING.—See Ear.

HEART.—" Blue lips and bulging eyes point to heart disease "—Look to Eye strain. Tobacco habit.

Ailments in general, Aur. *Aur bro 3x.* CACT. CRATAEGUS OX. *θ.* DIG. Kalmi. SCUT. Spo. Vis a *6.*

Angina Pectoris — " Heart Pang": — ANTIPYRIN 10 grs. Cact 1x. GLO 2x 1 drop, 5 minutes. Lat m. *Spig.* ALCOHOL, dilute one half, 1 teaspoonful, 5 minutes. CRATAEGUS OX. *θ,* 10 drops. (See AMYL.)

Sweat of agony, ACO. Ars. Verat a.

Cold sweat upon the forehead, Verat a.

Attack renewed by every motion, *Ars.* Bry. Dig SPIG.

Fainting, Ars. Lach. LAUR. SPIG.

Violent palpitation, Cact Laur. SPIG.

Must sit bent forward, Ars. Lach.

Cannot endure throat touched, Lach.

Guard against attacks, ARS. Cact. *Dig.* Cup. NUX V.

Hot fomentations over heart region. (See *Amyl.*)

Carditis—Endocarditis—Pericarditis :—

First, ACO.

Acute stitch, ACO. Bry. Cact. SPIG.

Heart action tumultuous, ACO. *Ars* Cact. SPIG. *Verat v.*

Palpitation violent, ACO. *Ars.* Cact. Dig. SPIG.

Fainting, Ars. *Dig.* Laur.

Coldness, Collapse, Ars—Cold hands and feet, Lact.

Cold sweat, Verat a—Blue lips, Dig.

Constrictive pain, Aco. CACT — Cramp-like, Lach.

Effusion, Ars. Bry. *Cact. Dig.* Spig.

Hydropericardium : *Adon v θ. Apo c θ.* Ars.
Caffein 5 grs. CACT. DIG 1x 10 drops, 4 hours. Spig. Spartein 1x. Stigma *θ.*

Hypertrophy of the Heart : *Aco.* Arn. Brom.
Cact. Naj. Spig. VIS A *θ.*

From violent exertion, Arn. Sul 200.

Ossification of the valves : Cal fl. See Diet Q.

"Weak Heart"—"Heart Failure :" COCAINE
2x. APOC *θ.* ARS. Ars iod. Adon v. *Caffein* 1 gr. *Glo 3x.* HELO H 200. LACH 30. *Piper m θ* 10 drops. Stigma *θ,* 20 drops. See Coffee. Hydrogen. See apparent death.

Pains and sensations in the heart :—

In general, Cereus b. PASS *θ* 30 to 60 drops. Spig—Extending to left arm, Cimi—With numbness of arm and shoulder, Rhus.

From Rheumatism, Aco. Cact. Cimi. *Colch.* KALMI. SCUT. *Spig.* Vis a.

—Strong drink, APO C *θ.* Glo.

—Tobacco, APO C *θ.* Glo.

Coldness, Pet.

Dropping, Cann s.

Heat, Cann s. Glo. Rhod.

Heaviness, Spig. Lil t. ZN.

Shock, Con. Gel. Glo. Lith c. *Nux v*—At night, Agar.

Spasm, CACT. Coc. Mag p.

Squeezing, Arn. CACT. *Lil t*—Cramp-like, Lach.

Stitch, *Aco.* Bry. Cact. Rhus. SPIG. *Spo.* SUL.

Trembling, *Ars.* Cic. SPIG. *Rhus.*

Twisting, Tarent C.

Abnormal action of the heart :—

Action seems as if it would cease, Aur—Stops and starts, Aco. Cimi—Starts with a thump, Aur—Seems to stop if the body moves, DIG. Spig—Seems to stop if the body is still, *Gel.*

Excessive action, tumultuous, ACO. Ars. Amyl. Cact. Laur. SPIG. *Spong.* Verat a— Audible, Dig. SPIG. Sul. Thuj. Verat a.

Fluttering, Cact. Helo h 200. LAUR. *Lil l.* Spig—With gasping for breath, Helo h 200 Laur. CRATAEGUS OX *θ*, 10 drops.

Intermitting, DIG. Kal c. Lach. NAT M. Sep.

Palpitation : MELI. PASS *θ*—"Stoop forward, arms pendant." See Coffee.

From the least motion, DIG. NAT M. Pho. Sil. STAP—Audible, Ars. SPIG. Dig. *Thuj.*

With fear of death, Aco. Ars.

—Cold sweat, Verat a.

—Heart pain and gasping forbreath, Spo.

—Nervous Excitement, *Amb.* Asa. *Laur.* Mos. Val.

—Smothering, Ars. Lach. Laur. Spo.

—Syncope, Asa. Lach. Laur. Pul. (See Coffee).

Worse at night, Ars. Dig. Lil t. Spo. Sul—On

HEARTBURN.

first lying down at night, Alston c. Ox a—
Preventing sleep, Ant c. Lil t—Wakened by
it, Alu. *Spo.*
—Lying on the left side, Cact. Pul. Spig.
—Lying on the back, Ars.
—Sitting, Pho. Rhus. Spig—Bent forward,
Spig.
—Walking, Dig. *Nat m.* Spig. *Slap.*

Pulse :—

Almost imperceptible, Ars. Carb v. Verat a.
— Thready, DIG. *Hell.* Verat a.
Irregular, *Ars.* Cic. Cimi. *Cact.* DIG. Mur a.
Mer c. Nat m. Nit a. PASS *0.* Pho. SEC.
Intermittent—See Irregular, especially, *Mer c.*
Sec.
— Every third beat intermits, Dig Mur a.
— Every fourth beat, Nit a.
— Every fifth or seventh, Dig.
— Three beats of the pulse, to one throb of the
heart, Aco.
Rapid, hard full, bounding, *Aco. Bell.*
VERAT V.
Rapid and weak, Iod. Pho.
Slow and weak, Adon v. Cann I. *Cic.* DIG.
Kalmi. Laur. *Sec.* ZN.
Slow and irregular, Dig. Laur. Verat a.
Slow pulse, yet rapid heart action, Glo.
Weak pulse, *Cact 0 5 drops*—Fluttering Cuprum
ars. Laur. Stram.
— Trembling, Hell. *Tart e*—Vanishing when
pressed, *Cocain* 2x—See Hydrogen—See
" Weak heart."

HEARTBURN.—See Stomach.

HEAT—PYREXIA.—See Ague—See Fever—See
part affected. Recurring every night, Aco. Bell.

Gel—Every evening, Gel. Pul—Morning and evening, Gel.

Without thirst, APIS. *Gell. Hell.* Nux m. Pho PUL. Squil.

With Dread of uncovering, HEP. NUX V. PUL. Sam. Sil. Squil.

— Shivering, Bell. Cham. Hell. Mer—Alternating with shivering, Ars. Bry. Mer—Mingling heat and chill, Cham. Mer.

Flushes of heat: Grap. LACH. Lyc. Pho. Sil. SUL. Thuj—Rising flushes, Indigo. Helo h 200. *Lach.*

— At change of life, Sang. LACH. SEP. Sul.

— From every little excitement or pain, FERR.

— — The least exertion, Val.

— With burning soles, Cup. Sal.

— — Faintness, Sep. Sul.

— — Fiery red face, Amyl. *Ferr.* Meli.

— — Sweat, Amyl. Pilo. *Sep. Sul.*

— — Vertigo, Ustil.

Worse at night, Kal iod. Lach. (See Face.)

Hyper-Pyrexia—Excessive Fever Heat: Aco. ANTIFEBRIN 10 gr. ANTIPYRIN 10 gr— BELL. *Carbol a.* BROM. *Iod.* "Quinia in controlling doses." "THALLIN (Sulphate or Tartrate) 1 gr. 1 hour." "Musk (by rectal injection), adult 10 gr, suspended in an ounce of mucilage of acacia. This will reduce temperature, 3 degrees in 20 minutes."

HEAT RASH.—*Arn.* Rhus. Sul.

HECTIC FEVER.—See Fever—Hectic.

HEEL.—See Limb—Leg—*Foot.*

HEMORRHAGE.—See *Bleeding*—See the affection, or part affected.

HEPATIC.

HEPATIC.—See Liver.

HERNIA.—See Abdomen.

HERPES.—See Skin. See part affected.

HICCOUGH.—See Chest—See Stomach.

HIP-DISEASE.—See Limb—Leg—*Hip*.

HIVES.—See Skin.

HOARSENESS.—See Chest—Voice.

HOMESICKNESS.—Caps. Cup. PH A.

HOT WATER.—*Chronic Disease—Drink Habit:*—Hot water treatment.—*Quantity:*—1 to 1½ pints at one drinking, begin with smaller amount, and gradually increase the quantity, until all rank odor disappears from the urine, then continue with *that* quantity.—*Time:*—1 to 2 hours before each meal, and ½ hour before going to bed.—*Mode:*—Sip, not drink, the hot water, may consume 15 or 20 minutes in taking the draught.—*Course:*—6 months, in order to cleanse all the organism. As it makes well people better; may continue as long as you please. "This is the fundamental treatment for *all Chronic diseases*, and will break up all *hankering for strong drink.*"

If at first there should be diarrhœa, boil some pepper grains in the water. If there should be constipation, boil bran, tied up in a bag, in the water.

Pain, Sprain, Stiff neck, Stiff back :—Flannel wrung out of hot water. Apply and cover with dry compress, then over this pass slowly and lightly a hot sad-iron.

Lock-jaw :—Same to nape of neck and spine.

Lady's Ailments in General—(Uterine and Vaginal Congestion, Inflammation, Ulcera-

168

tion, *Painful Menstruation, Leucorrhœa, Sterility:*—Inject into the vagina hot salt water, three pints, twice a day; hotter each day; until as hot as can be borne by patient's hand. Persevere and cure.

Convulsions of Children:—Put patient naked into warm water; retain in bath 10 minutes, with cold wet cloth to the head. If very feeble infant, retain in bath only about 3 minutes. Give as a stimulant some gin in hot water, sweetened. Warm water containing a few drops of Camphor spirits should be injected into the bowel.

Colic of Any Kind—Dysmenorrhœa—Pains of Dysentery:—Frequent copious injections of hot water. To be retained as long as possible patient lying on the left side. Also hot fomentations to the abdomen. Hot sitz bath excellent; especially for *Kidney Colic, Amenorrhœa* and *Dysmenorrhœa.*

Injury to the Head—from fall or blow, Croup, Cold in the Chest, Congestion of the Lungs, Pleurisy, Pneumonia, Engorgement of the Breasts, Piles, Inflammation and Enlargement of the Prostate Gland:—Hot fomentations, and hot foot baths. (Hot mustard seed tea may be used instead of the plain hot water in some such cases, often to great advantage.)

Quinsy:—Gargle frequently, and freely with hot water in which black pepper grains, or whole mustard seed. have been boiled; and apply fomentations of the same, and cover with compress. Steam received into the mouth and throat, from *baked oats*, steeping in hot water, is a charming thing in quinsy in the last stage to hasten it to break.

HOUSEMAID'S KNEE.

Apparent Death, from Convulsions or other cause: Pour hot water, not scalding hot, from a height upon the heart region; or place scalding hot cloths over the heart. Heating the bowl of a spoon hot, and making with spoon repeated quick light taps over the heart, will sometimes excite the heart to action in case of apparent death.

Wound bleeding: Hot water on cloth or sponge; continually renew, hot; or a stream of hot water—130° to 140° F.—let flow upon it.

Ague, even Chronic: "After the chill and during the heat, before it reaches its height, get into bath tub, in luke warm water, submerge to the chin, keeping the while a cold wet cloth on the head; when the fever goes off, get out of the bath and wipe dry and dress No more Ague."

Local Sweat: Bathe part with hot water, hot as can be borne, until red and tingling, several times a day.

HOUSEMAID'S KNEE.—Sil. See Seaton. See Iodoform.

HUNGER, CANINE.—See Stomach—Appetite.

HURRIED FEELING.—See Mind. See Nerve.

HURT.—See Wound. See Cause—Injury.

HYDRASTIS. — *Ophthalmia — Granular lids:* Sulphate of Hydrastis 2 grains, in distilled water, 1 ounce; apply the solution several times a day.

Baby's Sore Mouth: Hydras. 1x trit, 5 gr, in a wineglassful of water; of this give a teaspoonful every 2 hours. Wash the mouth also with same each time. The same remedy for *Nurse's sore mouth,* or *any ulcerated condition of the mouth.*

Chafing of infants—Rawness in the folds of the skin: Powder with common starch medicated lightly with Hydras. θ; or sprinkle the parts well with Hydras. root, triturated, 10 per cent, with cornstarch. Same for *Chafing and abrasion of adults.*

Sore Nipples (Chapped, cracked, ulcerated): Successful when all other means fail. Hydras. 1x trit, 10 grains in a wineglassful of tepid water; wash the nipples gently, but thoroughly with this solution, each time after child nurses. If baby has *sore mouth*, leave the lotion on the nipple, if not wash it off before offering the breast.

Ulcers: Very successfully treated by frequently renewed applications of bread soaked in this solution.

HYDROCELE.—See Male—Scrotum.

HYDROCEPHALOID.—See Head.

HYDROCEPHALUS.—See Head.

HYDROGEN PEROXIDE. —*Diphtheria:* Swab with Hydrogen per., diluted one-half with water, as often as seems needful to dissolve the patches.

Foul Ulcers, Caries, Gangrene, Cancer, Purulent Ophthalmia, Otorrhœa, Carbuncle: Hydrogen per. in 12 vol; saturate cloths or pledgets and apply; when admissible cover with gutta percha tissue. Perfectly harmless.

Granulated Eyelids " Crumby margins." Any Inflammation or Ulceration of the Eyelids: "Cleanse well with warm water; then wind some cotton on a toothpick and dip it into the solution 12 vol. of the Hydrogen per. and apply it to the whole extent of the margin.

HYDROPERICARDIUM.

Apply until the parts "bubble," every day until the cure is effected.

Ozæna : "Moisten sponge with the Hydrogen per. (1:3 water) and insert into the nostril and allow it to remain for an hour, first in one then the other, and thus cause to inhale thereof several times a day. This is a wonderful remedy."

Gonorrhœa : ' Inject Hydro per. diluted one half with water; from beginning of second stage, ½ oz. 3 times a day, for 3 days; then in full strength, 2 drachms, once a day, until cure effected.

Freckle, Moth Spot, Tan : Anoint with unguent made of Hydro per and Lanolin equal parts.

Lady's Moustache and "side burns" : After washing the growth with a solution of Borax in water, apply Hydro per. 12 or 15 vol. This bleaches the down so that it is invisible. No harm.

Internally: Hydro per. adult 1 vol, 10 drops in water sweetened has been found useful in cases of *Indigestion, Asthma, Cough, Whooping Cough, Croup. "Internal weakness" of Ladies. Nervousness, Debility, Fainting, Collapse, " Death's door" conditions from any cause.*

HYDROPERICARDIUM.—See Heart.

HYDROPHOBIA :—(Dread of water: Bell. Canth. Hyo. Stram.) Guard, ARS 2x trit 3 times a day. Bell *θ* dilute. CEDRON *θ*. Gel *θ*. HYDROPHOBIN 30:200. Stram *θ* dilut. "Bleed in the mouth (pull a tooth) and direct patient to swallow some of the blood, on the third day after being bitten." " In Russia whole packs of bitten hounds are rescued from rabies, by smearing their chops with the bleeding flesh of the biter.''

'' Have the patient eat the American Aloe, stem and leaf, and nothing else for days, or until the craving for it ceases, and the patient rejects it.''

Credon θ is said to have cured rabies, even after spasms have set in. *Bufo* should be thought of, also *Scuttellaria*. I think however I should place my main reliance upon HYDROHOBIN 30-200.

Retention in hot air, until heat reaches 57° Centigrade, is reported to have cured many cases after spasms had set in. Also steam baths as hot and as long as can be borne

A case reported cured, in the convulsion stage, by throwing the patient into deep water, and permitting him to drown, apparently— sinking the third time—then coming to the rescue.

HYDROTHORAX.—See Chest.

HYPERÆMIA.—See Congestion.

HYPEREXIA.—See Fever.

HYPERPYREXIA.—See Heat.

HYPERTROPHY.—See the part affected.

HYPOCHONDRIASIS.—See Mind.

HYPOPYON.—See Eye.

HYSTERIA.—

In general, Amb. Aur. Aur bro 3x. ASA. *Cimi*. *Ig*. *Mos*. ZN p. ZN V. NUX M θ. TARENT C. Amyl, inhale. (See Celery, Hydro per).

'' Fits,'' Asa. *Con*. IG. Mag p. MOS. NUX M θ. Plat. TARENT C. Val.

'' Globus,'' ASA Cimi. Con. *Gel*. *Ig*. Lach. PB. VAL. ZN V.

173

ICE.

Laughing, Aur. Cimi. Coff. HYO. *Ig.* Mos. NUX M *0*.

Crying, Aur. Coff. Ig. *Pul.*

Screaming, Ig. Plat.

Lascivious, *Hyo.* Mos. Pho. *Plat.*

Sighing, Ig.

Thoughts of suicide, Aur.

During a fit, dash cold water in the face. Hold ice to nape of neck. Amyl, inhale.

Guard: Nux m 0. 5 drops on sugar.

ICE.—*Quinsy :*—Crushed ice in rubber bag, bladder, or flannel cloth, to the throat, apply.

Cramp in Stomach or Bowel:—Ice to spine, *opposite* the seat of pain.

Vomiting in Typhoid Fever:—Ice to lower part of spine. Eating crushed ice, or drinking iced champagne, controls nausea and vomiting sometimes even of pregnancy.

Menses Scanty or Suppressed:—Ice to the back, low down, ½ hour at a time, once or twice a day.

Falling of the Womb. Leucorrhœa: Ice to the back, low down, one or two hours at a times daily.

Shrunken breasts: Ice to the back, in rubber bag, opposite to the breast, two hours at a time, twice a day, for several weeks. " Hot water applied in the same way will *diminish* the size of the breasts."

Local anæsthesia. Insensibility to pain: Mix pounded ice or snow with salt, equal parts, and apply this mixture, enveloped in a soft cloth, to the part to be operated upon, until it becomes numb.

Opium poisoning, Profound stupor:—Ice, reduced to small pieces, a pint or more, insert into the rectum. Also apply ice to spine of the neck, and in the arm pits. "Restoration in 10 minutes."

Sudden sinking from Hæmorrhage: Ice to the spine and hot sand bags, frequently renewed, under the back of the head. Cordage.

Stranguary: Plug the rectum with small pieces of ice; in twenty minutes the urine will flow. Sitting upon a chamber vessel containing chopped onions steeping in hot water will also excite the flow.

Spasms:—Ice to back of the neck, near the base of the brain, not directly to the head.

Cold feet. (Chronic condition): Ice in rubber bag, to spine low down, an hour at a time, once a day for a week

ICHTHYOL.—Dose, adult 2 gr pill, 2 or 3 times a day. "For *any pain*, or for any *blood or skin disease.*"

By combining, when practicable, the internal and external use of Ichthyol, we become armed with the most efficient means yet devised for the treatment of *Blood and Skin Diseases. Eczema in all forms, acute or chronic, Pruritus, Prurigo, Acne, Psoriasis, Erysipelas Lipoma, Lepra, Rheumatism acute and chronic, Gout, Tumefaction of the joints, Catarrh of Nose or Throat,* (gargle) *Gastric Catarrh, Chronic Constipation, Piles, Fractures, Cuts, Lesions, Wounds, Poisoned wounds, as by cut of a dissecting knife; Abscess, Bruise, Burn, Boil, Carbuncle. External Inflammation, Local Redness, Red Nose, Local Itching, Local pain. Neuralgia. Sciatica:* Apply Ichthyol pure, or 75 or 50 per cent. ointment. If very moderate

175

ICHTHYOSIS.

strength desired mix Ichthyol 2 parts, and water 4 parts, and Lanolin 5 parts.

ICHTHYOSIS.—See Skin.

ICTERUS.—See Liver—jaundice.

ILEUS.—See Abdomen—Bowel obstruction.

IMBECILITY.—Bacill 30-200. See Mind.

IMPETIGO.—See Skin.

IMPOTENCE.—See Male.

INDIGESTION.—See Stomach.

INDURATION OF TISSUE.—Aur. *Con.* Fl ac. Ham. Iod. Kali m. SIL.

After inflammation, *Bell.* China. Mag m. SIL. See Organ Affected.

INFANT.—(See Cold Water. Olive Oil. Diet Z. (1:12)

Averse to being washed, Ant c SUL.

Cross, CHAM—Cries all day, Jalap—Day and night, Ig. Stram— Before passing water, Lyc—Quiet only when carried, CHAM— Rapidly, Ars.

Fretful, peevish, Cina. Kal p. *Pul*—Cannot bear to be touched or looked at, *Ant c. Cina.* Tart e—Suddenly lets go the nipple and cries, Tart e—Afraid of strangers, Bar c.

Dull, will not play, *Bar c.* Thuj—Late learning to talk, *Nux m;* or walk, Cal c. Nux m.

Dreads doward motion, Borax—Will not be rocked, Borax—Wakens when laid down, Borax.

Emaciated, Abrotan. Arg n. Cal c. Cal p. Iod—With large abdomen, Bar c. Cal c— Weak ankles, Sil—Ceasing to walk, Cal c— Head large, Cal c. Sil. Sul—Skull bones thin, Cal p—Head sweat in sleep, CAL C.

Too fat, folds of the skin raw, Cal c. Grap
Lyc. Sul.

Jaundiced, Cham. *Chel.* Op. POD.

"Sour," Cal c. *Cham.* Mag m. Nat p. RHEU.
ROBIN. Sal a

Face pale, and blue around the eyes and nose,
Cina. Laur—One cheek red, CHAM.

Neck thin, emaciated, Nat m—Weak, Cal p.
Verat a.

Mouth hot, Borax—Sore, Borax. Bism—Dry,
with brain trouble, Pilo. 2x.

Nose stopped up, Am c. Sam—Boring finger
into the nose, Cina.

Stomach pit bulging out, CAL C—Vomiting
breast milk in thick curds, ÆTH—Gagging,
Ant c. Cina. Hell *Pod.*

Bowels constipated, Alu 200. Op 200. Nat m
2x—Too loose, *Pod*—Green stools, *Cham.*
Ip. *Mag p*—Ash gray, DIG—White, Cal c.
Pod.

Sleep unquiet, Aco. Gel—Crying out in sleep,
Bell. Sul—Shrill screams, *Apis*—Twitching
in sleep, *Bell.* Hell. Ig—Gnashing of teeth,
Cina. Cic. *Pod.*

Teething painful, *Kreo. Mer.*—Slow, Cal p—
Head affected, MAG P. *Bell.* Pod—Spasms,
Agar. Bell. Cic. Mag p. MELI θ. PASS θ.

INFECTION.—See Contagion.

INFLAMMATION. — See part affected. (See
ACONITE. Arnica. Calendula. *Ichthyol. Mullein
oil.* Poultice.)

In general—In the *first stage*, before effusion
takes place, Aco. Cact. Ferr p—In the *second
stage*, Engorgement, Effusion, Exudation,
"Patch": Bry. Kali m. Nat s—In the *third*

INFLUENZA.

stage, Abscess, Suppuration, Ulceration :
Cal p. *Hep.* Iod. Mer. *Sil.* Sul.

Burning, Aco. *Ars.* Caps. Canth. *Rhus.* Sul—
With Stinging, *Apis.* Mer.

Blue, Asa. Lach.

Hard, Bell. Chin. *Sil.*

Heavy and tight, Bry.

Red, shining, Aco. *Bell.* Ichthy. in. and ex.

Suppurating, Ulceration, Fl a. *Hep.* Iod·
Mer. Nat p. *Sil.* Sul.

Gangrenous, Ars. Crotal. *Lach. Thuj.* in. and
ex. (See Logwood.)

INFLUENZA.—See Nose.

INFRA-MAMMARY PAIN.—CIMI. Pul. RAN
B. Ustil.

INGROWING NAIL.—See Limb—Nail.

INJECTION OF FOOD.—See Food.

INJURY, MECHANICAL.—See Cause—Injury.

INGUINAL HERNIA.—See Abdomen—*Hernia.*

INSANITY—"*Dumb-Thumb.*"—See Mind.

INSECT BITE.—See Bite.

INSOMNIA.—See Sleep.

INTER-COSTAL NEURALGIA.—*Cimi.* Pho.
RAN B.

INTERMITTENT FEVER.—See Ague.

INTERTRIGO.—See Skin.

INTESTINES.—See Abdomen. See Bowel.

INTOXICATION.—See Alcoholism.

INUNCTION.—See *Glycerine.* Olive Oil. Lard.

INVOLUNTARY PASSAGES.—See Bowel.—
See Urinary Organs.

"INWARD WEAKNESS." — See Female—
Uterus—Displacement.

IODINE.

IODINE.—ALSO BROMINE.—*Bronchitis, Catarrh of Air Passages, Membranous Croup, Hay Asthma:* Inhale Iodine or Bromine. A convenient way to administer the vapor is to put into a drachm vial, half full of pure water, 4 or 5 drops of the tincture of Iodine or Bromine, a part only of which will be dissolved, whilst the rest will fall to the bottom and be taken up as fast as that already in solution passes off by its excessive volatility. Thus the solution may be kept of uniform strength from 24 to 36 hours. For administration the vial is to be held with the uncorked end in the mouth, so that the vapor will be inhaled through the mouth. The first few inhalations will cause some resistance on the part of children, but by having them take two or three, and then wait a moment, this is easily overcome. Most little patients will inhale it while sleeping.

In Croup give inhalations every two or three hours, about twenty inhalations each time, or until it causes severe coughing and vomiting.

In Chronic Bronchitis and Chronic Catarrh of the Air Passages give to inhale five minutes at a time, four or five times a day.

Tartar on Teeth, Ulcerated Gums, Ulcerated Mouth or Throat : Tincture of Iodine, apply.

Photophobia : Tincture, paint around the eye.

Goitre : A woolen cloth sprinkled on one side with a tincture of Iodine: wear as a collar, with saturated side next to the skin. With camel-hair brush paint the tumor with tincture of Iodine of such strength as to make the skin a dark orange color: do this in the evening, and in the morning wash it off with Aqua Ammoniæ diluted. If the Iodine be applied too

179

IODOFORM.

strong it will fail, not otherwise. If the goitre
contains fluid, let it out by trochar and inject
a solution of Iodine and water equal parts. If
it originates from the heart, is vascular, eyes
project, administer a few gentle inhalations of
Amyl, several times a day. APIS. Bell. Thuj.

Enlarged Glands, Lumps in the breast, Orchitis:
Tincture of Iodine iu water—1 ounce to the
pint—keep constantly applied.

Hydrarthrosis:—Inject into it Tincture of Iodine,
1 ounce.

Hydrocele: Inject into it Iodine θ, 1 to 4 drachms.
Three thicknesses of thread saturated with
Iodine θ, and drawn through the part as a
seaton, also cures.

Asthma: "Paint to a blister the front of the
neck from ear to ear, and from jaw bone to
collar bone, with Tincture of Iodine. This
masters the most desperate cases. The same
for *Croup.*"

Erysipelas—Especially of the Scalp: Paint with
Iodine tincture.

Carbuncle, Boil, Sty: In the forming stage:
Paint with Iodine θ. This will abort them.

Smallpox pustules kept off the face: "Paint
the inside of the thighs with Iodine tincture,
at the onset of the disease, and all the pustules
will form on the parts painted, none on the
face."

IODOFORM. — *Goitre, Tumor, lymphatic or
glandular, Tubercular inflammation of joints:*
Iodoform in Glycerine, inject once a week.

Pruritus, Acrid Ulceration, Cancerous Ulcer:
Iodoform in Glycerine, or cocoa butter, apply
freely.

Breast Lumps, Mammary growths, House-

Maid's Knee, Purulent Ophthalmia: Iodoform
lotion, 1 part to 15 water, constantly applied.

Chest pain of Consumption, Pleurisy pain:
Iodoform 1 part, with Collodion 15 parts, mix,
and apply night and morning.

Onychia, Enlargement of prostate gland: Iodoform Ointment.

*External ulceration, Fetid sores, Syphilitic
ulcers:* Iodoform powder; the standard dressing. Being considered the safest and best of
all antiseptics. *Iodol* is however an admirable
substitute, having none of the odor or poisonous
properties of the Iodoform. See *Acetanilide.*

IRITIS.—See Eye.

IRON.—*Ingrowing nail:* Perchloride of Iron dry,
insinuate as deeply as possible between the free
edge of the nail and the sore surface. May
render the parts insensible first with Cocaine 4
per cent applied on cotton. One thorough application is enough.

Sweating of the feet: Bathe the feet night and
morning for three days with tar water, half an
hour at a time, then stop the foot baths, and
paint the soles once a day with perchloride of
iron. In four days the soles will be found
hard and dry. Simple and speedy cure.

Bleeding from any accessible part: Dust with
dry persulphate of iron: or moisten lint, and
roll it in the same and apply: or apply perchloride solution on cotton or lint.

ITCH.—See Skin.

ITCHING, LOCAL.—See Skin—Pruritus.

JAUNDICE.—See Liver.

Jaw stiff from a cold.—Dul. Gel. Kreo.
— Symptoms of the jaw. See Face.

JERKING.

JERKING. TWITCHING.—See Nerve. See the part affected.

JOINT AFFECTIONS. See Limb.

Chalky concretions, Bacill 200 — "Sul for a month, then Sil, to complete the cure"
Creaking. Agn. CAL FL. Lyc. *Pet.* Sil. Sul.
Stiffness, Caust. Pet. Rhus. Sabin. ZN.
Swelling and Tenderness—See Acetan. *Clay.* Ichthy. Iodine. Vinegar. Verat oint.

KELOID.—Fl. ac. Grap. Nit a—See Resorcin.

KEROSENE.—*Cold in the Chest, Sore throat, Quinsy, Croup, Diphtheria, Diphtheritic Croup, Any pain,* as of *Gout, Rheumatism, Neuralgia:* Apply Kerosene on flannel, kept constantly saturated, and covered with compress.
Felon: Submerge it in a bowl of Kerosene: repeat the dip as often as pain returns.
Orchitis: The same.
Lice: One application suffices.

KERATITIS. See Eye—Inflammation.

KIDNEY.—See Urinary Organs.

KNEE.—See Limb—Leg.

LABOR.—See Female—Labor.

LACHRYMATION.—See Eye.

LACTIC ACID.—*Moth, Freckle:*—Lactic acid and glycerine, equal parts mix: lave
Fungus Caries, Epithelioma, Tubercular inflammation and ulceration of pharynx or larynx, Lupus: Apply in solution, at first from 20 to 30 per cent, and afterwards from 50 to 75 per cent, and some times full strength on cotton or spong.

LADY'S MUSTACHE.—See Face.

LA GRIPPE.—Aco. Am bro. EUP PER. Ferr p. GEL. Nux v. "Ferr p 3x and Nat m 2x trit alt, for 3 days; then Kali m 3x and Kal s 3x alt. to perfect the cure."

Dregs of La Grippe, Kali m. Kal s. NAT S. PASS *0.*

LAMENESS.—See Limb—Leg.

LARD.—*Fever:* Anoint the body all over with lard several times a day. This mode of treatment will conduct almost any inflammatory or eruptive fever through its course successfully to the end."

Scarlet Fever: "Rub the body all over twice a day with warm lard, and *no dropsy* will supervene, and *no contagious elements* remain."

Itch: "Lard alone, by thorough inunction three times a day will cure the itch."

Seat Worms: Lard applied inside the anus, night and morning, will destroy them.

Burns or Scalds: Apply lard and flour in equal parts mixed.

Gathering speedily to head: The same as for *Burns.*

Constipation of infants: Anoint the abdomen well with warm lard, or castor oil at bed time.

Baby's Colic: Anoint the abdomen with hot lard and laudanum mixed.

Lumbago—Sore Throat: "A plaster, 4 by 6 inches, of bacon, fat side in. Wonderful relief." A bandage of enameled cloth, or silk oil-cloth around the loins, outside a flannel skirt, produces perspiration on the parts, and thus greatly relieves the pain of lumbago.

LARYNGISMUS STRIDULUS.—See Chest—Croup, *false.*

LARYNGITIS.

LARYNGITIS.—Arg n. Pho. Sang. Spo. See Chest—Cough, *with hoarseness.*

LEAD.—*Burn, Scald, Erysipelas, Carbuncle, Eczema, Birth Mark :* Cover with white lead mixed thick as cream with linseed oil; renew the coating occasionally,

Maliguant Onychia : Cut away the dead part, and cover thickly with nitrate of lead powder. In a few days the slough will come off, leaving a sound surface.

Iugrowing toe nail : Dust the diseased parts with nitrate of lead powder, every three days. This will soon effect a cure. Sang θ, 10 drops to an ounce of water, frequently applied, is said to cure.

Ring worm: Compound Citrine ointment, one thorough application.

Mechanical iujury—Pain and inflammation from a *wound, Bruise, Sprain, Laceration, Compound fracture:* Lead water and laudanum equal parts, mix, and apply ice cold.

LEMON.—*To check diarrhœa:* Drink *hot* lemonade.

To arrest immoderate flow of menses: Suck the juice of lemon.

To harden the nipples before coufinement: "Begin two weeks in advance, and lave them with lemon juice."

To arrest flooding: Inject the juice of half dozen lemons into the womb.

Sweating Rheumatism. Scurvy: Partake of lemon juice, or lemonade freely.

To Cure Biliousness: Instead of calomel, take the juice of one two, or three lemons, according as the appetite craves, in as much water as will render it pleasant to drink, without sugar,

before going to bed: and in the morning half
hour before breakfast, take the juice of *one* in
a goblet of water.

Cough: Lemon juice and sugar.

Chilblain: Dilute Citric acid and Peppermint
water in equal parts, mix, and apply twice a
day.

Cancer pain:—Citric acid 1 drachm in water 8
ounces, mix, and apply the solution with
camel hair brush. Renew the application as
often as needful. Pledgets of lint saturated
with the same, and applied answers the purpose.

Impure water rendered innoxious: By making
it into lemonade. "Stagnant water touched
with citric acid, becomes harmless to drink."

Diarrhœa caused by bad water: "Is best con-
trolled by essence of ginger."

LEPRA-LEPROSY: Ana. ARS. *Bacill* 30–200,
CANTH. *Dul.* ICHTHYOL 2 gr pills 12 hours:
also Ichthyol ointment. HYDROCT. Pip m—
"Oleate of copper apply nightly."

LEUCORRHŒA.—See Female.

LEUKÆMIA.—See ix, Ergot. hypoderm.

LICHEN.—See Skin.

LICE.—See Kerosene—See Parasite.

LIENTERY.—See Bowel—Stool, *undigested.*

LIGHTNING STROKE.—Nux v. See Cold
water.

**LIMB—UPPER AND LOWER—HAND AND
FOOT.**

Arm including shoulder :—

Pain in general, Kalmi. PHYT. Stict—Stitches,
Bry. Kal c. Ran b—Shoulders, Phyt. Kalmi
—Right shoulder, Sang — Left shoulder.
Ferr.

Aching and bruise-like soreness, Apis, *Arn*, Cimi. EUP PER.

Boring in *joints*, Thuj.

Burning, Agar—Left arm, Carb v.

Coldness, Am bro. Am m. Hep Helo. h. 200.

Cramp, Cal c. Cup m. Lyc—In shoulders, Plat. Lyc. (See Sulphur.)

Cracking *joints*, Cal fl. Lyc. Nit a. Thuj. See Joints.

Creeping like ants, Sul.

Creeping like a mouse, Bell. Lach—before spasm, Sul.

Crooked by rheumatism, Caust. Grap. Guai *θ*. Nat m. Lyc.

Cutting, Bell—Transverse, ZN.

Drawing in the right arm, Bell—Left at night, Rhus.

Enlarged *joints*, Cal c. Carb a. Thuj—(See Clay. Ichthyol.)

Fuzzy feeling, Sec.

Heaviness, *Alu*. Cro. Mur a. *Nat m*. Sil—Left arm, Arg n.

Hot *joints*, Apis—*Hot, red, swollen*, LYC. Kalmi. Mer.

Humming, buzzing, Op.

Jumping, life-like, Cro.

Jerking, starting, Cic. Cina. Stram.

Lameness, Aco. Bell. Bry. Rhus. Ruta. Sul—Paralytic, Aco. Bell. Caust. *Cann I. Sil*—Right, Cann I—Left, Bell. Caust. *Colch*—Left at night, *Rhus*—From rheumatism, Colch. Rhus. Ruta. Phyt.

Motion involuntary of an arm or leg in brain affections, Agar. Apoc. Hell—Left arm, Bry—Right, Gel—Restless motion constant, Lyc. Rhus—Even in sleep, Caust.

Numbness, Aco. Lyc. Nux v. Pho—After
diphtheria, Nux v 2x — With coldness,
Nux m—Left arm numb, *Aco.* Amb. Cimi.
Hyper. *Lach.* Rhus—Numbness, as when
"gone to sleep," Amb. *Coc.* Grap. Kal c—
When lying on the arm, Rhus. Sil.

Pressure in the left arm, Kalmi—On top of the
shoulder with cutting, Bell.

Shocks in the arms, Agar, Nux v.

Shortened feeling, Æth.

Stiffness, Caust. Kal c. *Nux v—Elbow*, Kal c.
Lyc—Shoulder, Phyt.

Throbbing, Cann I.

Trembling, *Alu.* Arg. n *Con.* Mer. Rhus. Stram.
Thuj—Left arm, Hyper. Rhus. Spo.—After
exertion, Rhus

Twitching, Cic. Cina. Stram—In the shoulder,
Dros. Sul.

Twisting. Bell.

Weakness, weariness, *Bell.* Mer. *Nat m.* Pho.
Rhus. Sep. Sil. *Sul.*

Weight, Bell. Nat m. Pul. Stram.

Under the Arm. Axilla :—

Eczema exuding, Sep.

Lump, Tumor, Bar c—Hard blue, Cal p.

Pimples, Lyc. Pet. Sep.

Scurf, Nat m.

Sweat offensive, Hep. Nit a. Pet. *Sul.* Thuj—
Odor of garlic or onion, BOVIS. Lach. (See
Chlorine. Potash.)

Tetter, *Carb a.* Dul. Lyc. *Sep.*

Hand including Wrist :—

Pain in general, Agn. Led. Ruta—Cold pain,
Led.

—In finger joints, Ant c. Led. Phyt.

—In the wrist, *Caul.* Kalmi. *Viol o*—Sprain-like, Arn. *Led* EUP PER. Rhus. *Ruta.*

In the thumb, sprain-like, Kreo.

Blue hands, Arn. Nux v—Blue and cold, Cap. Verat a.

Burning, Sep. *Sul*—In the evening, Pul—Palms, Æs. Caps. Sang *Sep. Sul*—Child, hot palms, Borax—Hot dry palms, BISM—Hot hands at night, Lach—*Finger* ends burn, Apis—Burning blisters on finger ends, Canth.

Coldness, *Cup.* Hep. MER. Nat m. *Sec.* VERAT A—Icy cold and blue, Cup *Helo h 200.* Pho. *Verat a*—Cold or hot, Sep—Hands always cold and blue in winter—Cup a—Cold hands and feet with hot head, Bell. ZN—One hand cold the other hot, Dios. Ipe. *Mos.*

Cracks, fissures, *Alu.* GRAPH. *Hep.* Lyc. PET. SIL—Finger tips crack and bleed, Pet 30.

Cramp, Amb. Grap. Lyc—Thumb cramp, Spo—"Artist's cramp," Nux v. Mag p. (See Sulphur.)

Deadness of the fingers, CAL C. Calad. *Sep.* Thuj—"Gone to sleep," Coc. Nux v.

Drawn crooked, Kal c. Lyc.

Dryness, BISM. LYC. SUL. *Thuj*—Dry palms, *Bism.* Lyc.

Enlarged feeling, Bap. DIAD. Calad

Enlarged joints painful, Ant c. *Benz a.* LITH LAC 2x—Nodes in joints, Sabin. See Gout. (See Ichthyol. Iodoform.)

Excoriation between fingers, Grap.

Felon (Onychia. Whitlow): *Apis.* Ars. FL AC. *Hep.* SIL.

—Burning intensely, Apis. *Anthra. Ars.*

—Stinging, *Apis.* Mer.

—Throbbing, Bell. *Hep.* Mer. *Sil.*

—Terrific pain, *Stram.*

—Worse at night, Mer.

—Gangrenous, Anthraxin 200, Ars. *Lach.*

Saturate cloth with Lobelia tincture and apply. This at an early stage, assuages the pain, and aborts the abscess. Keep constantly applied Aqua ammoniæ and water equal parts. Immediate relief of pain, see *Kerosene.* Salt. (See Poultice). Open without pain, see Anæthesia—*Local.* See Alcohol.

Formication, Nat m. Sil. Sul.

Heat of the hands, AGAR. BELL. Carb v. Pho. Pul—Palms, Sul.

Hot joints, Apis—Red hot swollen, LYC. Mer.

Hardness of the palms, *Grap. Sul.*

Heaviness, *Alu.* Bry. Pul. *Nat m.*

Itching, AGAR. Sil. SUL.

Jerking, Cap. Stram—Of the tendons, Hyper. Iod.

Numbness, Apis. *Lyc.* PHO. *Sec* — Numb *thumb*, *Apis.* Kal c—*Fingers* numb, Ana. *Cal c.* Lyc. *Nat m.* Sec. Sul—Numb *finger ends*, Arg n. *Ox a.* Pho.

Nodes on finger joints, *Cal c.* Grap. Lyc.

Peeling palms, Am c. Grap. Red Fl a.

Pricking like needles, Nux v. Rhus.

Shrivelled look, Ph a. Sec.

Spots brown, Pet—Copper colored on palms, Coral.

Stiff fingers, Carb a. Agar. Colch. Lyc. Rhus. Sep—Wrists, Ruta.

Sweating hands, PILO 1x—Palms, Cou. Sul—Cold sweat on palms, RHEU. Cham. Sep—Damp sticky hands, Spig.

Swollen, Cal c. *Sabin*—After washing, Æs—
Swollen red, Sabin. Thuj.

Tetter on palms, Kreo. Nit a.

Thrilling, Cann I.

Tender joints, *Lith lac* 2x—See Gout. See
Joints.

Tingling thumb, Amb—Finger ends, *Aco.* Am.
m. Nat m. Thuj.

Trembling, AGAR. *Arg n.* Ars. MER. Nat m-
Kal p. Pho.

— While eating, Coc.

Ulcer on finger, Sep—ends, ARS—on back of
finger joints, Borax. Sep—gangrenous, Sec.

Wasting away, paralytic, PB.

Warts, Lyc. Thuj—on palms, Caust.

Weary hands, Mer Sars—when writing, Mez.

" Wrist drop " PB. 200. Nux v.

" Wrist puff," *Carb a 200.* Sil.

Leg, including Hip and Thigh:—

Hip-Disease—Coxalgia—Coxarthrocace;—

First stage, knee pain, limping, APIS. Bell.
Kal c. Rhus.

Second stage—Suppurating, Cal c. Cist. Hep.
Iod. Mer. Pho. *Sil.* Sul.

Left joint caries, STRAM.

Cham θ dilute, or Chamomile Tea, arrests sup-
puration, and there is no better tonic than
Cham tea. (See Clay. Carbol a—See Diet
—R.)

Sciatica:—APO C θ. Cini. Colo. GLON 2x. VIS
A. ZN v.

— Left side, Colo. Rhus. Stram—SUL 30,
Right Dios.

— Pains insupportable, CHAM—Especially at
night, *Aco. Ars.* Cham. PB—Come and go
suddenly, *Bell.* Colo.

— Burning, Ars.

— Formication, Lyc. Rhus.

— Numbness, Nux v. Rhus.

— Worse during the day, Colo—When lying quiet, Rhus—From motion, Bry. Colo.

— Senile, Sep 200. (See Chloroform. Hot water. Ichthyol. Sulphur—See Pain.)

Pains, Sensations and Conditions of Lower Limbs:—

In the bones. See Bone.

Aching, Rhus—More at night, Aur. *Mer. Pod* —Still, *Verat a.*

Bruised feeling, Apis. Arn. EUP PER. Chin. Cimi—In the Calf, Arg n. EUP PER. Pic ac.

Burning, Agar. Sang. Sul—In hollow of the knee, Bar c.

Coldness, Ars. iod. Am m. *Hep.* Helo h 200. Ox a—"Legs cold and heavy as lead," Pic a—Cold up to the knees, Carb v. Sil—Cold and Clammy, Cal c. Mer. Pic ac—Cold knees, Berb. Laur. Stan —Cold knees at night in bed, Carb v. Pho—Cold damp thighs at night, Cal c. Mer—Coldness and creeping like a mouse, Sil.

Cracking knee joints, Cal fl. Coc. Ig.

Creeping as of a mouse, Sep. Sil—As of ants in the calf, Sul—In the soles, Sep.

Cramp in the Calves, Cup m. Mag p. Lyc. Pod. Verat a.

—At night in bed, *Colo.* Rhus. Sep. Sul. VIBURN PRU θ 10 drop doses, during the day. "Sleep with garters on." Cramp during day, Pet—When dancing, Sul—Sitting, Rhus—Walking, Sul. (See Sulphur.)

Crooked by rheumatism, Caust. Grap. Guai. Lyc. Nat m.

Dropsy in the joints, Thuj—Knee dropsy,
Dig—"White Swelling" of the Knee, Apis.
Iod—"Knee Puff," Arn. in. and ex.

Elephantiasis : Canth—See Lepra.

Enlarged joints, Berb. Cal fl. Kal iod. Led.
See Gout.

Heaviness, ALU. Mer. Nux v. Rhus. Sep.
Sul—"Heavy as lead," Pic ac—Heavy and
weak, *Alu.* Apis. Chin.

" *House-maid's Knee,*" Slag.—See Seaton. Iodoform.

Humming, Buzzing, Ol.

Jerking, Cic. Stram—Of the gluteal muscles,
Agar.

" *Milk-Leg.*"—See Female—Child bed.

Motion, involuntary of leg or arm in brain
affections, Agar. Apo c. Bry. Hell—When
walking one foot shoots out, Stram—The
step is too high, Euphorb. Rhus—The foot
circles round, Cyc—Drags, Pho—The gait is
unsteady, Agar. ZN—Staggering in the
dark, Stram—Restlessness of the legs, Ars.
Apis. Ig. Rhus. Sul. *ZN.*

Numbness, Hyper. Lyc. Nux v. — Of the
thigh, Grap—After sitting, Aco. Rhus—
"Going to sleep," Amb. Diad. *Coc*—Numb
calf, Aco. *Sil*—Paralytic numbness, Coc.
Con. Tarant. ZN—In old age, Bar c. Con.

Pricking as of needles, Hyper. Nux v.

Shocks, Agar. Nux v. Sec.

Soreness from chafing between thighs, *Lyc.*
Sep. Sul. See Skin—Chafing.

Sprain-like pain, Led. Rhus—At the groin,
Am m. ZN.

Stiffness, Apis. Bry. Rhus—After sitting,
Rhus—From shortening of tendons, Colo—

Stiff calf, *Arg n*—Stiff knee, Bry. Rhus. Lyc. Sul.

Stitching pain in the joints, *Kal c.* Sil—On motion, *Bry*—In the thigh, Sil.

Swelling of the knee, inflammatory, Bry. LYC. Pul.Rhus.SUL 3x to 200 C—Red hot swelling, Aco. Ferr p. *Lyc.*—Tight, Bry—Dropsical, Apis. *Dig.* Iod. Sul.

Thrilling sensation in the knee, Cann I.

Trembling, *Alu.* Arg n. Con. Mer.

Weakness, ALU. Ars. Con. Mer. Rhus. Sil. Sul—Weariness, *Bry.* Cal c. Chin. COC—When sitting, Alu. Rhus.

Weak knees, Chin. COC—Giving out, Coc. Tab 200—More on descending stairs or hill, Stan—Must crawl, Pul — "Knock-knee," Arg m.

Feet, including Ankles :—

Aching heels, Cyc. Phyt.

Boring in the heels, Pul.

Bruised sore feeling in the *heels*, CYC. *Led.* Mang. Mur a—In ankles, as if sprained, LED. *Rhus.* RUTA. Kalmi. *Val.*

Bunion : Arnica in. and ex. Hyper. in. and ex. Soap plaster. Verat. ointment—See Ointment.

Burning feet, Cal c. Fl a. Pho. *Sul*—With cold hands, Sep—Soles burn, Æs. Amb. Cal c. *Canth. Cham. Cup m.* Ph a. Pul. *Sang.* Sil. SUL—Soles burn at night, Cham. *Canth.* SUL—Toe tips burn, SARS—Blisters on toes, Ars. Grap.

Chilblains : AGAR 2x. Abrotan. *Urtica.* ZINC OINT.

—Burning blisters, Ars. Rhus.

—Blue, Pho. *Pul.*

—Ulcerating, Hep. *Sil.* Sul.

(See Eucalyp. Glycerine. Lemon—See Ointment.)

Coldness, HEP. HELO H 200. LYC. *Mer. Pho.* Pic ac. Sep. SIL. Verat a—Preventing sleep, Am m—Cold and damp, CAL C. Hep. Helo. *Sil.* Sul—As if in cold water up to the knees, Mag c. Sep—Cold and numb, Ig—One foot cold, Lyc—Right foot cold, Sabin. (See Ice.)

Corns: ANT C.

—Inflamed, tender, *Sil.* LYC 30.

—Smarting, Ig. Sep.

Pare away the hard part, at bed time, and apply fresh slaked lime paste; or salt and tallow, well rubbed together. Saturate cloth with linseed oil and bind on every night. Soon cure. Ichthy Ex.

        (See Turpen. Vinegar.)

To remove the corn without pain. See Alcohol—See Anæsthesia—*local.*

Cramp, Am c. *Caust.* Pod. SUL—In soles at night, Agar—In toes, *Cal c.* Lyc—Toes spread out, Sec. (See Sulpur.)

Cracking ankles, *Cal fl.* Caust. Lyc. Nit a. *Pet.*

Crawling sensation, Æth. ZN—On the toes, Sul.

Enlarged joints, Arn—Big toe joint, Sabin. See Gout.

"Fidgety feet," APIS. ZN.

Hard soles, *Ant c.*

Heavy feeling, Nat m. Pic ac. Sec.

Light feeling, Stict. See Nerves.

Itching feet at night, Led—Soles itch, *Hydroct.*

Numbness, ALU. Ig. Pho—Numb and cold, Con—Numb when sitting, *Alu.* Plat—

.Numb heels, ALU—"Going to sleep," Coc. Nux v—Numb toes, Sec.

Offensive odor, Grap. Thuj in. and ex.,—As of old cheese, PB—Sour, Sil—(See Bism. Iron. Potash. Tann.) See Sweat offensive.

Paralytic lameness, Ol. Tarant c. ZN—When sitting, Rhus—Dragging the foot, Pho. PB —In the evening cannot walk because of a paralytic condition of the ankles, Cham.

Pricking sensation, Bry. *Cep.* Nit a.

Restlessness, Ars. APIS. Ph a. *Rhus.* Sul. ZN.

Stitches, Bry. Kal c.

Sweat—profuse, Pilo 1x—Cold and clammy, CAL C. Lyc. Sil—Sour, Thuj in. and ex. Kreo. Sep. *Sil*—Soles sore and raw, Cal c. Pet. Lyc. Nit a. *Sil.*

Sweat offensive—(See odor offensive), *Bar c.* Kreo. Nat m. Nit a Pet. Sep. SIL. Thuj in. and ex.

(See Alum. Bism Borax. Chloral. Chlorine. Iron. Potash.)

Swelling, *soft, puffy, Ferr. Helon, Nat m.* Sep —*Dropsical,* APIS. *Ars. China.* Dig. Kal c. *Nat s.* ZN—Inflammatory Bry. Lyc Pul. Rhus—See Rheumatism and Gout—Stiff, Lyc., *Apis.* Rhus—Tight, Bry—In the morning, Led—During the day, Bry.

Tearing in the joints at night, Colch.

Tender soles, hurt to stand, *Alu.* Ant c. *Led*— Tender heels, Am c. *Cyc.* Mang. *Mur a*— Tender joints, Arg n. See Gout. Tingling, Aco.

Trembling, Am c. Apis. *Mur.* Pul.

Ulcers, *Ars.* HYDROCT. Sep—On the soles, Ars—Toes, Ars. Grap. Pet. Sep—Gangre nous, Sec.

Weak ankles, *Carb a. Caust.* Cal p. Nat m.
SIL.—Giving way when walking, Carb a—
Foot turns under, Agn—Walking on edge of
foot, Cic.

Nails :—

Discolored, Thuj—Black, Ars. Thuj—Blue,
Chel Dig. Nux v—Yellow, Con. Sep.

Deformed, Cal c. Cal fl. Fl ac. *Graph*—Brittle,
Alu. Grap—Indented, Lyc. Thuj—Soft,
Thuj—Split, Ant c. Sil—Thick, Alu. GRAP.
Falling off, Hell. Grap Ustil.

Under the nails burning, Sars—Redness and
soreness under and around, Caust. Grap⁻
Nat s.

" Run round," Cal c. Cal fl. Fl ac.

" Hang nails," Nat m. Sul.

Ingrowing nail: Mag pol aust 200. Sil. Thuj.
" Tannic acid, concentrated solution, fresh, 1
ounce to 6 drachms of water, gently heat
and paint it upon the soft part twice a day.
Able to go about work at once with com-
fort, effectual cure "—(See IRON. Lead·
Potash.)

LIME.—*Pimple:* Lime water and Rose water,
equal parts.   Apply at bed time.

Piles: Lime water and Olive oil, equal parts.
Apply.

Burns and Scalds: Lime water and Linseed oil,
equal parts.   Apply.

Open Cancer—Bleeding at slightest touch: Dress
it with powdered quick lime.

*Bite of dog, or other animal—even mad dog
bite:* Slaked Lime, fresh, thick as mush; apply;
renew as often as it becomes *green.*

Skin poisoning—Ivy poisoning: Slaked Lime
paste, thick as cream; apply every half hour.

Congestion, Congestive Chill, Inflammation, Gout, Rheumatism, Neuralgia, Dropsy: Lime sweat. Take two lumps of fresh lime, half the size of a man's fist, and wrap each in a *moist* cloth, and this again with a dry one, well secured with cord. Place one on each side of the body of the patient while in bed. With sweat comes relief.

For *Dropsy* take sweat two or three times a week.

LIPS.—See Face.

LIPOMA.—See Ichthyol. See Seaton. See Tumor.

LITHEOSIS.—See Urinary Organs—gravel.

LIVER.—(See Fever—Bilious.)

Pains in general:—CARD *o.* *Chel.* HOMAR. *Mer. Nux v.* Phyt. *Pod.*

Burning, *Kal c.* LACH. Mag m. Mer. STAN.

Cramp, Ph a.

Cutting, Carb a. Lach.

Drawing, Bry. Con. Nat m.

Pressing, *Carb v.* Dig. Nux. *Sul a.*

Sore pain, Arn. *Carb v.* Lyc.

Sprain-like, Kal c. Lyc.

Stitches, Aco. *Bry.* CHIN. CARB V. Kal c. *Mer.* Nux v.

Tearing, Con.

Throbbing, *Nux v.* Sep.

Tenderness, Æs. CHIN. *Mer.* Nux v. *Eup per.* PHO.

Better by rubbing, Pod; or standing, Chel.

Worse by standing upright, Lyc; or turning, Rhus.

Ailments of the Liver—"Liver Complaint:"
Abscess: Hep. *Lach.* Lyc. Mer. *Sil.*

Atrophy: Pho. Phyt.

Biliousness: Bry. *Card θ.* Cham. EUP PER. *Euony.* HOMAR 3x. Ipe. Mer. MER PRO 2x. Nat s. Nux v. POD. (See Lemon.)

— Bilious vomiting especially, Bry. IPE. *Pod. Euony.* NAT S.

Cirrhosis: Aco. Ars. Pho.

Congestion or Inflammation. Hepatitis.—See Fever—bilious.

Enlargement:—Aur. Bursa p *θ.* CAL. C. CHIN. *Fl ac.* Homar. Lyc. MER PRO. NIT A. *Nux v.* PHO. POD. *Sep.* Sil. Sul—Painful swelling, Chel. Ptelea 2x. Belladon. plaster.

Fatty degeneration:—Pho. Phyt.

Heaviness, Lyc. *Nux m. Ph a.* Pod.

Induration:—CAL. C. CHIN. *Lyc.* MAG M. NIT A. Nux v. *Sil.*

Inflammation. Hepatitis:—See Fever—bilious.

Gall-stone, Lodged—Hepatic Colic:—CAL C 30 ¼ hour. IPE 6. Dios *θ* 60 drops. Olive oil, gill doses, ½ hour. Glycerine 6 drachms at one dose. Podo. purge 1 to 3 grains; followed in 6 hours by 3 ounces of Olive oil; and during interval until bowels moved, Chloroform by inhalation from time to time, to subdue pain. Euony 2 grains. Nux v—Cold sweat, Ars. (See Amyl. Chloroform. Ether. Hot Water. Turpentine—See Poultice.)

—*Preventive treatment, of gall stone:* Berb. Chel. Mer. Pod. CHINA 2x 5 grains daily for a week, then three times a week for a month, then once a week for three months. Chloroform 3 drops on sugar, 3 times a day for a month. Olive oil, 1 pint once a month. Glycerine 3 drachms, 3 times a week.

Jaundice:—

In general, CARD θ. Chion θ. *Homar* 3x.
Lept. Mag m. MER PROT. Nat s. (See Infant.)

—Black, *Ars.* ARS IOD. AUR. *Crotal.* Iod.
Pho—With stupor, Pho.

—Chronic, Aur. IOD. Lept. *Lyc.* Nat s. NIT A.
Pod. Sul.

—Malarial, Ars. CHIN. Iod.

—Of infants, Cham. CHIN. *Ipe.* MER. *Pod*
—With stupor, Pho. *Pod.*

—From gall stones, Cal c. Pod—See Preventive treatment of gall stone.

—*With* itching intense, *Card*—DOLI θ 5 drop
doses. Pilo 1x.

— —Clean tongue, CHEL. *Dig.*

—Green tongue, Nat s.

—Red tongue, Chel.

—Yellow tongue, Mer. MER PROT.

Sinking at the stomach and palpitation,
Hydras.

—Vomiting, Aco. *Ipe.* Saug. *Mer.*

—Diarrhœa, *Mer.* Pod—Stools white, Aco.
CHEL. *Mer. Pod*—Gray, DIG. Mer.

—Constipation, Lyc. NIT A. Nux v.

—Urine fetid, Nit a—Red, *Aco.* Mer. *Chel.*

LIVER SPOTS.—See Skin—spots.

LOCHIA.—See Female—Child bed.

LOCKJAW — TRISMUS — TETANUS.— *Aco.*
Arn. *Angus. Gel.* HYPER. 1x. *Nux v.* PASS θ
60 drops (See Ether—Hot Water—Onion.)

First, HYPER 1x.

Renewed by slightest touch, *Nux v*—By attempting to drink, Bell.

From fright, Aco. *Ig*—Injury to the head,
Cic—Wound of joint, Rhus.

Opisthotonos, *Aco. Ig.* Laur *Nux v*—With

LCCOMOTOR ATAXIA.

cold sweat on face, Aco—Stiff jaw from a cold. See Face—jaw.

LOCOMOTOR ATAXIA.—("Cannot walk backwards. Cannot walk in the dark or with eyes closed without staggering"), *Agar.* Arg n. Alu. Bell. Con *Helo h 200.* Pho. PHYSOS. ZN p. *Stram.* (See Sulphur.)

From a fall on the back, Hyper.

For the fidgets, ZN.

For the severe pain, Hyoscin hypoderm.

LOGWOOD.—*Fetid ulcer, Hospital gangrene, Open cancer, Erysipelas from amputation:* Logwood pulv. thick coat; or pomade of equal parts of Logwood pulv. and Lard, apply. It removes all fetor in a few hours.

LOINS.—See Urinary Organs—Kidney.

LUMBAGO.—See Back.

LUMBAR CARIES.— Bacill 200. Cal c. Sil. See Bone Caries.

LUMP. — See part affected. See Node. See Tumor.

LUNGS.—See Chest.

LUPUS.—See Face.

MAD DOG BITE.—See Hydrophobia.

MALARIA.—See Ague. See Contagion.

MALE.—

Balanitis—Balanorrhœa—Sore glans: Mer. Mez. *Nit a.* Sep. *Thuj.*

Blenorrhœa: See Gonorrhœa—*Gleet.*

Bubo: See Syphilis.

Chancre: See Syphilis.

Condylomata: Nit a. Pso. Sabin. THUJ.

Cracks in the glans, Ars. *Kal c*—Prepuce, Mer. Sul.

Dampness of glans, Mer. Nit a. *Thuj*—Scrotum, *Pet.* Sil. Sul. *Thuj*

Drawing up of the testicle—Retraction, PB. Pul. *Thuj.* ZN.

Eczema: Grap. *Hydrocl.* Skook—Scabs on the prepuce, Nit a. Thuj.

Fetid odor: Nat m. Sars. *Sul.*

Gangrene: ARS. Canth. Rhus.

Gonorrhœa: See Gonorrhœa in separate section.

Herpes: Dul. *Nat m. Pet.* Sep.

Hydrocele: *Chel.* Dig. Grap. Pul. RHOD 1x. Sil —Infant, Arn. in. and ex.—See cold water, Iodoform, Thuj.

Impotence: AGN. *Arg n.* Avena θ, 20 drops in water at bed time. Bacill 30-200. COCA. *Con.* "Damiana fl. ex. 3 drachms 3 times a day." Mer. SABAL S θ 10 drops, 12 hours. Sang. STAP θ 5 drops, 12 hours. Ustil 2x—No erections, Con. Kal iod—Penis cold and relaxed, *Gel.* Hep. *Lyc.* Sil. Sul—Cold scrotum, *Caps*— Spinal exhaustion, Nux v. *Stryc.*

Induration of testicles: *Agn.* Arg n. Aur. Cal fl. CLEM. CON. Iod. RHOD. Sil.

Inflammation of testicles. Orchitis: *Aco.* APIS. Bell. CLEM. Con. HAM. Mer. PUL. *Rhod.* *Spo.* Stap. (See Clay. Iodine. Kerosene. Mullein oil. Poultice.)

— Chronic, PB.

— Right especially, Apis. Aur. Bell. Clem. Urti.

—Left, Grap. Lach.

From contusion, Arn. Con. *Ham.* θ dilute in. and ex.

Onanism—Masturbation. Sexual excess: Avena θ 10 drops in water, 12 hours. Cal c. PH A. 1x. Plat. 30. Tarent. 200.

Paraphimosis:—Mer c. Introduce the loop ends of three or four hair pins underneath the constricting ring, at regular intervals, and over the bridge thus formed, the prepuce may be drawn down.

Phimosis:—*Cann I. Mer.* Nit a. *Sul.* THU—Reduce œdema by hot local bath, in mug.

Pollutions. Emissions, Seminal, in Sleep—Spermatorrhœa: Agn. Avena *θ* 10 drops in water at bed time. Bar c. China. Canth. *Dig* 3x. *Dios* ix. Gel. Kal bro pure, 5 to 20 gr. *Kal p.* Nux v. PH A ix. STAP *θ* 5 drop doses. Uran n. Urti. Ustil 2x. Thuj. ZN.

— First, STAP *θ*: or Dios ix.

— Very exhausting, *Alu.* China. Ph a ix.

— Without erections, Con. Gel.

— Prostatic fluid with urine, Sabal s ix. *Thuj.*

Priapism:—CANTH. *Nux v.* Nat m. PIC AC. Sil. *Plat.* Stap. (See Gonorrhœa.)

Prostate enlarged:—*Benz a.* Lith c. Mullein oil. Pul. SABAL S *θ* 10 drops 6 hours. Stigm. fl. ex. 20 drop dose. Thuj. *Pass. θ* full doses. (See Hot water. Iodoform. See Suppository. See Poultice.)

Prostatic fluid discharged, Cal c. CON. *Pet.* Ph a—During stool, Alu. *Hep. Sep.* Sil—While urinating, *Ana.* Cal c. Sep. *Thuj.*

Pruritus: CROTON. Grap. *Hydroct*—Itching glans, Sul.

atyriasis: Canth. Coca *θ.* 5 drop doses. Myo. *Nux v. Pho.* Stap.

Spermatorrhœa: See Pollutions.

Sweat on scrotum: Con. Daphne. *Hep.* Sep. SIL. *Thuj*—Cold sweat, Caps—Oily, Fl a.

Stricture. Clem. Lith c. *Sabal s θ.* Sil. Thuj. See Urinary Organs.

Ulcer: See Syphilis-- *Chancre.*

Veneral ailments:—See Gonorrhœa. See Syphilis.

Pains and sensations in genitals.

In general, Aur. Clem. Ham. Tereb. Urti. ZN.

Aching, Aur. Nux v. Thuj.

Bruise-like pain, ARN. CON. Clem. *Hom. Rhod.*

Burning, *Ars.* Amb. Mer. *Plat. Stap.*

Cramp-like squeezing, Graph. *Spo.*

Cutting in glans, Lyc—Penis, Oleum a—Testicles, Berb. Sep. Tereb.

Gnawing in testicles, Ph a. *Plat.*

Numbness, Amb.

Stinging in glans, Mer. Rhod—Penis, Mer. Mez. Thuj. *Vio t*—Prepuce, *Ars.* Euph. Pul —Scrotum, Mer. Sul. Thuj—Testicles, Arn. *Caust.* Rhod. Stap.

Stitching, Nit a. Sul.

Tearing in penis, Clem. Mez—Spermatic cord, Bell. *Colch.* Pul—Testicles, Euph. Pul. *Stap.*

MALFORMATION PREVENTIVE.—PHOS.

To mother during gestation.

MAMMÆ.—See Female—Breasts.

MANIA.—See Mind—*Insanity.*

MARASMUS.—See Atrophy.

MASTITIS.—See Female—Breasts.

MASTODYNIA.—Cimi. Con. Ham. Phyt.

MASTURBATION—ONANISM.—Cal c. PH A. *Plat.* TARENT C—Sad gloomy, Cal c. Chin. Stap—Irritable nervous, Nux v. (See Male.)

MEASLES—MORBILLI—RUBEOLA :—

In general, *Aco.* Gel. Pul.

Fever high, *Aco.* Bell. Gel.

MEDICATION BY INUNCTION.

Eyes bad, Euph. *Pul.*

Throat sore, Apis. Bell. Mer.

Croupy cough, Aco. Dros. KALI M. Pho.

Eruptions fade, Ars. *Bry.* Ip—Skin cold, *Camp θ*—Spasms threatening, Cup m. ZN. DREG: Cough, Eup per *Kali m.* Pul. STICT. Sul.

— Glands swollen, MER PROT. Sul.

— Dysentery, Mer c. Ipe. and Pet. See Cold Water. Lard.

MEDICATION BY INUNCTION.—See Glycerine.

MELANCHOLY.—See Mind.

MEMORY DEFECTIVE.—See Mind.

MENINGITIS.—See Fever—*Brain.*

MENORRHAGIA.—See Female—*Menses.*

MENSES.—See Female.

MENTAGRA.—(Chin scab), Cic. Kali m—See Face.

MERCURY—ILL EFFECTS.—Aur. Clem. Hep. Iod. Kal iod. Phyt. See Cause—drug.

MESENTERIC GLANDS AFFECTED.—Cal c. Iod. See Atrophy.

METEORISM.—See Abdomen—Bloat.

METRITIS.— See Female—Uterus—(*Inflammation*).

METRORRHAGIA. — See Female — *Uterus* — (*Hæmorrhage*).

MIASM.—See Contagion.

MICTURITION.—See Urinary Organs.

MIGRAIN.—See Head—Headache.

MILIARIA.—*Aco.* Ars. *Bry.* Led.

MILK.—See Female—Breasts.

MILK FEVER.

MILK FEVER.—See Female—Child bed (Fever).

MILK-LEG.—See Female—Child bed.

MILK CRUST.—See Head—Scalp (Favus).

MILK DISAGREES.—See Diet—G. H.   See
Stomach—Things that disagree.

MIND.—

Anguish, Aco. ARS. Cimi. Cup m. Kal iod.
MER. Stan. Verat a—"Horrid thoughts,"
Plat—Indescribable uneasiness, Mer. Stan.

Apprehension of misfortune, Aco. *Cal c.* Dig.

Confusion and stupidity, *Arg n.* BAP. GEL.
Lyc. NUX M. Ph a. Sil—Worse when constipated, Lyc.

Inability to think, *Arg n.* Bap. Gel. *Nux m.*
Lach. *Nat m.* Sil—To will, Pic ac. Sil—
Brain Fag, Kal p. ZN p—Cannot think, talk
or walk, Arg n.

Lost, well known places seem strange, Glo.

Slow speech, Ars. Mer. Pho. Sec. Thuj. ZN.

Stammering, Bovis. *Bell.* Mer. *Stram.*

Unconsciousness, Cann I. Bell. Hyo. Laur.
Ph a.

"Wild feeling," Lil t—"As if going crazy,"
Cimi. Plat.

Fear:—

Fear in general, ACO. Alu. ARS. *Camp.* Ig.
Pso. Xanth—Of death, ACO. Ars. Cal c.
Grap. Plat—Of insanity, Aco. Alu. CAL C.
Cimi. Lil t. MER.

— Frightened feeling, *Aco.* Ig. *Xanth*—In the
dark, Camp. Stram. Verat a—In a crowd,
Aco. Plat—When alone. *Ars. Lyc.* Pho—
Horror before rain, Elaps.

—Shrinking from presence of others, Amb.
Bar c. Cup m.

205

—"Stage fright"—Students fright, Ana. Copai.
GEL.

—Terror, *Aco.* Bell. Sec—"Night terror,"
Aco. Aur bro 3x. Sul—On waking, Stram.

Imbecility :—

In general, Æth Bell. HELL. Hyo. *Mer.*
Nux m. *Ph a*—From onanism, Plat 30.

— Idiocy—Cretinism, Bacill 30-200, one dose a
week. Bar c. Thuj.

—Undeveloped mind, *Bar c.* Cal p. Nux m.
Thuj.

— Memory undeveloped, Hell.

— Loss of decency, AM C—In epileptics, Ran
b.

— Weak mind—Look for adhesions of clitoris,
or prepuce, or constriction of urethra.

Insanity ("Dumb Thumb") :—

In general, Ars. *Atrop.* Aur bro 3x. Cann I 1x
3 gr. Hyo. Kali bro. pure, 20 gr. *Kal p.*
Laur. Lyc. *Nat m 2x. Stram.* Verat a—
"VERAT A and MELI alt."

— From bodily disease, ZN p—Hard study,
Cimi. Cup m. Nux v. ZN p—Strong drink,
Cimi. Nux v. ZN p.

Mania a potu: See Delirium.

Monomania: Cann I. Cic. Hyo. Stram—Re-
ligious, *Ars.* Hyo. Lach. Pul. *Sil.* Stram.
Verat a.

Nymphomania—Erotomania: CANTH. Camp.
COCA 1x 3 drops. Dul. HYO. PB. Pho. *Pic ac.*
Stram.

Puerperal mania: See Female — Child bed.
(Mania).

Sudden violent insanity: CANN I. 1x. 5 gr.
HYOSCIN. hypoderm. MELI 0. *Nat m 2x*
trit.

With intense congestion, face and hands dark
red, *Meli θ*. USTIL ɪx.

— Conduct boisterous, loud laughing at trifles,
Cann I. Hyo—Laughing at serious things,
Ana — Sardonic laughter, Ig — Lascivious,
Canth. Camp. Hyo—Biting, tearing, Bell.
Stram. VERAT A.

— Habit filthy, no sense of decency, *Am c 30*.
Diad.

— Language profane, *Ana*. Nit a—Unintelli-
gible, Solan n.

— Temper raging, Hyo. Stram. Verat a—Obstinate, unmanageable, Am c. Ars. Dig.
Nit a.

— Propensity to wander, Verat a.

Absence of mind :

In general, AGN. *Alu*. *Apis*. CANN I. Caust.
Nux m. Ol. Pul. Verat a.

— Lost in thought, Cann I.

— Letting things fall from the hand, Hell.

— Fixed thought, Ig.

Clairvoyance, Aco. Pho.

Swoon, Mos.

Trance, *Cann I*. Mos.

Loss of Memory:—

In general, AGN. Alu. ANA. CON. *Hell*.
Hyo. Lach. Lyc. MER. Nat m. Nux m. PB.
Pho. SUL. ZN p.

For dates, Fl ac.

For names, Lyc. Sil. Sul.

Using wrong words, Alu. Ana. Lyc. PB.

Cannot think of the right word, *Arg n*. Coc.
Dul. Kal bro. pure 20 gr. Lyc. *Sil*. Sul.
Thuj.

Saying one thing and meaning another,
Cann I.

Loss of speech and memory, Arg n. *Lach.*

"Forgets how to talk," Kal bro. pure 20 gr.

Inability to sustain any mental effort, CON. Pic ac. *Ph a.* Sep.

Disposition :—

Changeable, *Aco.* Alu. *Ig.* Nux m. Plat. ZN.

Contemptuous to self, Agn—Toward others, Ars Lach. PLAT.

Despairing of recovery, Ars Cal c. Grap. Pso.

Domineering, *Lyc.* Plat. Sul.

Ecstatic, Lach. Op.

Grieving, Ig. Ph a—About trifles, Grap—Sighing, Bry. *Ig.*

Happy, cheerful, *Cann I.* CRO. Hyo. Lach. *Spo.* SUL.

Haughty, *Lyc.* PLAT. Lach. Stram. *Verat a.*

Hypochondriac, Aur. Con. NUX V. PB. Pul. Verat a.

Impatient, *Aco*—Vehement, Nat m.

Indignant, Colo. *Stap.*

Indifferent, Am m. *Arn.* Ig. *Pho. Ph a.* Pul. *Sep.*

Irritable (See Infant), Borax *Bry.* CHAM. Cimi. *Kal p.* NUX V. *Nat m.* Pho—Easily vexed, Grap. Nat m. Sep—Cannot endure contradiction, Aur. Mer—Scolding, Pet. *Mos.*

Irresolute, Aur. IG. Nux m. Lach. Pet. *Sil.*

Jealous, APIS. Camp. Hyo. LACH.

Jolly, Cro. Spo

Lascivious, Cann I. CANTH. Cal c. *Cro. Hyo.* LACH. *Pho.* Stap. Verat a—Shameless, *Hyo.* Stram. Verat a.

Loquacious, Bell. Lach. Stram.

Morose, sullen, Cimi. *Nux v.* Viol t.

Murderous, Ars. Mer. *Nux v.* Hyo. Lach.

Petulant, Colo. Spo. Stap.

Peevish (See Infant), Alu. Aur. *Cina*. KAL P. Nit a. PUL. SUL. Stap—Resents a touch (adult), Kal p. Thuj.

Retiring—wanting to be alone, Bar c. Carb a. Cimi. *Nux v*—Avoids society yet feels lonely, Con.

Sad, gloomy, ARS. Ana. Arg n. AUR. *Am bro* 3x. *Cardu*. HELON. Kal p. Lyc. NAT M. Nux v. *Pul*. Plat. Stan. Thuj—Sad and irritable, Ars. *Aur*. CIMI. Kal iod. Kreo. Thuj.

Suicidal gloom, AUR. Ig. Lach. Grap. *Nux v*.

Suspicious, Aco. Ars BAR C. *Cic*. Hyo. LACH. Lyc. Pul.

Taciturn, Carb a. *Con. Ph a*.

Tearful, Iod. Kal p. PUL. *Lil t*. Sep—Sobbing, Hell. Lob i—Whole nights in tears, Indig 2x—Music causes weeping, Thuj.

" Touchy," Asa. Plat. Stap.

Uncivil, Cham.

Propensity to:—

Groan or moan, *Bell*. Chim. Cic. CHAM. IG. ZN.

Hurry, Amb. *Arg n*. Ars. LIL T. *Sul a*.

Hurry others, *Aco*. Alu. *Arg n*. Cann I. *Nux m*.

Speak hurriedly, Ars. Bell. *Hep*. Hyo. LACH. MER. Stram.

Scream, Bell. Cham. *Cina*. IG. Sil.

Scold, Dul. *Mos*.

Swear, ANA. Cann I. *Lil t*. NIT A. Verat a.

Touch everything, Bell.

Try to touch inaccessible things, Sul. Thuj.

Toy with pins or needles, Sil—Break them, Bell.

Vulgarize, Nit a.

Imagination of being :—

G*　　　　　　　209

Away from home, Bry. Bell. Op.—In a strange
    land, Bry. Plat. Verat a.

Brittle, friable, Thuj.

Dead, Apis. Lach—Dying, Mos.

Double, Ana. Mos—In two places, Lyc—Soul
    and body separated, Ana. Cann I. Thuj—
    Having two contending wills, Ana.

In pieces scattered about, Bap.

In three pieces, Ars.

In bed with another person, Pet.

Made of wood, Rhus—Of glass, Thuj.

Obsessed, Ana. Lach.

Poisoned, Hyo.

Pursued, Ana.

Not one's self, Alu.

Taller, Stram.

Imagination of hearing :—

Bells or music, Cann I.

Reiterating chorus, Lyc.

Voices, Ana Cham—Quarreling, Naj.

Imagination of Seeing :—

Bugs, spiders, or bats, Op—Mice, Cal c.

Faces, Chin. Cup a.

Images, Amb. Arg n.—On closing the eyes,
    Cal c. Cimi. Hyper.

Skeletons, Op.

Sharp points directed to the eye, Sil.

Living creatures rising up from the corners of
    the room, Pho—Jumping things, Stram—
. Prowling wolves, Bell.

Things diminished in size, shorter, Camp.
    Carb v. Nit a. *Plat*—Narrower, *Plat.*

Things increased in size—longer, taller, Camp.
    Dros. Nit a.

Delirium :—

In general, AGAR 1x trit, 1 gr. Am c. Ars. *Bell.* Carbol a. Hyo. Stram. *Pass θ.*

Nightly, Aco. Bell.

Furious, Bell. Hyo. Stram. PB.

Showing great strength, Agar.

Tearing things, Verat a.

Barking, Bell. Canth.

Biting, Bell. Canth. Stram. Verat a.

Chewing, Bell. Hell.

Spitting, Bell. Cann I. Cup m.

Muttering, Arn. *Ars.* Apis. *Bap. Lach* Mur a. Pho. Ph a. *Rhus.* Tarent. Tereb. *Pass θ.*

Picking at bed clothes or grasping at flocks, Ars. Hyo. Op. Pho. *Pass θ.*

Uncovering, immodest, Canth. *Hyo.* Verat a.

Talking constant, Bell. Cimi. Hyo. *Lach.* Stram—About going home, *Bry.* Bell. Op.

Speech hurried, Hyo. Lach. Mer. Stram. Verat a.

Slow speech, PB. Ph a. ZN—Falling asleep while answering, Bap.

Lost of speech and memory, Lach.

Wholly unconscious, Ail. Apis. Arn. *Bell.* Cic. Gell. Hell. *Hyo.* Mur a. OP. Pho. PH A. Rhus. Stram.

Delirium Tremens :—CANN I 1x trit, 2 gr, ½ hour. "HEMP EXTRACT, ¼ or ½ gr. pill 3 hours, until effective, then 12 hours as long as needful." Cimi *θ.* Gel *θ* 3 drops, ¼ hour. Hyo. NUX V 1x. STRYCH 2x, 1 gr, ½ hour. PASSIF *θ* 60 drops, ½ hour. "Jamaica dogwood fl. ex. 60 drops ½ hour." Sumbul. *Beef tea* red hot with cayenne peper, frequent copious draughts.

Cold sweat, Camp. *Hyo*—Profuse, Tart e.

MISCARRIAGE.

Delirium, furious, Bell. *Hyo.* Stram—Loquacious, Hyo. Lach—Muttering, Hyo—With frothing mouth, Camp. Hyo—Grinding teeth, Stram.

Difficult deglutition, Bell. Lach.

Prostration extreme, Ars. Camp.

Profound stupor, Op.

Tremor, Ars. Hyo. *Nux v.*

Retention of urine, Camp.

Guard against Delirium Tremens, Apo c *θ*. See Alcoholism. (See Coffee—Cold water, Musk.)

To control patient in Cases of Violent Mania:—"Place your left hand behind patient's head, and your right upon the front of the throat, with thumb upon the upper rings of the trachea and make a sudden firm, but momentary pressure. The result will be unconsciousness to the patient for a while."

Forced Feeding:—Firmly close patient's nostrils with your thumb and finger; must open mouth to breathe; pour the liquid food into the mouth; cannot resist swallowing it.

Colored Glass Cure:—

For violent mania, *blue* glass room.

For melancholy, *red* glass room

MISCARRIAGE.—See Female—Pregnancy.

MOLE.—See Skin.

MONOMANIA.—See Mind.

MORNING SICKNESS.— See Female -Pregnancy.

MORPHIA POISONING.—See Antidote.

MORPHINE HABIT.—Avena 30 drops in water morning and evening. Passif *θ* 60 drops at bed time. "Take the opium in the usual quantity, with Gamboge added, 1 part to 3. Disgust soon follows and no after hankering. Cure effectual."

MOTH PATCH.—See Face.

MOTION INVOLUNTARY.—See Limb or part affected.

MOUTH, CAVITY INCLUDING PALATE:—

Foul breath (See Charcoal, Chlorine, Potash): Ana. Ars. Fl ac. *Kal p. Kreo.* MER. Mur a. *Nit a.* Pet. Phyt. Pod—As from spoiled egg, Arn—Old cheese, Aur—Musty, Alu. Kal bi. Led—Sour, Cham. Mag c. Sul—Urinous, Grap. — From ulcerated gums—Stomacace: Caps. Carb v. Dul. Mer. Nux v.

Salivation:—"The Alkalies" IRIS V. MER. *Pilo.* Kali iod. *Sang n* 2x. TAB. Tereb. Trif p. —very offensive, MER. Nit a— Sickening, Colch. *Ipe.* Iris v.

From abuse of Mercury, Hep. Iod. Nit a.

Saliva acrid, Arum. Mer. Nit a.
— Bitter, *Ars.* Sul. *Thuj.* See Taste.
— Bloody, Kal iod. Mag c. MER. Nat m. NIT A. *Nux v.* Sul.
— Clammy, Pul. Phyt—in the morning, Bell.
— Cool, Asa. Cist.
— Frothy, *Canth.* Bry. *Dig.* PB—"Like cotton," Coc. Nux m. *Pul*—Green froth, Sec— Red froth, Bell.
— Glairy dribble, Stram
— Oily, Cubeb.
— Ropy, Carb v. *Hydros. Kal bi.*
— Sickening, Colch. *Ipe.* Iris v.
— Salty, Sul—See Taste.
— Sour, Cal c. Ig—See Taste.
— Soapy, Bry.
— Sweetish, *Dig.* PB. *Pul.* Sabin.—See Taste.

— Yellow, Gel. *Kal bi.* Rhus—When sleeping pillow wet with saliva, Mer—Staining yellow, Nit a.

Sore mouth — Ulcerated:—BORAX. Sinap. HYDRAS θ dilute in. and ex. *Hydrocl.* KAL BI. Kal iod. Kal m. Lach. *Mer.* MER PROT. Nat m. Nit a. Nux v. Ph a. *Phyt. Sang n. 3x. Sul a.* (See Alcohol. Alum. *Bism. Borax.* Chlorine. Cold water. *Hydras.* Iodine. Sugar. *Myrrh.*)

Baby's sore mouth:—Any of the remedies for sore mouth, but especially *Borax. Hydras.* Kal bi. See Infant. (See Alcohol. *Borax. Bism.* Cold water. *Hydrs.* Sugar.)

Nurse's Sore Mouth: Any of the remedies for sore mouth, especially the acids. Mur a. Nit a. Ph a. Sul a. (See Alum. Hydras. Myrrh.) "Argent nit, 6 gr. put in water 1 pint, and with this wash and gargle, 5 or 6 times a day. No need to wean the baby."

Syphilitic sore mouth, Kal iod. Mer. Nit a. *Phyt.* Pod.

Pain, Sensation and Condition of Mouth and Palate:—

Bleeding, Borax. *Ph a.* Nit a. Sul a. *Arum*—Bleeding sore corners of mouth, *Ant c. Arum.* Grap. Mer. Rhus.

Blisters, *Caps. Hell.* Rhod. RHUS. Phos. SUL. Stap.

Burning, ARS. ARUM. *Canth. Caps.* MEZ. Tereb. Verat a—Burning and dry, Borax. Mos—Burning and raw, *Arum.* Pho—Palate, Lach. Ran b. Sil.

Dryness, ALU. *Ars. Ig.* Lyc. NAT M. PILO 1x. Sil—In the morning on waking, Grap. NUX M. Pul. Sul—Too dry to swallow, *Bell.*

Lach. Lyc—Palate, *Cal c. Carb v.* Hell.
Stram.

Gangrene, *Ars.* Lach. Sec. Sul a.

Heat, Cham. Carb v. Nat m—Palate, Camp.
Dul.

Inflammation, *Aco.* Bell. Mer—Palate, Cal c.
Lach. Mer.

Pimples, Dulc—On palate, Pho.

Relaxation of membrane. *Biting cheek when
chewing*, Caust. Ig. Pet. Ph a.

Relaxation of palate—Elongated uvula, *Brom.
Cal c. Iod.* LACH. Lyc. MER C. Sil. Sul—
Uvula bloated like a sac, Bap. *Kal bi. Rhus.*
(See *Alum. Mustard.* Tannin.)

Color of Mouth Cavity:—

Blue, Mer—Spots, PB.

Pale, Nit a—White, Kal iod.

Red, See Inflamed—Glossy red, Apis—Raw
red, Arum.

Yellow, Gel. Kal b. Rhus—Yellow spots, Lach.
Lyc. Nit a.

Tongue—Pain. Sensation. Condition:—

Aphthæ, Ars. *Borax.* Mer. Nux v. *Sul a.*

Atrophy, Mur a.

Biting tongue when chewing or talking, Caust.
Ig. Pet. Ph a. Lach.

Blister, Am m. APIS. Ars. HELL. *Grap.*
NAT M. Nit a. Thuj. *ZN*—At the tip,
Canth. LACH—Edge, Grap.

Burning, *Ars.* CAUST. *Lach. Mer c.* PH A.
Sul—At the tip, Cyc. *Kal c.* Teucr.

Crack, fissure, *Ail. Apis.* ARS. BELL.
CONDU. FL AC. Lyc. *Rhus. Spig.* SUL.
Verat a—Lip, Lach.

Coldness, *Bell.* CARB V. Camp. VERAT A—
Tip, Colch. *Cup m.*

Dryness, ACO. ARS. Arg n. *Ail.* Dul. Lyc. MUR A. NUX M. PILO ix. RHUS. Sul. Verat a. *All the fever remedies.*

—On waking in the morning, NUX M. Pul. Rhus. Sul—Seems dry when not so, Nat m.

Gangrene, *Ars.* Lach. Sec. *Sul a.*

Heaviness, *Bell.* Lach. Mur a. PB—with slow speech, *Carb v.* Lach.

Indentation by the teeth, Ars. MER. Mer prot. Pod.

Induration Aur. *Bar c.* Mer. *Sil. Semper t.* 3x in. and ex.

Inflammation, ACO. *Apis.* BELL. Lach. *Mer.* Ox a.

Itching, Alu. Sul.

Large broad flabby tongue, HYDRAS. Kreo. Mer. Pod.

Moving out and in, Cup a. *Hell.* Lyc. *Sul*— Darting out, Lyc. Sul—*Protruding*, Lach— Hanging out, Lyc. Stram.

Numbness, *Aco.* Agar. Amb. COLCH. *Gel.* NAT M. NUX M.

Pain at the root when swallowing, Phyt.

Papillæ prominent, Arg n.

Paralysis, lameness, *Bell.* CAUST. Coc. *Diad.* Dul. Gel. LACH. PB. *Nux m.*

Peeling, Ran s—In patches, Tarax.

Pimples, Lyc. Mur a. Nux v.

Ranula: Amb. *Cal c. Mer.* Mez. Nit a—Blue, *Thuj.*

Sensation, as if scalded, *Iris v.* Mer. *Phyto.* Pod. Sep—Elongated, Æth—Hairy, Therid—As if a hair lying on it, Kal bi. Nat m. Sil—Or loose skin, Rhus.

Soreness, Lach. *Mer. Nux v. Sil.* Tarax—Tip,

Rhus. Sep. Thuj—Rawness, *Arum*. Gel.
Kal bi. Rhus—Left side, Jac.

Stiffness, Hell. Lach. Rhus.

Stinging, *Aco. Nit a*. Tarax.

Stitching, Kalmi.

Swelling, APIS. ARS. *Bell*. DUL. LACH.
MER.

Tingling, Aco. Sec. ZN.

Trembling, *Agar*. Apis. Bell. Gel. Hell. LACH
Lyc. Mer—And pointed, Cimi.

Ulceration, Arg n. *Canth. Hydroct*. MER.
Nit a. Semper t, 3x, in. and ex—Under the
tongue, Agar. Sep—Edge of tongue, Phyt.
Withered tongue, Kreo.

Color of the tongue:

Black, ARS. *Carb v. Chin*. Canth. LACH.
Mer. Pho. Verat v.

Blue, Ars. Dig — Bluish white coating,
Gymnoclad 2x.

Brown, ARS. BAP. *Bell. Bry*. Crotal. *Kal p*.
Lach. RHUS. *Sil*—In the middle, *Bap*. Kal
bi. Pyrogen.

Green, Mag c. NAT S. *Nit a. PB*. Rhus.

Red, "The Acids." APIS. ARS. BELL. Hyo.
Kal bi. Lach. Mer. Pod. Rhus. Tart e—Beet
red, Arum—Red row, ARUM. Kal bi. Rhus—
Scarlet red, Crotal—Shining red, *Lach*. Nux
v. *Tereb*--Red in streaks, Tart e—Red middle,
Arg n. Ars. Tart e. Verat a—Red edges, *Ars.
Bell*. Cina. *Rhus*. Verat a—Red tip, Arg n.
Apis. Ars. Phyt. Verat a—"Triangular red
tip," RHUS—Red spots, Mer. *Tarax*.

White, "The Alkalies." ANT C. *Bry. Bism*.
CARBOL A. China. *Dig. Kali m*. Mer. NUX
V. Pet. PUL—Slimy white, Cardu θ. Chel.
Kali m. Pul—"Mapped," Nat m.

Yellow, Chin. CHEL. Colo. Bry. Kal bi. *Lept.*
MER. MER PROT. *Nux v.* Verat a—
Slimy yellow, Hydras. KAL S. Pul—Yellow
at the root, Kal bi. MER PROT. Nux v—In
the middle, Bap. Verat v.

Taste :—

Lost, *Alu.* IRIS V. Lyc. *Nat m.* PUL. Sil—
Taste of food, as of wood, Ars; or straw,
Stram.

Bitter, CARDU *θ.* Cham. CHEL. NAT S.
Nux v. Pul. Sul —In the morning, Cal c.
Nux v—Everything tastes bitter, Aco. *Bry.*
Colo—Persistent bitterness in the fauces, ZN.

Bloody, *Ipe. Nux v.* Lil t—In the morning,
Sil.

Chalky, Nux m.

Cheesy, Æth. Pho.

Coppery, metallic, Bis. COC. CUP M *Kal bi.*
Nat m. Nux v. Phyt. RHUS. Sul. ZN.

Foul, Fl ac. *Kal p*—From catarrh, LEMNA.
Pet. Pul. Sul—When hawking, Nux v—Like
spoiled egg, *Arn.* Grap. Sil—In the morning, Ana. Nat m. NUX V. PUL. Sul.

Greasy, Asa. Caust. Pul. Val. See oily.

Inky or irony, Alo.

Musty, Kali bi. Led.

Oily, Æs. Cubeb.

Onion-like, Æth.

Salty, Carb v. Chin. Cyc. IOD. *Mer. Pho. Pul.
Sep.* ZN.

Soapy, Iod.

Sour, *Cal c.* Ig. Kal c. *Lyc.* NAT P. Nat m.
Nux v. Sul—In the morning, Nux v.

Sweet, *Alu.* Dig. *Mer.* Nit a. PB. Pho *Pul.*
Sul. *Stan.*

ARS. Crotal. NAT M.

Thirst:—

Constant, intense, Aco. ARS. Crotal. NAT M.
Sec. Stram—For cold drinks, Pho. Verat a—
Yet tongue moist, Mer—Constant sipping
small drinks, ARS. Apis Chin.

Craving drink, but dread of strangling, Canth.
Cann I.

Greedy drinking, Hell—Nervous haste, Ig—
But must stop between sips to take breath,
Ana. Nitr—Sight or thought of water sickens
the stomach, Ham. Pho.

Night thirst, Ant c.

No thirst, though mouth dry, *Apis.* Hell.
Pul. Nux m. Tart e.

Gums:—

Gum-Boil: Bell. Cal fl. HEC L. Hep. Mer. *Sil.*
— Hard, Cal fl. Hec l. Sil.

Aching gums, Arn. Stap.

Bleeding (*scorbutic*), *Am c. Carb a.* CARB V.
Kal p. Kreo. Lach. MER. Nit a. *Pho.* Ph a.
Sep—Black blood, Ars. *Grap.* Kal p. *Kreo.*
See Myrrh.

Blistered, Bell. Mez. *Nat m.*

Burning, Bell. *Caps.* Lach, *Mez.*

Blue, Con. *Ol.* Sabi—Blue line, PB.

Cracked, Plat.

Fistula: CAL FL. Caust. FL AC. Nat m. *Sil.*

Foul, putrid, *Grap.* Hep. *Kal p.* Kali m. Kreo.
MER. *Mer prol.* Nat m. Nux v.

Loose—retracted, *Carb a.* Kal iod. Mer. *Pet.*

Sore, Mer. Nit a. Sil—Raw, Lach. Sep—Pain-
fully sensitive when chewing, Cal c. Carb v
—Sensitive to cold water, Sil.

Spongy, *Carb v.* Kreo. Lach. Mer. Nit a.

Throbbing, Cal c. Sul.

Unhealthy—ulcerated: *Cal c.* Kal iod. Kali m.

Mer Stap (See Alum. Iodine. Myrrh. Potash. Vinegar.)

White, *Acet a. Carb a. Ferr.* Mer. Nit a. *Stap.*

Teeth :—

Black, Mer. Stap—Black crust, Chin. Con.

Covered with *sordes*, Ail. *Ars.* BAP. Hyo. Mur a. RHUS Stram—Black sordes, Chin. Con— Brown, Sul a—Yellow, Iod. PB—Putrid, Mez.

Decayed, Ant c. Kreo. Mer—At the root, Mez. Thuj.

— At the crown, Cal p. Fl ac—Notched, Lach. PB.

— Enamel rough, Cal fl—Syphilitic decay, Fl ac.

Loose, Alu. Am c. Cal fl. Caust. Carb v. Mer. Nit a. ZN—with salivation, Mer. Sang.

Sensitive—tender, Ant c. Fl a. Kal mi. *Lyc. Mer.* Nat m. *Plantago*—To cold air, Cal c. Sil.

Sensation of being cold, Ph a. Sep—Loose, Alu. Am c. Caust 2x—Too long, Alu. Caust. Mer. *Mez.* Plant. Rhus—Numb, Chin. Ig. Plat— "On edge," Mer—Itching, Kal c. ZN—Smooth, Carb a. Pho. Selen—Soft, *Alu. Caust. Ig. Lyc. Nux m.*

Tartar on teeth, Sil. Sul. See Iodine. Vinegar,

Teething: Kreo. Pod. SCUT—Head trouble, Bell. MAG P. Pod—Delayed, Cal p. See Infant.

Toothache: (See *Aconite.* Benzo.)

In general, GLO 2x. KREO and MER. PLANT in. and ex.

Pains boring, Sil. Sul — Throbbing, Glo— Furious, PIP M θ 10 drops.

Causing anger, *Cham.* Nux v—Cold sweat, Verat a—Swelling of the cheek, Cham. Lyc.

Involving the ear, Lach. Mer. *Plant.* Pip m *θ*
—The eye, Caust.

Better by cold drink, Bry—Warm drink, Lyc.
Nux v. Sul—Pressing teeth together, Ars.
Chin. *Coff*—Rubbing the teeth, Mer—Sucking
the teeth, Clem—Sucking in cold air, Pul.

Worse at night, Cal c. Grap. *Mer*—Before a
storm, Rhod—In cold air, Cal c. Hyo. Nux v
—In open air, Con. Nux v—When eating,
Kal c. Nat c. ZN—After eating, Cham. Kal c.

Renewed by cold food or drink, Cal c. Carb v.
Cham—Warm food, Cham. Coff. Nux v. *Pul.*
Toothache in " plugged teeth," Am c. Cic.
Saturate a pledget of cotton with Passiflora
tincture and insert it in the cavity, if any, or
pack it round the tooth. See Benzo.

MUCOUS DISCHARGES.—

Acrid. Kreo. Sul.
Green, Kal iod Nat s. Stann.
Ropy, Hydras Kal bi.
Watery, Alu. Ars. *Nat m.*
Yellow, Kal p, Kal s. Lyc.

MULLEIN OIL.—*Pain, Swelling, Inflammation, Piles, Sore Eyes, Earache, Deafness, Orchitis:* Mullein Oil pure, or diluted with a little water. Apply as the case may require.

MUMPS—PAROTITIS:—

In general, Aco. *Bell.* Con. PILO ix. *Rhus.*
Kali m. MER PROT 2x.
Shifting to brain, Bell.
—To female breast, Pul. Belladon ointment.
—To testicles, Phyt in and ex. Belladon ointment. See CAMPHOR.

MUSK.—*Exhaustion of vital power, Giving out of nerve centres, Extreme degree of cold or heat,*

MUSTARD.

Sudden collapse—Death-door condition in typhoid fever, Adynamic pyæmia—Delirium tremens:—"Musk, by rectal injection, for adult 10 grains, with Laudanum 20 drops, suspended in an ounce of Mucilage of acacia, effects marvelous results. In hyperpyrexia it reduces temperature 3 degrees in 20 minutes. In no case repeat the injection until emergency demands it."

MUSTARD.—*Congestive headache:*—Induce nosebleed by inserting into the nostril a small roll of mustard paper, and leaving it *in situ* for a few minutes. When the nose bleeds the headache ceases.

Headache in fever or diphtheria:—Mustardwater foot bath; hot as can be borne.

Relaxed throat—" palate down "—Cough caused by elongated uvula : Mustard seed tea gargle.

Cold in the chest and cough :—Mustard plaster to the breast—Mustard mixed with flour and vinegar, or white of egg, or molasses.

Sore throat, Quinsy:—Saturate bread with vinegar, and sprinkle it with mustard flour and apply to the throat.

Nausea and vomiting :—Mustard plaster to the stomach.

MYALGIA.—Cimi. Gel. Stict. (See Chloroform.)
—Pain as if bruised, *Arn.* Bap. CIMI. *Eup per.* Phyt. Rhus—From violent exertion, Rhus. SUL 200. Arnica oil ex.
—Sore all over, *Arn.* Bap.
Lameness in groups of muscles, *Gel.* Arnica oil ex.

MYELITIS.—Agar. Ars. Bell. Ox a. PB. Physos. Sec. See Fever—Brain and Spotted.

MYOPIA.—Physos. See Eye—Sight.

MYRRH.—*Sore Mouth, Diseased Gums, Ulcerated Thoat:* Into a 4-ounce bottle put three drachms of Tincture of Myrrh, and fill the bottle with water; gargle therewith several times a day, holding it in the month each time a short while, also swallow some.

NÆVUS—BIRTH-MARK.—Thuj, in. and ex. "Insert into the nævus the point of a needle immediately after having dipped it into pure Nitric acid. This will effect its removal, leaving but little scar." (See Collodion. Lead. Vinegar.)

NAILS.—See Limb—(Last notation).

NAIL, INGROWING.—See Limb—Nail.

NAPHTHALIN.—*Itch, Ichthyosis, Eczema, Psoriasis, Prurigo, Ulcer:* Naphthalin 1 part to 10 parts Vaseline. Apply.

NARCOTIC POISONING.—See Antidote.

NAUSEA.—See Stomach. See Diet C. See Ice. Mustard.
> — In the throat, Cyc. *Phyt.* Stan.
> — After surgical operation, Glo — *Vinegar dilute.*

NECK.—
> **Pain in general:**—Bell. Bry. Cal p. CIMI. Guai θ. Dul—From slight draught, Cal p—Terrible pain in spine of the neck, Stram.
> Aching, Bar c.
> Boring, Coc. Thuj.
> Bruise-like, Croton. Sabin—Nape, *Agar.* Nux v. ZN.
> Burning, *Caust.* Cal c. Ig. *Mer*—Nape, *Ig.* Lach.
> Cramp, Iod. *Plat. ZN*—Nape, Arn. Sil. Thuj.
> Drawing in the nape, Lyc. Nux v. Sul.
> Jerking pain, Caps. Ph a. *Sep.*

Pressing, *Lach. Ol.* Spong. Sep—Nape, Ana. Laur. Nat m.

Shooting, Bar c.

Sprain-like, Sars—Nape, Agar. Sul—Easily sprained, Cal c.

Stitches, Alu. Nat m. Sul.

Tearing, Nux v. Lyc. Sul—Nape, ACO.

Conditions and Sensations of Neck :—

Boil, Nat m. Sep. Sil.

Bloat, Con—See Swelling.

" Crick " : From sudden chill, Aco—Drench in rain, Rhus—With sore throat, Bell— Worse by motion, Bry—Better by motion, Rhus.

Coldness, Sil.

Creeping, Spo.

Emaciation, NAT M. See Infant.

Eruption, Lyc. Pet. Sil.

Glands: Inflamed, Bell. Rhus—Enlarged, BAR C. Cal c. Cist—Back of the neck, Rhus—Nape, Sil—Suppurating, CIST. Hep. Sil. Sul. See Gland.

Goitre : Cal c. *Fl ac.* IOD. Nat p. SPO—Exophthalmic, Naj. Thuj in. and ex. See *Iodine* —With suffocative attacks at night, Spo— Small, hard goitre, Cal fl.

Greasiness, Apis. Lyc. *Thuj.*

Heaviness, weight, *Paris.* Rhus—Nape, Caps. Pet. *Pho.*

Heat, Sil—Nape, Ig. Lach.

Itching, Alu. NAT M. Rhus. *Sep.* Thuj.

Lameness, Spig.

Lumps, Nodes, Ig. *Lach.* Lyc—Nape, Caust, ZN.

Numbness, Dig. PLAT. Spig.

Palsy, Lyc.

Pimples, Lyc. Nat m. Pet. Sep. Sil.

Sensitiveness, Lach. See Tenderness.

Spasm, Fl ac.

Spots, Carb v—Livid, Lyc.

Stiffness, *Bell.* Bry. CHEL. Cimi. *Dul. Ferr p.* Lyc. Pho. RHUS. SIL—In the morning, ZN—From draught of cold air, Cal p—In cool, damp weather, *Dul*—With headache, Sil—With stiff jaw, Dul. Kreo. " Aco and Bell alt."

Swelling, BAR C. *Con.* Iod. Pho—Inflammatory, Apis. Bell. Lach. Rhus—Hard swelling on one side, Lyc—Neck and jaw swollen on one side, Thuj.

Throbbing carotids, BELL. *Glo.* Hyo.

Tenderness, *Apis.* Bell. LACH — Of neck, spine, CHIN S. Stram—Lowermost vertebra, Con. Sil.

Tightness, Tension, Con. Sul. Thuj.

Tumor, Bar c. Grap. Sil—Fatty, Bar c.

Twisted neck, Ars. Caust. Hyo.

Ulcers, Lach—Sores or scars from gatherings, CIST.

Wasted—"Scrawny neck," Cal p. NAT M. Sec.

Weak neck, Chel. Lyc. VERAT A. Plat. Sul—Weak nape, *Plat.* Nit a. Sil—So weak that the head trembles, *Coc.* Mer—Head falls forward, Cup m.; or to one side, Cal p.

" Weary neck," ZN.

" Wry neck," Lyc—See stiff—See Twisted.

NECROSIS.—See Bone.

NEPHRITIS.—See Urinary Organs.

NERVE.—(See Mind).

Nervousness (See Coffee. See Diet S.), Amb. *Asa. Aur bro.* Avena θ. *Camp bro.* Cic. Coc.

NERVE.

Coff. *Ig.* Kal p. "*Kola tablets.*" Mag p.
Meli θ. *Mos.* NUX M θ. PASS θ. *Val.* ZN.
ZN p. ZN v—Laughing and crying. See
Hysteria.

Nervous excitement verging upon hysteria,
PASS θ, 30 to 60 drop doses. *Nux m* θ, 30
drops in ½ glass of water, teaspoonful doses.
"Tincture of Nux m secures results, in every
way about equal to that of Passiflora. It also
cures *sick headache.*"

Nervous irritabillty, threatening insanity:
Cann I extract ¼ to ½ gr. pill, 12 hours.
Cimi 2x.

Nerves "on edge," cannot endure a scraping
scratching sound, Asar.

"Fidgets," *Caust.* Ig. Sil. *Val.* ZN—Uneasy
hands, Bell—Rubbing the hands together,
Tarant—Uneasy feet, APIS. ZN—Not still a
moment, Aco. Caust. Ig. ZN—Pushing and
pulling when in pain, Lyc.; or scratching
upon something, Arn—Wandering about,
Apis. *Mer.* Nit a. *Stan. Verat a.*

Hurried feeling, *Lil t.* Sul a—Doing everything in a hurry, Sep. *Sul a*—Cannot wait
for others, Aco. *Arg n*—Rapid speech, Hep.
Mer. Stram—Greedy haste, Ars. Sep.

Jerking, twitching, Arg n. Bell. Cic. Hyo. *Ig.*
Nux v. *Sul.* Tarant. *Val.* ZN.

Pulsations, Pul. Nat m.

"Shivers" nervous, Cimi. Gel. Plat.

Shocks, Cimi. *Nux v*—From surgical operation, Glo. *Atrop.* Hyper.

Sensation of distension all over, Lil t. Lyc
—Feeling of *lightness,* Asa. Nux m—As if
flying, Cann I. Mauc. Thuj—As if could fly,
Gel. Mos—Legs seem to have no weight, Pul

—When lying down feet seem to float, *Stict.*

" Stage fright " — " Examination scare," *Ana.* Copai. *Gel*—Urging to urinate, Copai.

Starts, Nat m. Sil. ZN—When touched, Kal c.

Thrills, *Cann I.* Sil.

Throbbing all over, Glo. Iod. Grap.

Trembling, Agar. *Con.* Cup m. Hyo. *Mer. Mos. ZN*—Internal trembling, Camp. Sul a
—Feeling as if trembling, but not, Sul a.

NETTLE RASH.—See Skin—Hives.

NEURALGIA.—(See Face. Seè Part Affected. See PAIN. See Diet S)

In general, GAULTHERIA θ, dose not less than 10 drops; if pain very severe 20 drops, or even 30, always on sugar; repeat the dose in half an hour if needful. *Gel θ* and *Kalmi θ.* SPIG. Vis a. ZN v. *Breathe vinegar vapor.*

With camel-hair brush apply, along the track of pain, the *Oil of Peppermint*, or tincture of Aconite, or Cimicifuga or Veratrum v. (See Aconite. Amyl. Chloroform. Ether. Ichthyol. Lime-*sweat.* Turpentine.)

" First," SPIG 3x. or *Meli* 2x, or *Pass θ.*

Periodical, *Ars.* Chin *Cedron. Diad.* Spig—In head and face with sick stomach, Iris v.

Pain driving to desperation, Aco. Cham. Stram—Started by the least touch, Chin. Spig—Located in old scars, Hyper.

Burning, Ars.

Cramp-like, *Plat.* Sep.

Darting, Aco. BELL. Mag p.

Jerking, Chin. Pul.

Tearing, Colo. Spig. VIS A.

With hot head sweat, Cham.

— Cold sweat, Mer. Verat a.

NIGHTMARE.

—Coldness, shivering, Pul. Verat a.

Worse by motion, Bry. Bell. Colo. *Spig*—At night, Mer. Rhus.

NIGHTMARE.—See Sleep.

"NIGHT TERRORS."—See Sleep.

NIPPLES.—See Female—Breasts.

NODES.—Aur. Mer. Mez. Nit a. Sil. Still.

NOMA.—ARS. Lach. Mer. (See Bismuth.) See Mouth.

NOSE.—

Nosebleed:—Grasp the nose with thumb and finger, breathe only through the mouth. Inhale into the nose hot water, or hot ashes, or hop dust, or Camphor, or, *best of all, fumes of boiling vinegar*. Apply ice to root of nose, or back of head, or, in a cloth, to genitals. *Put the feet in hot water to the knees.* "Stuff a pledget of cotton inside the lip, and hold it firmly in place by passing a cord around under the nose and over the ear, and securing it tightly behind the head." Plug the nostrils. *Ligate the limbs at arm-pit and groin.* "Snuff Hamamelis extract. Sure cure."

Habit of nose-bleeding, ARN and PHO. Ferr. Ham. *Mill. Trill.* Urti—Chronic, frequent, profuse, Kal c. *Kreo 30.*

"Specific," MELI θ.

"Monthly," Bry. Ham.

At night in sleep, Grap. Rhus. Mer.

In the morning on rising, Amb. Bry — On washing the face, *Am c.* Kal c.

In low fever, Ars. Rhus. Pho. Ph a.

In measles, Ipe.

With red face, Aco. Ferr p. *Meli*—Pale face, Carb v. Chin. *Cro.* Sec—Fainting, CRO.

When blowing the nose, Pho. Sul.

(See Alum. Cold Water. Iron. Vinegar.)

Catarrh—Acute Coryza—Influenza :—

In general, *Am bro* 2x. Camp θ 1 drop, ½ hour.
Ccp 2x. EUP PER. Gel. Hydras. Kal bi.
LEMNA 3x. NAT M 2x trit. Sang n 2x.

"Colds of all kinds, acute or chronic, ACO 2x
and SUL 2x."

"Sneezing cold," LEMNA 2x. NAT M 2x.

Flowing nose, *clear water*, *Aco. Cep*. Euphr.
Kal iod. Mer. *Nat m*—With headache, Eup
per—Hot, excoriating liquid, *Ars iod*
—Thick mucus, Mer iod. Lemna. Kal bi—
Tough, stringy, Hydras. Kal bi.

"Stopped-up" nose, Ambrosia. LEMNA 2x.
Sam—More indoors, Sul—More at night,
Nux v.

"Snuffles," Cup m. *Lemna* 3x. *Sam*.

Racking cough, Aco. CEP 2x. MER. Sang 2x.

Catarrh, Chronic—Ozæna :—

In general, " *Am bro and Nat m*." " *Kal bi
and Mer bin*." " *Pet and Sep*." " No better
general remedies than KAL BI and KAL C."
" Of all remedies, ARG N, in varying attenu-
ations, has survived as the fittest."

(See Alum. *Carbol a*. CHLORIN. *Eucalyp*. Hydras. Hydrogen. Iodine. Ichthyol. Potash. Resorcin. Tann. Thuj. Turpentine.)

" Try Aurum mur and Oleum j; Aurum, morning and evening, and Oleum j, 5 drops
salted, after meals; if this does not master
the case, follow with Lemna 3x or Skook 3x;
or with Calc fl; or perhaps with Bacill. 200,
or Psor 200, one dose a week."

Mind gloomy, thoughts of suicide, AUR.

Pain in the forehead, *Aur. Nux v*—At the

root of the nose, Alu. Pet. (Relieved by·
pressure, Kal bi)—Extending over the eye,
Kal bi—With attacks of sick headache,
Sang.

Eyes weak, Arg n—Watery eyes, lids puffed,
Ars iod.

Ears cracking or roaring, Ars iod. *Grap.* Sil—
Deafness, Ars iod. Sang. Sul.

Neck glands enlarged, Ars iod—Hard but not
painful, Nit a.

Mouth ulcerated, Hydroct. Mer. Nit a.

Tonsils enlarged, Ars iod. Mer prot.

Hawking constant, Ars iod. Cal c. Nat c.

Hoarseness when walking against the wind,
Pho.

Cough and altered voice, Kal bi. *Sang*.
SANG N 3x—Cough when reading aloud or
laughing, Pho.

Skin unhealthy, subject to boils, or eruptions,
Hep. Sul—Especially festering easily, Grap.
Hep. Sul—Yellow, Sang.

Feet cold and damp, Cal c.

Malaria in the system, Ars iod.

Summer Catarrh, "Hay Fever," "Rose Cold":—

In general, Ars iod. Arum. KAL IOD. Naph.
Naj. Pso 30. STICT. (See *Quinia*, Iodine.
Sulphur.)

Sneezing constant, *Sabad*.

Stopped up nose, watery eyes, wheeze cough
Ambros.

Discharge from the nose:—

Acrid corroding, making nose and lips sore,
Æs. Alu. Am m. Aur iod. ARUM. Cep.
Euphr. KAL IOD. Mer. Sul.

Bloody, Ail. Arg n. Arum. Pho. Sul. Thuj.

Burning, Æs. Am c. *Ars*. Ars iod. Cep. Kal iod. Pul.

Brown, Kre. Thuj.

Green, Asa. Aur. Cal fl. Kal bi. Kal p. *Nat p*. Pho. *Pul. Sep*. Thuj—Green, dripping back into throat, Kal p. *Sep*.

Yellow, Aur. Asa. Cal fl. Grap. Kali m. KAL S. Mer. Nat p. PUL. Sep—Ropy, Hydras. Kal bi.

Fetid, Arg n. Ars. ASA. AUR. Grap. Kal bi. Kro. MEZ. Sep. Thuj—From decay of bone, Asa. *Aur. Cal fl*. Fl ac. Nit a. Therid— Odor of herring brine, Elap.

Transparent, Nat m—*Dripping back* into the throat, HYDRAS.

Watery, dripping, *Aco*. Ail. Æs. *Agar*. Ambros. Aur iod. Am m. Cep. Iod. Kal iod — In low fever, Mur a.

Odor in the nose as of:—

Blood, Nux v. Sil.

Brimstone, Ars. Cal c. Grap. Nux v.

Burnt horn, Pul.

Burnt sponge, Ana.

Chalk or lime, Cal c.

Egg, spoiled, Cal c.

Gun powder, Cal c.

Herring brine, Elaps.

Musk, Agn.

Old catarrh, Grap. Pul. Sul.

Pitch, Ars. Con.

Smoke, Sul.

Sour, Alu. Bell.

Sweet, Aur. Nit a. Sil.

Urinous, Grap.

Sense of Smell:—

Too acute, *Bell.* Coff. Grap. Lyc. *Nux v.*
Pho. Sep—Odor of flowers intolerable, Grap.
Lost, Ana. Aur. Caust. *Nat m.* Pho. PUL.
Sep. SIL. Sul—From catarrh, Grap. *Lemna*
2x. Nat m. Nux v. Mez. Pul. Sep.

Pains, Sensations and Condition of the Nose:—

Pains in the bones, Aur. Hep. Mer. Thuj—Relieved by pressure, Kal bi.—Boring, Nat m.
Spig. Sul—Burning, Aurum mur. Kal c.
Kal iod—Cramp-like, Arn. Plat. ZN—Drawing, ZN—Gnawing, Kal iod.

—Pressing, Lach. Stict. ZN—Shooting, Spig
—Pricking, like splinter, Arg n. Hep.
Nit a—Throbbing, Kal bi. Kal iod. Sil—
Tightness, Mer. Thuj.

Outer Nose:—

Blackish, Mer—Black pores, *Grap.* Nit a Sul.
Bluish, Verat a. Laur.
Burning, Carb an.
Chapped, Ant c. Arum. Grap.
Coffee color, Ars. Carb an.
Cracked, Ant c. Alu. Arum. Grap. Sul—*Tip,*
Alu. Carb an.
Cold, Arn. Verat a.
Fanning, wings, LYC.
Hard wings, Thuj.
Numb, Asa. Nat m. *Plat.* Viol o—*Tip,* Viol o.
Pale, Nat m—Pale and pointed, Ars. Verat a.
Peeling, Canth. Carb an—Scaly, Ars. Aur.
Grap.
Pimply, Cal c. Kal c. Pet. Sil—Tip, Caust.
Sep.
Red, Agar. Alu. Aur. Lach—Red and swollen,
Apis. Ambros. Ars. Kal bi. Kal c. Kal iod.

Rhus. Phos. Thuj—*Tip*, Aur. Cal c.
Carb an. Nit a—Wings, PB. (See *Ichthyol.*)
Swollen, Grap. Hep. Pho. Rhus—One side,
ZN—Tip swollen, "Knobby," Aur.
Sweaty, Rheu.
Tettery, Æth. Alu. Sep. Skook—Tip, Æth.
Ulcerated, Aur. *Cal p*.
Warty, Caust. Nit a. Thuj.

Inner Nose :—

To cleanse the nose: Stuff the nostrils with
twists of cotton; the moisture of the nose,
in the course of half an hour, will bring off
the crusts and leave a free surface on remov-
ing the cotton.
Burning, Ars. Aur. Kal c.
Cold, Kal bi—Cold when inhaling, Ant c—
"Cold to the brain" when inhaling, Cimi.
Cracked and crusty, *Ant c*. Hep. Grap. *Stict*.
Dry, Alu. Hyper. Kal c. Sil. STICT.
Dark "sooty," Ars. Hell.
Plugs—"Clinkers," KAL BI. *Lemna* 3x. Sep.
Sil—Bloody, Sep—Hard and dry high up,
Lemna 30. Lyc.
Stopped up, Ambros. AM C. Arum. LEMNA
—As if the nostrils were gummed together,
Aur. Nit a. Lyc. Pho—In the morning, Con.
Lyc—At night, Lyc. Nux v—Child wakens
smothering, face blue, SAM. Lemna. See
Infant.
Scabby, *Grap*. KAL C. Lyc. Nit a. Thuj.
Scurfy, Alu. Ant c. Arum. *Grap*. KAL C.
Sore, Ars. *Ars iod*. Mer iod. Lemn. KAL BI.
Pimply, Ox a. Teuc. Thuj.
Polypus: CAL P. *Lemna* 3x. Teuc. Thuj.
Snuff pulv. Sang root. Snuff salt. Snuff Re-
sorcin. (See Resorcin.) "Have patient close

NUMBNESS.

the free nostril and blow the nose until the polypus comes down well, then with hypoderm. syringe inject 15 or 20 drops of a solution of Tannin in water. In a few days the polypus will shrink up and can be blown out."—(See Vinegar.)

Ulcer, *Aur.* Asa. CAL P. *Kal bi.* KAL C. *Kal iod. Lyc.* Mer. Nit a. Pul. Sul. Thuj.

NUMBNESS.—(Insensibility of parts affected), *Aco.* Cann I. Kal bro. *low. Nux v.* Sec.

All over, preventing sleep, *Cimi.* See Parts affected.

NYCTALOPIA.—See Eye—Sight.

NYMPHOMANIA. — Amb. *Canth. Camphor bro.* Coca θ 5 drops. Nuph l. Pho. *Plat.* Tarent C.

OBESITY.—Cal c. Caps. Grap. PHYT θ 2 drops, 6 hours. " Phytolacca berry tablets " (B. & T.), Two tablets before each meal, or immediately after. See *Diet* Y.

ODOR OF THE BODY OFFENSIVE.—Ars bro Bacill 30–200. Psor 30–200 *Sul.*

ŒDEMA.—See the part affected, as Face, Eyelid, Throat, Lung, Scrotum, Feet, &c.

ŒSOPHAGUS.—See Throat Symptoms—swallowing.

Burning, Ars. Canth. Mer c. Pho.

Coldness, Meny.

Closure, Convulsive, Arg n. Mer c.

OFFENSIVE ODOR.—See the Affection, or *part* affected.

OINTMENTS.—(Boericke & Tafel.)

Bed sore, Arnica. Boracic acid.

Bite, Ledum—Venomous, Plantago.

Boil, Arnica. Lycopersicum.

Breasts, "Caking," Phytolacca — "Gathering," Phytolacca.

Bruise, Arnica. Hamamelis — Bruised, sore feeling, Arnica.

Bunion, Arnica.

Burn or Scald, Urtica urens—The skin broken, raw, Urtica urens—The skin unbroken, Cantharis.

Cancer pain, Belladonna.

Carbuncle, Cantharis. Lycopersicum.

Chafing, Arnica. Calendula.

Chapped skin, Calendula.

Chilblain, Arnica. Urtica urens.

Corns, Arnica.

Cracks, Calendula. Graphites. Hamamelis.

Cuts, Hamamelis.

Eczema, Iris. Graphites. Skookum chuck.

Eruption, Iris—Scurfy, Hamamelis. Rhus— Itching, Naphthalin Phytolacca—About the rectum and scrotum, Yellow ox. Mercury.

Excrescences, Thuj.

Eye sore, Graphites. Hydrastis. Yellow ox. Mercury.

Favus, Phytolacca.

Felon, Lycopersicum.

Fungus, Thuja.

Gangrene, Eucalyptol.

Gland enlarged, Bryonia. Rhus.

Gout, Ledum.

Herpes, Chrysophanic acid. Graphites. Hamamelis. Thuja.

Hives, Urtica urens.

Inflammation, Aconite—Pale, Apis—Malignant, Plantago.

Joint enlarged, painful, Bryonia, Ledum.

Lepra, Cantharis.

OINTMENTS.

Lupus, Cantharis.

Neuralgia, Aconite.

Nipples, cracked, sore, Graphites. Hamamelis.

Nodes, Ledum.

Pain pleuritic, Bryonia—Rheumatic, Arnica. Rhus tox. Stramonium—Stinging, Apis. Ledum.

Piles, Æsculus. Hamamelis—Blind, Æsculus—Bleeding, Hamamelis—"Old," Phytolacca—With rectal pain, Stramonium.

Pimples, Arnica. Ledum. Sulphur.

Prairie itch, Phytolacca.

Prurigo, Naphthol. Phytolacca.

Psoriasis, Cantharis. Chrysophanic acid.

Rigid os, Belladonna.

Ringworm, Chrysophanic acid. Phytolacca.

Scald head, Iris. Yellow ox. Mercury.

Scars, painful, Graphites.

Shingles, Phytolacca.

Schirrus tumor, Belladonna.

Sores, Graphites. Hamamelis—Old, indolent, Pine pitch—Scrofulous, Phytolacca—Soreness back of the ears, or between the toes, Graphites.

Sprain, Rhus tox.

Sting, Arnica. Apis. Ledum.

Stricture, spasmodic, Belladonna.

Sycosis, Phytolacca.

Testicle, swollen, tender, Apis. Hamamelis.

Tetter, Chrysophanic acid. Graphites. Hamamelis. Thuja.

Tinea capitis, Iris. Phytolacca.

Ulcer, Calendula. Hamamelis. Hydrastis. Lycopodium—Foul, Boracic acid. Graphites. Lycopodium—Indolent, Cantharis. Lyco-

podium—Itching, Hamamelis—Malignant
Plantago.

Warts, Thuj.

White swelling, Bryonia. Hamamelis.

Zoster, Graphites.

OLIVE OIL.—*Ailments of infants:* Anoint with
Olive oil *hot*, several times a day.

Earache: Wrap a little black pepper in raw cotton, saturate the cotton with Sweet oil and insert it into the ear. Instant relief.

ONION.—*Lockjaw from a wound, especially from
a nail:* Apply raw onion pulp mixed with salt.

Ague: "Bind to the feet and wrists, for several
days, raw onion pulp."

Obstruction of urine: Apply raw onion pulp
to region of bladder; or sit twenty minutes
upon a chamber vessel containing bruised
onions steeping in hot water. .

Falling of the hair: "Apply onion juice to the
scalp twice a week."

Abscess, Carbuncle, Boil: Apply onion roasted.

Nervous Croup: Hold to the nose a bruised
onion.

Baby's Colic: Onion tea.

Bilious Colic: Eat a raw onion—Drink onion
tea.

Kidney Colic: Apply to seat of pain raw onion
pulp. Eat raw onion.

Painful Piles: Raw onion pulp. Apply.

ONYCHIA.—See Limb—Arm—Hand (*felon*).

OPACITY.—See Eye—Ball.

OPIUM, POISONING.—See Antidote. HABIT.
See Morphine.

OPHTHALMIA.—See Eye.

ORCHITIS.—See Male.

OSSIFICATION.

OSSIFICATION.—Bacill. See Diet Q.

OS UTERI.—See Female—Uterus.

OTITIS.—See Bone.

OTALGIA.—See Ear.

OSTITIS.—See Ear.

OTORRHŒA.—See Ear—discharge.

OVARY.—See Female.

OZÆNA.—See Nose—Catarrh, Chronic.

PAIN.—

Sedative Treatment External — Topical Treatment of Pain :—ACETANILID 30 gr, to Vaseline ½ oz. Mix. Apply.—*Soap liniment and oil of winter green*, equal parts. Mix and apply. Apply by camel-hair pencil the *oil of peppermint*, or tincture of Aconite, or Cimicifuga, or Veratrum v. (See Aconite. Arnica. Belladonna. Alcohol. Chloroform. Coca. Ether. Hot Water. Hydrogen. Ice. *Ichthyol.* Kerosene. Lime (*sweat*). Mullein oil. *Poultice.* Resorcin. Sulphur. Turpentine—See Ointment.)

Treatment by Inhalation :—

See Amyl. Chloroform. Ether. Turpentine. Fumes of boiling vinegar.

Hypnotic Treatment :—

Fix the eye of the patient upon a small shining object close to the face, so that the eyes have to slightly squint in looking at it. After a few minutes the patient will become insensible to pain. Available in labor. In order to awaken the patient, blow your breath upon the eyelids, or rub them with your thumbs, or apply hartshorn to the nose.

Internal Treatment of Pain :—

Sedative: ANTIPYRINE 5 to 10 gr. " Antikam-nia " 10 gr. Atrop s 3x. *Ichthyol* 2 gr, 3 hours. Croton chloral 10 gr, in water 1 ounce bottle, adult 1 teaspoonful every hour until relief then *stop.* Cannabis Indica (Hemp) extract ¼ to ½ gr pill every 6 to 12 hours. Hemp fl ex 5 to 15 drops. "Jamaica dogwood, 30 drops, induces natural sleep and relief of pain." Piper m *θ* ½ drachm in ½ glass of water, adult ¼ of this at one draught, then 2 teaspoonfuls every 10 minutes. " Kava. Kava fl ex. 8 drops in 2 tablespoonfuls of water, every 3 hours; in extreme cases of exhausting pain, 30 drop dose." Codeia, adult 1 gr, 12 hours, or ½ gr 6 hours, or ¼ gr 3 hours. " Acetate of morphine 1 gr, in water 1 ounce bottle, adult 1 teaspoonful, every ¼ hour until pain ceases, or sleep is induced." Opium adult ½ grain, 4 hours. Passiflor, adult 30 to 60 drops in hot water, ¼ to ½ hour. Viscum album *θ* 20 to 30 drops, especially for *tearing* pains. Chamomile tea controls pain. " First thought " MELI 2x.

Estop to pain at once: " Direct a bright beam of arc-light upon the scene of suffering by means of a powerful reflector; or by application of direct illumination by means of a condenser."

Pains come on slowly, increase gradually to a high degree, then as gradually subside, *Stann;* or suddenly cease, Sul a.

Pains come suddenly and as suddenly cease, *Bell.* Cimi. Mag p.

Periodical pains, Ars. Chin. Spig—Exactly on time, Cedron. Diad.

Shifting, Kalmi. *Pul*—From joint to joint, Bry. Caul. Kalmia. Pul.

Extending from right to left, Lyc; or diagonally, Agar.

Intolerable pain, Aco. Cham. Coff.

Bruise-like, Arn. Cimi—In the bones, Ruta—As of bones broken, Eup per—or flesh pulled off the bones, Bry. Rhus—Tenderness of part in pain, BELLIS P—Tender spots, Nux v—Chronic soreness of all muscles, Guai.

Binding, squeezing pain, *Cact*. Colo. Sabad.

Boring, Aur. Mer. Mez. Thuj.

Bursting, Bry. Nat m.

Burning, Aco. Ars. Canth. Caps. Rhus—Like pepper, Caps. Mez—Like fire, Aco. *Ars*. Kreo—Fiery darts, Mez — Sparks, Sec—Spots, Fl ac — Burning stinging, *Apis*. Therid.

Cold pain, Led.

Clutching, as with claws, *Bell*. Cact; or hot pincers, Ars.

Cramp, Cup m. Colo. Plat. Mag p.

Cutting, as with knives, Bell. Ig. Spig.

Crushing, Cact. Glo.

Darting, like lightning, Cup m. Mag p—or electric shocks, Nux v. Pul.

Drawing flesh from bone, Bry. Rhus. *Thuj*.

Gnawing, Kal iod. Mer. Sil.

Humming, Caust. Grap. Ol.

Jerking, Chin. Pul.

Numbing, Aco. Asa. Nux v—Under the skin, ZN.

Packing, like a *plug*, Ana. Plat. Sep.

Pricking, like a splinter, Alu. Hep. Nit a.

Spasm-like, Am c. Led. Rhus. Ruta.

Stinging, *Apis*. Bell. Mer.

Stitching, Bry. Canth. Kal c. Spig.

Tearing, Chel. *Colch*. Led. Pul. Sul. *Vis a*.

Throbbing, *Bell.* Cal c. Glo. Hell. *Mer.*

During Pains :—

Coldness, Pul. Verat a.

Cold sweat, Ars. Puls. Mer—On the forehead, Verat a—Sweat without relief, Mer.

Delirium, Agar. Bell. Verat a—Colic with delirium, PB.

Face red, Aco. Ferr p. Meli θ—One cheek red, Cham.

Fainting, Aco. Hep. Nux m.

Pushing and pulling with the hands, Lyc.

Scratching with the nails, Arn.

Tossing and moaning. Aco. Pip m.

Pains start by thinking of them, Aur. Bar c. Hell. Ox a.

Pains depart by thinking of them, Camp. Cic.

Pains Better When :—(See Amelioration.)

Cold, Asa. Iod.

Cold water applied, Asa. Apis.

Head uncovered, Led.

Warm, Ars. Mag p.

Wrapping head up, Sil.

Riding in a carriage, Nit a.

Rubbing the part, Asa—Back, Nux v—Side, Pod.

Lying still, Bry.

Moving, Rhus—Slowly walking, Ferr. Verat a.

Walking rapidly, Gel. *Ig. Sep.*

Pains Worse by :—(See Aggravation.)

Arousing from sleep, Lach.

Contact, touch, Aco. Asa. *Chin.* Hep. *Spig.*

Jar, jolt, *Bell.* Bry. Spig. Sil.

Knock, *Arn.* Spig.

Motion, Bry. Ferr p.

Noise, Aco. *Bell.* Nux v. THERID.

Odor of tobacco, Aco. Gel. *Ig.* Thuj.

PALATE DOWN.

Mental exertion, Nux v.
Music, Amb. Ferr. Spig.
Warmth, Bry. *Led.* Pul.

PALATE DOWN.—See Mouth—Relaxation.

PALMS.—See Limb—Arm (*hand*).

PALPITATION.—See Heart.

PALSY.—See Paralysis.

PANCREATIC AILMENTS.—Bacill 200. Iod. Iris v. Mer bin.

PANNIS.—*Sul.* See Eye.

PARAPHIMOSIS.—See Male.

PARALYSIS.—See parts affected—is Face. Eyelids. Throat. Tongue. Sphincter. Limb, &c.

In general (See Vinegar), Aco. ARG N. Arn. Avena θ 10 drops, 6 hours. Bell. Cham. CAUST. Cal p. "*Mer and Lach, and Sulphur ointment to spine.*" PB Physos. Pho. Tarent C 200—Complete, PB—Better and worse, Tarent C 200—With insanity, Bufo. Hell. Op. PHYSOS. Stram—Death like coldness, Helo 200.

Agitans: Arg n. Avena θ. *Cocaine* 2x. CON. *Helo* 200. Hyo. *Mer.* TARENT C 200—One side, Bell. Stram.

Cause of Paralysis :—

Apoplexy, Lach. Op.
Diphtheria, Caust, GEL. Helo 200. NUX V 2x. ZN P.
Fall on the back, Arn. *Hyper.*
Intemperance, Nux v. op.
Night watching and grief, Ig.
Pressure, as for example a weight on the arm, *Aco* 2x.
Rheumatism, Colch. PHYT. Rhus. Ruta.
Suppressed eruption, Caust. Dul. Sul.

Old age, *Con.* Op.
See Person.

PEMPHIGUS.—See Skin.

PERICARDITIS.—See Heart.

PERIOSTITIS.—See Bone.

PERITONITIS.—See Abdomen.

PERSON.—(See Infant.) (See Mind.)

Aged decrepit, Cal p. Carb v. *Con.* Kal c. Nit a. Sec.

Childish, Bar c—Prematurely old, Agn—"Old maid," Bar c. Con. *Sec*—"Scrawny old maid," Sec—"Old maid dwarf," Bar c—"Old look," Arg n. Fl a.

Awkward, Apis. Caps—Clumsy, Asa. Caps—Dropping things, Apis. Hell—Stumbling gait, Pho.

Corpulent—Fleshy—Fat—*Pale, Cal c. Grap.* Kal bro—Large abdomen, Cal c. Lyc—Slender legs, Am m—Weak ankles, Sil. (Youth, Ant c. Cal c)—Sluggish, Am m. Caps. Grap—Phlegmy, Kal bi—Florid, Ferr. Sul—Gaining flesh, Ant c. Cal c. Sul.

Dwarfish, Bar c. Thuj—Stunted growth, undeveloped, Bar c. Cal p. Thuj.

Dark complexion, Caust. Nit a. Thuj—Dark hair, Aco. Alu. Nit a. Nux v. Plat. Sep. Thuj—Dark hair, firm fibre, irritable, Bry—Dark hair, rigid fibre, sensitive to cold air, Sep—Dark hair and eyes, Aco. Iod. Nit a—*Brownish* complexion, Iod—*Sallow*, Caust. Sep. Lyc.

Emaciated, Agn. Iod. Nit a. Pho—Losing flesh, Ars. Chin. Pho—Losing flesh while living well, Cal c. Nat m—"Skeleton," Ars. Pho. Lyc. Sabal s—Rapid emaciation,

PERSPIRATION.

Ars—Above the waist, Lyc—Harsh course hair, stooping gait, Sul—Shrivelled, withered, Ars. Alu. *Sars. Sec.* Sul a.

Florid, plethoric, *Aco.* Arn. Aur. Bell. *Ferr.* Sabin. Sul. Verat v—Crimson flush, Ferr.

Firm flesh, rigid fibre, Aco. Arn. Bry. Con. Thuj.

Flabby, lax muscle, Agar. Am c. Borax. Cal c. Sec. Spo.

Growth too rapid, Ph ac.

Light complexion—Fair, Kal bi. Pho—Red hair, Pho—Light hair, Agar. Aur. Brom. Kal bi. Sul a—Light hair and blue eyes, Brom. Caps. Pul—Fair and plump, Cal c. Kal bi. Pul.

Nervous, Aco. Amb. Ana. Asa—Restless, Aco. Ars—Easily startled, Kal c—Sensitive, Ail. Asar. Cham. Coff. Hyo. Lyc—Cannot endure pain, Arn. Cham. Coff—During pain furious, Aco. Cham.

Phlegmatic, Alu. *Cal c.* Stram.

Slim—slender—thin, Arg n. Alu. Amb. Kreo. Nux v. Pho. Plat. Sec. Thuj—Stooping shoulders, Sul—Thin body, bulky legs, Lyc.

Withered, dried up, Alu. Arg n.

See Habits.

PERSPIRATION.—See Sweat.

PERTUSSIS.—See Chest—Whooping cough.

PETECHIÆ.—See Skin—Blood specks.

PETIT MAL.—Kal bro pure 10 to 20 gr doses. Kal p. Op. Pho. Nux v— See Epilepsy—See Spasm.

PHARYNGITIS.—Aco. Apis *Tart e.*

" Follicular, tubercular, ulcerative; Sprinkle the diseased surface copiously, by insufflation, daily, with Pepsin mixed with aromatic powder (10 gr to 1 gr). After 3 days take the same internally, in 10 grain doses after each meal."

(See *Lactic acid*. Hamamel. Iodine. *Sulphur*—See Throat symptoms.)

PHIMOSIS.—See Male.

PHLEBITIS.—HAM in. and ex. *Ferr p*. Kali m. *Lith c*. Pul. *Tart e*.

PHOTOPHOBIA.—See Eye—Sight.

PHOTOMANIA.—See Eye—Sight.

PHRENITIS.—See Head. See Fever—Brain.

PHTHISIS. — See Chest — Consumption. See Atrophy.

PILES.—See Anus.

PIMPLES.—See Skin. See *Face*.

PITYRIASIS.—See Skin—Scale.

PLEURISY.—See Chest.

PLEURODYNIA.—See Chest—pain.

PLICA POLONICA.—See Head—Hair—tangle.

PNEUMONIA.—See Chest.

POISONING.—See Anttidote.

POLYPUS.—*Calc c*. CAL P. Con. Pho. Stap. TEUC. Thuj.

In the ear, nose, or os uteri, Cal c. *Cal p*. Thuj in. and ex.

Nasal, especially, Cal c. CAL P. *Lemna* 3x. TEUCR.

Uterine, *Cal iod*. CAL C. Sec. Thuj.

Mucous polypus, *Lemna*. "Apply Elixir of Opium, full strength; soon gone."

POLYURIA.—See Urinary Organs — Flow of urine.

PORRIGO.

PORRIGO.—See Head—Scalp (*scab*).

POTASH.—*Foul Breath, Diseased Gums :* Permanganate of Potash, 1 gr, in 1 ounce of water; rinse frequently.

Sore Mouth : Chlorate of Potash, 1 drachm in rose water 4 ounces; lave several times a day.

Ulcerated Sore Throat, Gangrene of the Mouth or Throat, Putrid Sore Throat, Fetid Diphtheria : Chlorate of Potash 5 grs, in water, 1 oz; gargle every hour.

Gonorrhœa : "Chlorate of Potash 1 drachm, in water 8 ounces; inject ½ ounce every hour, for 12 hours, then every 2 hours for 3 days."

Issue without the Knife—Opening of abscess, carbuncle, etc.: "Caustic Potash, lump size of a pea; apply under a compress."

Surgical dressing — After suppuration has ensued : Caustic Potash in very weak solution.

Ingrowing toe nail : Caustic Potash, 3 drachms, in 1 ounce of water.   Apply twice a day to the ulcerated surface.

Disinfectant: Chlorate of Potash, ½ ounce, dissolved in 1 gallon of water, and saturate towels or cloths in the solution and hang them about the room and dash some down the sewers and sinks.   A solution about this strength is suitable for injection into the vagina in cases of *offensive leucorrhœa;* and for irrigation of *fetid ulcers and cancer, and for offensive foot sweat, and foul sweat in the arm pits.*

POTT'S DISEASE OF THE SPINE.--*Carbol ac.* Cal p. See Bone and Back—Spine—Diet R.

POULTICE.--*Congestion* or *inflammation of internal parts:* Indian meal poultice, mixed with yeast, and saturated with Laudanum; or Flax seed poultice sprinkled with Laudanum; or Gum opium steeped in hot water, and the water thickened with cracker crust, especially for *painful sprains* and *violent orchitis.*

Chamomile flowers stewed in vinegar for *pain.*

For wounds to prevent lockjaw: Onion poultice. See Onion.

Failing labor pains: Hot mush poultice, hot as can be borne, over the fundus of the womb; as soon as a little cool, replace by a hot one; by the time that the third is applied, strong pains will set in.

PRAIRIE ITCH.—See Skin—Itch.

PREGNANCY.—See Female.

PREPUCE.—See Male.

PRIAPISM.—See Male—See Gonorrhœa.

PROCTITIS.—See Anus.

PROLAPSUS.—See Anus—See Female—Uterus.

PROSTATE GLAND.—See Male.

PROSTATITIS.—See Male.

PROSTRATION.—See Debility—See Diet A and I.

PROUD FLESH.—Sang root pulv. ex. Thuj in and ex. See Ulcer,

PRURIGO.—See Skin—Eruption.

PRURITUS.—See Skin—Itching.

PSORIASIS.—See Skin—Scab.

PTERYGION.—See Eye.

PTYALISM.—See Mouth—Salivation.

PUDENDA.—See Female—Local.

PUERPERAL.—See Female—Child-bed.

PULSE.—See Heart—Pulse.

PULSATION IN ALL THE ARTERIES.

PULSATION IN ALL THE ARTERIES—Iod. Glo. Nat m.

PURPLE RASH.—Aco. Ail. Am c. Rhus.

PURGATIVES.—See Constipation. See Castor Oil.

PURPURA HEMORRHAGICA.—See Skin.

PURULENT OPHTHALMIA.—See Eye.

PUS FORMATION, PREVENTIVE.--CHAM *θ* Hep. IOD. *Mer.* Sil.

PUSTULE.—See Skin.

PUTRIDITY.—See the affection and part affected.
> In general, *Bap.* Carb an. *Carb v. Carbol ac.* Crotal. Kreo. Lach. Mur a. Nit a. Sec.

PYÆMIA—SEPTICÆMIA(*Pus in the blood*).— Arrn. *Ars. Carbol ac.* Chin. Crotal. ECHIN. EUCALYP. *Kalp.* PYROGEN.

PYELITIS.--Uva. See Urinary Organs.

PYREXIA.—See Fever.

PYROSIS.—See Stomach--Heartburn.

QUINIA.—"*Hay Fever*," "*Rose Cold*" : "Prepare a weak solution of quinia in water. Lie down upon the back, and dip a small camel-hair brush into the solution and apply it to the inside of the nostrils, moving the head about gently, so as to make sure that the solution reaches all parts of the nostril, and is felt in the throat. Relief is experienced immediately. Three applications during the day, when there is threatening of return of the trouble, will prevent."
Itching in the Anus, or any local itching,
> *Pruritus :* Rub Quinia into Vaseline until as

rich as it can be made; and with this anoint the parts. It gives immediate relief.

Granular Eye Lids, Trachoma : Place, by camel-hair brush, Quinia on the underside of the lower lids.

QUINSY.—See Throat.

RABIES.—See Hydrophobia.

RACHITIS.—See Bone.

RANULA.—See Mouth.

RASH.—See Skin.

RATTLESNAKE BITE.—See Bite.

RECTUM.—See Anus and Rectum.

REDNESS.—See Inflammation. See Ichthyol—Alcohol.

REELING.—Bell. Bry. Nux v. Rhus. Stram. Verat a.—See Head—Vertigo.

REMITTENT FEVER.—See Fever—Bilious.

RESORCIN.—*Dandruff:*—Glycerole of Resorcin, 10 per cent apply.

Specks on the Cornea: Resorcin pulv. apply.

Ulcer in the Stomach:—" Resorcin 5 grs, in 1 oz. water, taken when the stomach is empty, stops the pain at once. Give predigested food; or restrict diet to milk."

Catarrh of the Bladder:—" Inject 1 per cent solution of Resorcin in water."

Cancer. Epithelioma:—" Resorcin ointment, 15 parts to 20 vaseline, twice a day apply; or 10 per cent in Cocoa butter."

Keloid:—"Resorcin, 1 per cent ointment, cured."

Cadaver poison:—Resorcin ointment.

Pain:—Resorcin ointment.

RESPIRATION.—See Chest.

RESTLESSNESS.—See Nerve.

RESUSCITATION.

RESUSCITATION.—See Apparent Death.

RETCHING.—*Ipe.* Bell *Kreo.* Phyt. VERAT V.

RETENTION OF URINE.—See Urinary Organs.

RETINA DETACHED.—Aur. Gel.   See Eye.

RETINITIS.—See Eye.

RHAGADES.—See Skin-crack.

RHEUMATISM.—

"Eat absolutely nothing, and drink only water, or lemonade, and all rheumatism acute or chronic will vanish in from 5 to 10 days.   Attest 40 cases."

"Remove the casters from the bed posts, and put thick pieces of plate glass under each post; this will produce calm and refreshing sleep."

"The outer part of my ankle joint was *red hot and swollen;* walking was exceedingly painful; and had been so for two months; when happening in a doctor's office, I chanced to take into my hand a stick of Rhus venenata (Root?), and directly I felt through my hand, although I had on silk gloves, a tingling sensation, as if from a very weak electric current.   I held the stick in my hand for a few moments, and directly after took my departure, but scarcely had I commenced to walk before I discovered that my ankle was entirely free from pain; the swelling also soon after subsided.   I was cured."

"In acute articular rheumatism, Antipyren, adult 30 to 60 grains, affords immediate and complete relief."

"I have the first case yet to see of Acute Rheumatism that would not yield to *Salicin.*

Suspend 4 drachms of Salicin, in 8 ounces of
hot water, and, adult, take 1 ounce of the
solution every 3 hours, until all taken; then
prepare fresh, and take ½ ounce every 3
hours, for 48 hours; then ¼ ounce, 3 times
a day until entirely well."

"In a case where the stomach rejected Salicylic
acid: A compress saturated with a 10 per
cent. solution of Salicylate of Soda, was applied to the joint affected, and covered with
oil-silk; next day the pain and swelling had
vanished, and power of motion was restored
to the joint."

Reported 250 cases in succession, of Inflammatory Rheumatism. Cured each case in 84
hours, with distilled *herring brine*, 20 drops,
every 2 hours. The same for *Lumbago*.

"In doses of 1 to 2 drachms of the tincture,
Cimicifuga has proved eminently curative in
Acute rheumatism and *Myalgia*, especially
when located in the neck, back, chest, hip,
ovary or uterus. After free sweat, rapid and
permanent cures ensue."

"For *Inflammatory Rheumatism*, and also for
Neuralgia, even in the stomach or bowels,
the specific remedy is the Oil of Winter-
green (Gaultheria); dose never less than 10
drops; if the pain is very severe 20 drops,
or even 30; always on sugar; repeat the dose
in ½ an hour if needful; then every 2 or 3
hours as long as some pain remains. The
cure is immediate and permanent."

Topical treatment. Try oil of Horse chestnut.
See Camphor. Ichthyol. Lime-sweat. Sulphur. (See Pain, Topical Treatment.)

Acute Rheumatism: ("Antipyrin hypoderm.")

Leading remedies, ACO. Bell. BRY. Caul. Chin. Cimi. Dul. Ferr p. GEL *θ* and KALMI. GAULTHERIA *θ* 10 to 20 drops on sugar. LACTIC ACID 2x. Led. Lyc. Mer. NATRUM SALI 1x, 10 gr, 1 hour. PASSIF *θ* 30 to 60 drops. Pul. Rhod. RHUS. *Spig.* Sul. Viol o.

Articular especially, Benz a. Lact a. *Lith lac.*

Muscular especially, Cimi. Stict.

Restless, ACO. Ars. Rhus. Lyc.

Quiet, BRY.

Fever remitting, Chin. Sul.

Chilly, Pul. Verat a.

Drowsy, Bell. Gel. Tart e.

Numb, Cham. *Nux v.* Lyc.

Sweating, Pilo 1x—*With* relief, Ars. Nux v— *Without* relief, Bry. Lach. MER. *Tart e—* Sour sweat, Colch. Mer—Hot head sweat, Cham—Cold sweat, Verat a. See Lemon.

Pains darting, Bell. Verat v—Furious, Aco. ·Cham. Colch—Tearing, Aco. Vis a—Shifting, Bry. Bell. *Caul. Pul.*

Better by continued motion, and warmth, Ars. Rhus.

Worse at night, *Mer.* Lyc. Rhus—Driving from bed, Cham. MER. *Verat a.*

Location; head, Gel—*Chest*, Bry. *Cimi.* Kalmi. Kal iod. RAN B—*Heart*, Cact. Colch. KALMI. *Spig.* SCUT—*Back*, Bell. *Cimi.* Nux v. *Lyc*— Ovary, Caul. Cimi— *Womb*, Caul. Cimi—*Shoulder*, Ferr. *Phyt. Sang.* Stict—*Anus*, Cimi, Sang. Stict—*Wrists—fingers—small joints*, Ant c. Caul. Lach. Viol o—Soles of the feet, *Ant c.*

Chronic Rheumatism.—See Pain.

"Obstinate rheumatic affections, with dry

skin, that would yield to no other remedy, were cured with "Fowler's Solution of Arsenic, 3 drops, 3 times a day, after meals."

"Ledum *θ* and Rhododendron *θ* in alternation 3 drops in water, every 3 hours. Cures obstinate cases of chronic rheumatism, in the joints, that has withstood all other treatment for years. It may take weeks, or even months, to effect the cure; but the cure will be effected."

"Ichthyol 2 gr pills, before meals and on going to bed, with application of Ichthyol ointment, 50 per cent in Lanolin, and compress of cotton; will master the most obstinate cases of chronic arthritis."

Limbs drawn crooked, Guai. Grap. Lyc. Nat m.

Joints stiff, BENZ AC 2x. COLCHICIN 1x, 1 gr. LITH LAC 1x Pet. *Rhus.* Sil. Sul—Wrist, Caul. Lith bro. Viol o—Hand, Ant c—Ankle, Led. Ruta—Foot, Ant c. Colch. Sabin—See Limb.

Paralytic condition, Phyt. Rhus. Ruta.

Syphilitic cause, Copai. *Kali iod.* Mer. *Phyt.* Thuj.

RICKETS.—See Bone-softening.

RIGIDITY, MUSCULAR.—Chel. Kalmia. Led. Rhus—See Joints.

RIGID OS.—See Female—Uterus.

RING WORM.—See Skin—See Head—Scalp.

ROSE COLD.—See Nose.

ROSEOLA.—Aco. Arn. Bry. Pul. Rhus.

RUBEOLA.—See Measles.

RUPIA.—See Skin—Scale.

RUPTURE.—See Abdomen—Hernia.

RUSH OF BLOOD.—Aco. Ferr p. Meli *ß*—See Congestion.

SALICYLIC ACID.—*Wound Dressing:*—Wipe the wound dry, and dust it thick with the acid and apply the bandage. Dust it every other day. "There will be no pain, fetor, pus or fever." Use the same for a *cut* or *abrasion*.

SALIVATION.—See Mouth.

SALT. *Ague:*—"Cure by putting a tablespoonful of fine salt in each shoe of the pair you are wearing."

"To stave off an ague chill, take a teaspoonful of salt at first warning."

Drowned:—"*Rub the naked patient all over with fine salt; or pack in salt for an hour;* or place patient upon the back on a board, or short ladder, across a suitable support and *see-saw*, now lifting the head and then the feet high up. Persevere."

Bee sting, spider bite:—Salt and soda, mixed in equal parts, apply."

Suppurating wound:—Strong salt water solution, apply.

Ulcer:—Bathe with weak solution of salt in hot water three evenings, twenty minutes at a time, then wait three evenings, and so on.

Sore eyes:—Bathe with hot salt water, of strength to suit sensation, morning and evening, and wipe them dry.

Seat worms:—Salt water: inject ½ teacupful at bed time.

SARCOCELE.—See Male.

SARCOMA.—See Tumor.

SATYRIASIS—EROTOMANIA.—See Mind.

SCABIES.—See Skin—Itch.

SCALD.—See Burn.

SCALD HEAD.—See Head—Scalp (*Favus*).

SCALP.—See Head.

SCAR.—Itching burning, Grap. Sul.

Painful, *Hyper*. Stap.

Re-opening, Crotal. Lach.

Removed: "Cut it cleanly off, and dress it daily, with perchloride of iron 1 drachm, and collodion 2 drachms, mixed; a barely perceptible line will be the result."

SCARLET FEVER.—See Fever—Scarlet.

SCARLET RASH.—Aco. Bell. Bry. Coff. Ig. Pul.

Restless, Aco.

Quiet, Bry.

Sore throat, Bell.

Rash slow coming out, Bry—Receding, Bry. *Ip*.

Wakeful and nervous, Coff.

Complication with measles, Pul.

SCIATICA.—See Limb—Leg.

SCIRRHOSIS.—Carb an.

SCIRRHUS.—Aco. *Con. Sil*. See Cancer.

SCLEROTITIS.—See Eye.

SCOBBUTUS.—See Mouth—Gums.

SCROFULA.—

In general, Ars iod. Bacill 30-200. Cal p. Carbol ac. CIST. Oleum j 2x trit, Iod. Still.

Growth stunted, Bacill. BAR C. Cal p.

Mind precocious, Bell.

Head large, Col c Sil. Sul.

Eye sore, mattery, Bell. CIST. Hep. Mer. Sul.

Bone Caries, *Cal fl*. Cal p. *Cist*. Mer. *Sil*. Sul.

Glands hard, Ars iod. Bell. CIST. Nit a. Sil—Bony hard, Cal fl—Suppurating, Bacill. CIST. *Hep*. Mer. Nit a. *Sil*.

SCROTUM.

Skin sore scabby, Ars iod. Dul. Sul.

Emaciation, Cal c. Iod—With large Abdomen, Bar c. Cal c. See Diet W.

SCROTUM.—See Male.

SCURVY.—See Mouth—Gums.

SEA SICKNESS.—APOMO 2x. *Coc.* Pet. Stap. Chloroform, 1 drop on sugar. (See *Amyl.* Ice).

"A cup or two of good strong coffee, without cream, taken upon an empty stomach, an hour or two before embarkation prevents sea sickness."

"Lie down and shut the eyes, and breathe *deeply, slowly, and regularly* for a few minutes." "Lie with hips higher than the head." "Watch the motion of the ship and make an effort with your foot, with every lurch of the ship, as if you were forcing it down on *that* side. Continue this for a short time, and the nausea will cease."

"Some people are sick and dizzy when riding in cars; this sickness may be prevented by placing a sheet of paper next to the skin over the stomach."

SEATON. — *Cystic Tumor, Solid hygrometous Ganglia, Atheroma of the scalp, Lipomatous Tumors, Sarcoma, House Maids' Knee:*—"Pass a double silk thread through the long diameter of the growth, and tie the end over the tumor; in large tumors another thread at right angles should be tied. After the sides have fallen in remove the thread."

SEAT-WORMS.—See Worms.

SEBORRHŒA.—See Skin—oily, flaky.

SEMINAL EMISSIONS.—See Male.

SEPTICÆMIA.—Arn. Ars. *Carbol a.* Crotal. Chin. *Euca.* ICHTHYOL. Kal p. LAPPA.

256

SHINGLES.—See Skin.

SHIVERS, NERVOUS.—See Nerve.

SHOCK.—From a hurt, or surgical operation, Glo 2x, 1 drop. Ammonia 10 drops, hypodermic. *Ether* 10 drops, hypodermic. *Hot* compress to the heart. Heat to feet. Head low. Brandy sips.

From a burn or scald, Camp *θ*. drop doses.

SHOULDER.—See Limb—Arm.

SHRIEKS.—Apis. Bell. Hell. See Spasms—See Fever—*brain*.

SICK-ROOM AIR KEPT PURE.—See Air.

SIGHT.—See Eye—Sight.

SILVER. *Purulent ophthalmia:*—Keep the eyes constantly cleansed, day and night, by sponging them with Boracic acid 4 per cent solution, and brush the everted lids daily with Nitrate of Silver solution in water, 1 gr, to the ounce. If the cornea is affected there may be need to use Atropia solution ⅛ gr, to the ounce of water, 1 drop in the eye every 3 hours. Besides the topical treatment, Arg n should be administered internally 3 times a day.

Gonorrhœal ophthalmia: — *Granular lids:* — Argent nit solution, 5 grs to the ounce of water, by camel hair brush, daily.

Fistula in Ano:—Apply a solution of Nitrate of Silver, 5 or 10 grs, to the ounce of water; make the application thorough; and if one application is not sufficient repeat it. The most obstinate cases may be cured in 3 weeks by this mode of treatment.

Ulcer. Bed sore:—Argent n, 5 to 20 grs in Nitrous Ether 1 ounce, apply by camel hair brush, daily. Rapid cure; or touch with *Lunar Caustic.*

I   257

SINKING OF STRENGTH.

To remove an ingrowing nail, with as little pain as possible:—Cover it with a thin layer of Nitrate of Silver, and then apply a poultice. After 24 hours this will loosen the nail; now continue the caustic and poultice, until the nail can be lifted off.

SINKING OF STRENGTH.—See Debility.

SINKING AT THE STOMACH—GONENESS.
—Chin. *Dig.* Dios. Gel. Hydros. *Ig. Sep.* Ustil—With deathly nausea, Dig. Gel—Not relieved by eating, Sep.

SKIN.—("Skin remedies should be externally applied while being taken internally.)

Abscess: Hep. Mer. Nit a. *Sil.*

Acne: See Face—Pimple.

Anthrax: ARS. *Anth.* Lach. Sil.

Barber's Itch: See Face.

Bed-sore: Ars. Lach. Arnica oil. Calendula oil —Maggoty, dust with Calomel—Air or water mattress—Buffalo robe beneath the under sheet, hair side up. (See Acetan. Alcohol. Bism. Clay. Silver.—See *Ointment.*)

Birth-mark—Nævus: Lach. previous to 6th month of age, Thuj. in. and ex—Dip needle point into pure nitric acid, and insert it into the nævus. (See Collodion—Lead—Vinegar.)

Bleeding pores—Blood oozing, Cup a. Lach. Tereb—In typhoid, Crotal. See Purpura hemorrhagica.

Blisters—vesicles: Ars. Canth. Croton. Euphorb. Rhus. Urti—Blood blisters, Crotal.

Blood specks under the skin—Petechiæ: Con. Led—In low fever, Ars. Pho.

Boil: Bell. *Hep. Sil.* BELLIS PER.—Crops,

ARN—All over, Viol t—Along the spine,
Lach—Blood boils, Led. Lyc. Thuj.

—Purple, Ail. Lach.

"*To abort a boil*, give Bry. Scrape the skin over
the spot where it is forming, with a sharp
knife; so that a drop or two of blood may be
pressed out. The boil will not develop."

(See Arnica. Camphor. Clay. Ham. Ichthyol.
Iodine. Sun Cautery. *Yeast*—See *Ointment*
—See Poultice.)

Burning in the skin, *Acet a.* ARS. *Caps.*
Lach. Mer. Pho. (See Acetan.)

Carbuncle: Arn. ARS. *Anth 200.* Bell. Cal fl.
Canth Carbol a. Hep. Hoang *0. Sil.*
TARANT C 3.

To allay pain, paint center of carbuncle with
fuming Nitric acid, but let none get on the
skin.

To abort a carbuncle, give Bry. See Camphor.
Iodine. *Dry Cup.*

To open carbuncle without the knife. See
Potash—*To open it without pain*, see Anæsthesia—Local.

(See Camphor. Dry Cup. Hydrogen. Ham.
Ichthy. Lard. Lead. Solar Cautery *Tannin*—
See *Ointment*—See Poultice.)

Chafe—Intertrigo: Arn. Cal c. Grap. Hep.
Lyc. Sul. Arnica oil ex. Calendula oil ex.

(See Benzo. Bism. Calend. Clay. Glycerine.
Ham. Hydrast. Salicyl. Starch. Tannin—See
Ointment.)

Chap—Crack—Fissure: Cal fl. Condu. Graph,
Hep. *Pet.* Skook—After washing, Sul.

(See Aloe. Benzo. Glycer. Hydrast. Starch—
See *Ointment.*)

Chloasma: Lyc. Pet. Sep.

Coldness: Ars. Ipe. Plat. Sec. Verat a—In spots as if touched by icicles, Agar; or a cold finger, Arn.

Desquamation, *Am c.* Arum. Ars. *Kal s. Mez*—Peeling palms, Am c. Mez Ol.

Discoloration—Off Color:—
— Blackish, Ars—Spots, Con.
— Blue. See Cyanosis—Spots, Arn. Ferr. Phos—In fever, *Ail.* Carb v. Lach. Pho. Sec. Sul a.
— Brown, Carbo an. Hydroct. Ustil—Spots, Con. Nit a Pho. Sep. Thuj—Copper brown, Croton. Mer. Nit a—Raised brown spots, Grap.
— Greenish, Ars—Spots, Ars. Con.
— Red Spots, Bell. Cal c. Pho. Sul—Itching, Con—Burning, Kal c.
— White, waxy, *Apis.* Ars—Ivory white, Pho—Spots, Sep. Sil. Sul. Thuj.
— Yellow (see Jaundice): Iod. Lyc Mer. Pso 200—Spots, Con. Crotal. Pho. Sep. Sul.

Ecchymosis: Arn. Crotal. Ferr. Lach. Sec.

Ecthyma: Ars. Lach. Mer. Tart e.

Eczema: Ars bro. Ars iod. Bacill 200. Bovis. Croton. Clem. DUL. Grap. Hep. HYDROCT 6-12. *Iris v ix. Mer.* Lyc. *Ol* 2x. *Pet. Rhus.* SKOOK 2x in. and ex. Sul 3x.

"Hydroct 6-12, followed if needful with Sulphur and Graphites in. and ex."
— Chronic, raw, *Canth.* Hydroct. Skook.
— Suppurating, *Dul.* Hep. Lyc.

Lime water for the itching—Skookum soap. (See Benzo. Bism. Borax. Camphor. Carbol a. Glycer. Hydrogn. *Ichthy.* Lead. Naph. Soda. See *Ointment.*)

Eruption : Ars bro. Ars iod. Aur bro. "Ichthy

2 grs, 12 hours, with Ichthy ointment."
LAPPA. NIT A 2x in. and ex. SUL. (See
Acetan. Ichthyol. Glycerine.)

— Only on *covered parts*, Led. Thuj—*Hairy
parts*, Mer. Nat m. Rhus—*Margin of hair*,
Nat m. Pet. Sul.

— Color *Black*, ARS. Mur a. Nit a. RHUS—
Blue, Arg n. Ars. Lach. Ran b—*White*, ARS.
Bry. Mer. Thuj. Sul.—*Yellow*, Cic. Mer.
Nit a. Sep.

— Sensation *Burning*, ARS. Carb v. *Hep.*
MER. *Sul—Itching*, Ars. DOLI 2x. Dul.
Mer. MEZ. Phyt. *Rhus.* RUMEX C. OL.
Sul.— *Stinging*, APIS. *Led.* LYC. *Mer.*
MUR A. SIL.

— Scaly: ARS. *Dul. Pho.* Skook. Sep. SUL—
Yellow, Kal s. Nat p. See SCALE.

— Scabby, crusty: Ant c. Cal c. Grap. Hep.
Mer. Ol. Skook. Sep. Sil. Sul — Green,
Nat p—Yellow, Kal s. Lyc. Nat p. Viol t—
Like dried honey, Cic. See SCAB.

Erythema: Aco. Apis. Arn. Bell. Rhus. Mez.
—Nodosum, Aps. Arn. Rhus. (See Acetan.
Benzo. Bism. Calend. Ham.)

Excoriation: *Cham.* Grap. Lyc. *Mer. Sul.*

Excrescence: Nit a. Stap. Thuj—Horny, Ant c.
Ran b. Sul.

Formication: Hyper. Nux v. *Plat.* Rhod.
Rhus. Sec. Urti—Under the skin, *ZN.*

Herpes — Tetter: (See Acetan. Ichthyol.
Glycerine. See *Ointment*) BOVIS. *Ars bro.*
Ars iod—In cold weather, Dul. Mez.

— Dry, *Ars.* Dul. *Graph. Nat m.* Sul.

— Moist, Dul. Lyc. Mer. Sep.

— Around the mouth—Labialis: *Hep.* Mer.

NAT M. *Rhus.* Under the knees, *Sal* and *Nat m.*

Hives—Urticaria: *Apis.* Ars. Croton 2x. Rhus. Ruta. URTI 1x—Burning, Croton, Rhus.

— Chronic: ARS. Bacill 200. *Skook.* Sul. *Ustil* —"Monthly," Dul. Nat m.

For the itching Menthol solution 5 grs. to the ounce of water; or Salicyl acid pulv. ex. or Vinegar dilute: *Ichthyosis.* See Scale. See Naphtha.

Impetigo: *Grap.* Hep. *Lyc.* Mer. *Mez.* Tart e. Thuj. (See Acetan. Glycerine.)

Intertrigo: Cham. Cal c. *Hep. Lyc. Mer. Sul.* (See Hydras—Starch—Samb).

Itch—Scabes—Psora: RUMEX C. in. and ex. *Sul. in.* and *ex.* "*Croton and Lobelia* alt." Pso 200—Bleeding, Mer. Lave with *Lyc.* dilute, 3 times a day. Petroleum apply, all over, 3 nights. Lard alone destroys the acarus. (See Alcohol. *Ichthy.* Naph—See Ointment.)

— Barber's Itch: See Face.

— Prairie Itch: PHYT. in. and ex. Kal c. "Wash the body thoroughly with soap suds, wipe dry, and anoint every night for a week with ointment made of Sulphur 3 parts, Carbonate of Potash 1 part, and Cosmoline 8 parts, and give Sulph." See *Ointment.*

Itching of the Skin, with or without eruption:— DOLI. 1x. RUM C. Phyt. Sul.

— Burning, Itching: *Ars. Crot. Rhus.* Sul— Burning after scratching, Mez. Ol. Rhus. Sul—or moist, Grap. Ol.

— When undressing, Ol. Rum c.

— At night in bed, Mer. Mez. Sul. Thuj.

— Voluptuous itching, Mer. *Plat. Sul.*

— *Local—Pruritus:* Apply Linseed oil; or
Lime water; or Peppermint water; or
Cocaine 4 per cent solution. (See Acetan.
Alcohol. Alum. Borax. Camp. *Glycer.*
Hydrogen. Ichthyl. *Quinia.* Soda.)

Lepra—Leprosy—(Scale): Ana. *Ars.* Bacill
200. *Canth.* Dul. *Ichthyol* 2 gr. pill, 12 hours;
and Ichthy ointment. Hoang θ 30 drops, 6
hours. HYDROCT 6–12. Pip m θ 10 drops,
6 hours. Hydrogen per. ox. 1 vol. 10 drops,
6 hours, in. and ex. Mer. SECALE COR-
NUTUM θ "has made some wonderful
cures." (See Ointment.)

Lichen—(pimple): *Apis.* Ant c. Ars. *Led.* Ol.
Sul—Brown, Card θ. (See Soda.)

Lump: See Node.

Lupus: See Face.

Mentagra: See Face.

Mole: Strangle with a silk thread. "Apply
by splinter of wood, a small quantity of acid
nitrate of mercury, carefully avoiding the
sound skin."

"Net work of veins:" Fl ac. (See Solar
Cautery.)

Node—Lump: Iod. Kal iod. *Led*—Blue, Nit a
—Brown, Bacill. Grap—Gummy, Kal iod.
Mer—On the bone, Aur. Nit a. Sil—With
night pain, Mez. Still.

Numbness: ACO. *Amb.* Gel. Hyper. *Nux v.*
Ol. PLAT. SEC.

Parasites—Lice: *Sul.* Stap. Apply Coal oil; or
oil of Anise; or Persian insect powder, or
Per. ox. Hydrogen 12 vol. Use Carbolic soap.

Pemphigus—(Blister): ARS. *Canth.* Dul.
Hydroct. RHUS. Thuj. See Blister.

Petechiæ: Ars. Bry. Con. Led. Pho. Rhus.

Pimple: Ars bro. Ars iod. Ant c. Apis. *Arn.* Gel. Kal iod. LED. NIT A ix in. and ex. SUL. THUJ. See Ointment. See Face.

Pityriasis (Scale): *Ars.* Fl ac. Mez. "Bathe frequently with hot water, rub hard, apply Borax glycerole. Give *Arsenic.*

Poisoning of the skin. Ivy poison: CYPR ix. Led. Rhus 200. Sang 2x. Apply slaked lime paste thick as cream; or Spirits of Nitre; or Camphor; or SANG θ dilute or *Soda.*

— Guard against ivy poisoning, or sumac, Ana 200.

Pricking, Lob i. Plat—As if sweat would break out, Sang.

Prickly heat: Aco. *Arn* Cham. Rhus. (See Acetan.)

Prurigo—Itching pimple: Ars. Cal c. Grap. *Mez. Nit a.* RHUS. *Sep.* Sul—Senile, Mez. (See Acetan—Ichthy. Glycer ointment.)

Psoriasis (Scale): *Ars.* Canth. *Cup m.* Grap. *Mer. Sep. Sul.*

Especially on the palms, Grap.

"Soak off the crusts, apply salve—Yellow Ox. of Mercury, 2 grs to the ounce of vaseline— Give Arsenic." (See Glycerine. Ichthy. *Naph*—See *Ointment.*)

Purpura hæmorrhagica, Crotal. *Cup a.* Ham. Kal p. Lach. PHO. TEREB. Acetate of Copper, adult, 10 drops, in cinnamon water 4 times a day, cured. Turpentine, 7 drops, 3 hours, in milk; cured a child 3 years old.

Pustule-pock: BAP. Bell. Cic. *Iris v.* Kal bi. Kal iod. Sil. TART E. THUJ. Ustil.

Rash: of infants, ACO. Bry. Cham. Ipe—*Lying-in women,* BRY. Ipe—*Miliary,* ACO.

Ail. *Agar.* Ars. Cal c. *Led—Purple*, Aco. *Ail.* Am c. Rhus—*Scarlet*, BELL. Rhus. Stram.

Ring worm—Herpes Circinatus: Bacill 200, one dose a week. *Bar c.* Phyt. *Sep.* TELL. (See Lead. Vinegar—See *Ointment.*)

Rupia (Scale): Ars. MER. Pet. Phyt. Sul. THUJ in and ex.

Scabies: See Itch.

Scab, Crust.—Ant c. Cal c. *Grap.* Hep. Iris v. Mer. Ol. Rhus. SARS 3x trit. Sil. *Skook.* Sul. Tart e—Hard dry, Ant c. *Hep.* Rhus. Sil—"Leathery," Mez—Green, Nat p—Yellow, Cic. Kal s. Lyc. Nat p. Viol t.

Scale:—ARS. Bacill. Canth. DUL. *Fl a.* Grap. *Hydroct. Ichthyol.* Mer. Mez. PHO. Phyt. *Sep. Skook. Sil.* SUL. Thuj—White scale, Ars. Nat m.—Yellow, Kal s. Nat p. ´

Scar painful, *Fl a.* Grap. HYPER. STAP—Breaking out, Crotal. Lach—Itching burning, Grap. (See Ointment.)

Scurf: ARS. Cal c. Rhus. Sul. (See Glycerine.)

Seborrhœa—Oily flaky skin: Bry. Nat m. PB. *Thuj in.* and *ex.*

Shingles— Herpes Zona — Zoster: Apis. Ars. CROTON. Phyt. RHUS. Mez—Brown, Mer. Sul—*To control the* pain, ARNICA in. and ex. *Ran b.* "Cantharis θ 1 drachm, in water 1 pint, apply 3 times a day. Cure in 3 days." (See *Ointment.*)

Spots: See Discoloration.

Sycosis: Hep. Kali m. Mer c. NIT A. PHYT. in. and ex. *Plat. Tart e.* THUJ. (See *Ointment.*)

Tenderness, excessive, CAPS. CHIN. Carb v. Con. Lach. Sil—Painful, Chin. *Spig.*

SLEEP. Prevented by.

Varicosus—Broken veins: Cal fl. CARD *θ.*
Collin *θ.* Fl ac. *Ham.* Lith c. *Pul.* ZN—Inject Ergot, 1 or 2 gr. in solution, near the
varicosus; or Ham *θ* dilute, a few drops.

Warts: Caust. *Ferr pic* 2x. Lyc. Nit a. *Sabin.*
Stap. THUJ in. and ex.—Fl ac, Caust—Stem,
Nit a. Thuj—Cancer wart, Ferr pic 3x. Thuj
in. and ex.—"Warty hands," Lyc. (See Solar
Cautery. Vinegar. Thuj Ointment.)

SLEEP.—(Sleeping room kept pure, see Air.)

Drowsiness with all ailments: ANT C. Alet.
Cann I. Coc. Op. PHEL. Pho. Tart e.

Drowsy fever, Apis. BAP. *Bell.* GEL. Tart e.

Drowsiness with voluptuousness, Cal c.

Irresistible drowsiness and pressure upon the
brain, ZN.

Uninterrupted sleep for days, Verat a.

Sleepiness but cannot sleep, *Bell.* Lach. Op.
Pul. Sil.

Stupor, Laur. Op.

Yawning, Chel. Ig. Plat. Stap.

Wakefulness, Insomnia: Aco. Amb. Ars. Cimi.
COFF. GEL. Mer. Thuj. Avena *θ* 10 drops in
water at bed time. *Cham θ* 3 drops. PASS *θ*
60 drops. STICTA *θ* 3 drops. A glass of hot
milk at bed time. A bath and brisk rubbing
at bed time. (See Amyl.)

—No sleep until 12, Pho. Rhus—Until 2 or 3
a. m., Cal c. Mer.

—None after once waking, Bellis p. Nat m. Sil—
none after 2 a. m., Kal c. Mag. Mer—None
after 3 a. m., Bellis p. Bry. Cal c. Mag c.
Nux v. Sep.

Sleep prevented by:—

Bone pains, Ana. Aur. *Mer.* Nit a.

Burning in the veins, Ars.

Burning itching skin, Agar. Bovis.

Coldness, Amb.

Cold feet, Am m. Carb v. Pho.

Colic, Coc. PB.

Cough, see Chest—Cough.

Fear of suffocation, Ars. Bap. Lach. S₁ o.

Feeling of lightness in the head, ZN—Wild feeling, *Lil t.*

Giddiness, Coc. Mer c.

Heat, Borax. Pul.

Hunger, Pho. Ph a. Lyc.

Itching all over, Arum. Stap.

Nervousness, Amb. Apis. CYPR θ. "Trional 5 grs."

Numbness, Cimi.

Palpitation, Ant c. Lil t—or oppression, Kal p. "Trional 5 grs."

Pulsations in the arteries, Nat m—In the head, Cyc—In the ears, Cact—In the stomach, Cact.

Restlessness, Aco. Ars. Rhus—"Hands and feet on the go," Caust—Fidgety feet, Apis. ZN.

Seat worms, Ferr. *Teucr.* URTI θ.

Sweat, Ars. Mer. Verat a—Driving from bed, Mer.

Vision of images, Arg n. Cimi—On closing the eyes, Cal c. Cimi.

During Sleep :—

Biting the tongue, *Ig.* Ph a. *Mez.* Therid. ZN.

Boring head into the pillow, Bell. Hell.

Cannot lie on the right side, Bry. *Mer*—Left side, Lyc. *Pho*—Either side, Aco. Ferr. Pho—Only on the stomach, Bell. *Cina.* Coc. STAN—Stomach and knees, Stram.

Chewing, Bell. *Bry.* Cal c. *Hell.* Ig. Mos.

Eyes half open, *Bell.* Bry. Ig. *Op.* Sam—Eye balls rolling, Æth. Coc—Rolled up, Bell—Fixed, Lyc. Tart e.

Grinding of the teeth, *Bell.* Cina. Ig. POD.

Groaning moaning, Aco. *Bell. Ig. Lyc.* Nux v. POD. Pul.

Head rolling, *Bell.* Hell. *Pod—Wet with sweat, Cal c.* Mer. Sil.

Hiccough, Cal c. Mer c.

Nightmare, *Aco.* Am c. Con. *Nux v. Pul.* Sil. *Sul.*

Nose bleed, Grap. *Mer.* Rhus. Sars.

Red face, Arn. GEL. Op. Stram.

Screaming, *Apis. Bell.* Cina. Hell. Ig. Sep. Stram. *ZN.*

Sighing, Ars. *Bell.* Ipe. Ph a.

Snoring, Bell. LEMNA 3x. Op.

Sobbing, *Aur.* Hyo. Nat m.

Spasms, Cup m. *Lach and Mer.* Sil Stram. Cal c. Caust.

Starting, BELL. Hell. *Ig.* Sul. *Stram.* ZN—When falling off to sleep, *Alston c.* Bell. *Ig.* Sul.

Talking, Ig. Sul. ZN.

Trembling, Ig. Rheu. Sam.

Twitching, Agar. *Ig. Hell. Sul.* Tart e. ZN.

Walking—Somnambulism: *Aur bro* 3x. *Bry.* Cic. Kal bro pure 20 gr. Nat m, *Pho.* ZN P—Leaping from bed and running around the room, Sul.

Weeping, *Cham.* Ig. Nat m. *Pul.*

On waking :—

Asthma: Aral r. AM C. *Bap.* Grap Kal bi. LACH. Nat s. Thuj—Smothering and Trembling, Sam.

SMALLPOX—VARIOLA.

Fear—fright: Cina. Stram. ZN—Screaming as
with fear, Kal p—Cross, Nux m. See
"Terror."

Palpitation, *Alu.* Benz a. Kal bi. Ox a—Also
smothering, Spo.

Shrieks, Apis, Sep.

Sore throat, HOMAR 3x *Lach.* Mer bin.

Strangling, Lach. Naj. Sep.

Sweat, *Agar* 2x trit. Dios. *Sam.*

"Terror," ACO. AUR BRO 3x. *Gel.* Kal p.
Kal bro pure 10 to 20 grs. *Sul.* Stram.

Weariness, Kal p. *Nux v.* Sep.

Worse after sleeping: Apis. LACH. Stram.
Verat a.

Dreams of:—

Falling, Chin. *Dig.* Pul. Sul. Thuj—Into
water, Am m. Dig.

Flying, *Apis.* Atrop. Indig. Xanth.

Swimming, Iod. Lyc. Ran b—Drowing, Mer
prot. Ran b. Ran c. Sil. ZN.

Urinating, Kreo. Lac c. Mer bin.

Wearying upon a journey, Rhus.

SMALLPOX—VARIOLA—Varioloid:—

In general, Carbol a 2x. BAPTIS. Merc Pho.
Sul. *Saracin. Tart e. Thuj.* VACCININ 30.
Variolin 30.

"At the onset, vaccinate the patient, this will
abort the disease. No other treatment
needed."

To prevent pits and scars, dust the scabs with
Calomel; or apply Glycerine freely; or which
is best of all, and sure of success, stab each
pustule, while its contents is fluid, with a
needle in several places around the base,
and with a cloth press out all the contained
lymph. See *Iodine.*

SMELL.

To guard against the infection, see Contagion.
Symptomatic indications:—
At the outset, Aco. Cimi. Tart e.

Backache severe, Cimi. Hydras.

Burning stinging, Apis. Mer.

Dark pock, Apis. *Ars.* Bell. Mer. SUL.

Eyes bad, Mer c. Sul.

Salivation, Mer.

Sore throat, Apis. *Bar m. Bell.* Hydras. *Mer.*

Stools bloody, Mer—Or other bleeding, Ars. Lach. Pho.

Repercussion of eruption, Ars. Camp. Sul.

Diet: well sustaining:—Broth, eggs, *Milk.*

Fresh ripe fruit, *Baked apples*, Grape juice.

Raspberry vinegar. (See Chlorine. Glycer. *Iodine.* Potash. Vinegar.)

SMELL.—See Nose.

SMOKING ESTOP.—Plantago 6–200.

SNAKE BITE.—See Bite.

SNEEZING.—See Nose.

SODA.—*Milk crust, Local itching, Pruritus, Itching eruptions, Itching Piles:* Baking Soda, saturated solution in water, frequent applications.

Burns or scalds:—Baking Soda, ½ lb, into a quart of cold water; saturate cloths and apply.

Dropsy after scarlet fever:—In hot water dissolve baking soda, enough to "feel slippery;" with this sponge the patient all over twice a day, a small surface at a time, and wipe the part dry as you proceed.

SOLAR CAUTERY.—"There is no cautery to compare with that of solar heat; it can be applied with perfect safety upon the most delicate tissue, and it is at all times under the control of the operator. The irritation and inflammation following is slight, and of short duration. Pain subsides immediately. I have burned the skin of nearly the whole side of the face, at one sitting, destroying the cuticle, and in five minutes after there was no pain."

Avoid blistering. The morbid tissue succumbs before the natural structure adjoining. This enables us to attack boldly the *malignant* or *morbid growth* without fear of injuring the healthy tissue.

In two minutes a *Chancre* or *Chancroid* is deprived of its contagion and changed into a simple ulcer. *Indolent ulcers* take on new life, granulate and heal. *Bleeding tissues* are changed to healthy condition. *Piles* bodily destroyed. *Moles and Warts* removed with perfect success; also *Boils and Carbuncles.* When necessary repeat the operation until every vestige of morbid material is destroyed. *Port wine colored spots on the face, removed* by two sittings; afterwards dressed with Zinc ointment.

In all cases Cocaine, or other anæsthetic may be used if preferred.

A 5-inch sun-glass, ¼ inch wide focus, answers the purpose. The parts to be burned should first be cleansed, and, if hairy, shaved.

SOLE.—See Limb—Leg (*foot*).

SOMNAMBULISM.—See Sleep. (During sleep-walking.)

SORE.—See Ulcer.

SORENESS, MUSCULAR.—*Arn.* Bap. Cimi Rhus. See Myalgia.

SORE MOUTH.—See Mouth.

SORE NIPPLES.

SORE NIPPLES.—See Female—breast.
SORE THROAT.—See Throat.
SPASMS—CONVULSIONS. — (Look to bad teeth, worms, constriction of penis or clitoris, etc.)

In general: ATROP. Bell. Cann I. Glo. *Lach. and Mer.* MELI θ. PASS θ. "Turn patient on left side." (See Amyl. Bandage. Chloroform. Ether. *Hot water.* Ice. Turpen.)

Renewed by light, or sight of mirror, or water, Stram—Thought of drinking, Canth—Sound of pouring or running water, Canth—Touch upon the larynx, Canth—Contact or noise, Nux v.

Local; see part affected—*Of the sphincters*, spasmodic tenesmus, Cup m. Gel. Mag p. *Nux v.*

Puerperal; see Female—Child-bed.

Uremic: CANTH. Carbol a. Op. Pilo. *Tereb.*

From fright, *Aco.* Bell. Hyo. *Ig.* Kal p. *Op.* Stram.

— Injury, Bell. Cic. Hyper. Led.

— Punishment, Ig.

— Rage, Cham.

— Teething, Aco. Agar. *Bell. Cham.* CYPR. IG. Mag p. MELI θ. PASS θ. *ZN.* (See Hot water. Olive oil.)

— Vaccine impure, *Sil.* Thuj.

— Worms, Aco. *Cic. Cina.* IG. INDIG 2x. Mer.

During spasm: Body bent back, stiff, Aco. CIC. Cap m. *Strych*—Dreadful distortion, Cic.

— Choking, Bell. Gel. Ig. Mag p.

— Cries—screams, *Cic.* Cal c. Cup m. *Hyo. Ig. Op.* Plat.

— Coldness, Camp. Hell. Verat a.

·— Eyes distorted, Bell—Turned down, Æth—
Half open, Cal c—Flooded with tears, Pul.

— Face blue, Camp. Cup m. Kal p. Verat a.
Verat v—Red, Meli *θ*.

— Fingers stretched out, Sec.

— Hands clenched on the thumbs, *Glo. Hyo.*
Mer. *Stram.*

— Happy feeling on coming out of spasm,
Sul.

— Laughter, Aur. Con. Ig.

— Mouth foaming, Bell. Cup m. Hyo. Laur.
Op. Stram.

— Motion constant between spasms, Cic.

— Motionless as if dead for a long time, after
spasm, Cic.

— Sweat profuse, Nux v. Op—Hot head, sweat,
Cham.

— Throbbing carotids, Bell. Glo. Meli *θ*.

— Trembling, Agar. Cham. Op. Verat v.

Night spasms: in sleep, Cal c. Cup m. *Lach.*
and Mer. Sil. Thuj.

"Monthly:" Spasms.   See Female—Menses
—(Ailments with).

St. Vitus' Dance: See Chorea.

Tetanus: See Lockjaw.

SPEECH.—Rapid, Hep. Mer. Stram. See Nerve.
Stammering, stuttering: Stram. Read aloud
with teeth closed for an hour daily; in a week
can open the mouth and read and talk without
difficulty. Keep time when speaking: at first
with the utterance of each syllable, and afterwards with each word; slowly at first then
more rapidly; persevere. Take a full breath
before beginning to speak. Speak in a whisper.

SPERMATORRHŒA.—See Male.

SPINE.

SPINE.—See Back—Spine.

"SPITTING BLOOD." — See Chest - - Hæmorrhage—See Bleeding.

SPLEEN.—(Congestion. Inflammation. Pain.)
> In general, Arn. ASA. Bry. CEANOTH. *Chin. Ig. Ran b.* Mag p. URTI U.
> Pain with every breath, Agar.
> Bruise-like pain, Apis. Asa. Sars. Ran b.
> Burning, *Ceanoth.* Bell. Ig. Sec.
> Cramp, Stan.
> Distension—Enlargement, Arn. CEANOTH. *Chin. Iod. Nat m.* Pho. Sec. URTICA U.
> Drawing pain, Cup m. Sul.
> Gurgling, Verb.
> Hardness, Induration, Agn. *Ars.* CAPS. CEANOTH. Chin. Ig. *Sul.*
> Sprain-like pain, Arn. Con. Nat m. ZN.
> Stitches, *Arn.* Bry. *Con. Nat m.* ZN.
> Tenderness, Apis. *Asa. Nat m.* Ran b.

SPLINTER.—Hyper. Led. See Cause—injury.

SPOTTED FEVER.—See Fever—spotted.

SPRAIN. — Arn. Hyper. *Led. Rhus. Ruta.* SYMPH.
> From lifting, Cal c. Rhus. Ruta.
> Nerve hurt, Hyper.
> Bone injured, Symph.
> (See Camphor. Clay. *Collodion.* Hama. Hot water. Lead. Verat. See Ointment. See Poultice.)

SQUINT.—See Eye.

ST. VITUS' DANCE.—See Chorea.

STAGGERING GAIT. — Coc. Ox a. Stram. Verat a.

STARCH.—*Chapped hands :*— Rub them with

starch powder, especially after taking them out of suds, or dish water. The same for *Erysipelas* to allay heat and pain.

Discoloration from a bruise—Raw surface:—
Moisten starch powder, or arrow root, with cold water, and lay it on the bruised or raw surface.

Dysentery—(Very painful with excessive straining): "Inject into the bowel from time to time, as occasion may seem to require, *boiled starch*, adult 2 ounces, containing 20 drops of Laudanum, or 5 grs of Chloral hydrate. The same greatly relieves the pain from *stone lodged in the ureter*.

STERILITY.—Alet θ. "Aletris Cordial." Borax 1x 5 gr. HELON. Con 2x. Iod. See Female—Ailments.

STING OF A BEE.—See Bee sting

STOMACH.—Pains, Sensations, Conditions :—
Aching pain: *Arg n.* Bry. *Con.* IG. KAL C. Mer. Nux v. *Oenanth θ.* Sul.

Acidity: Borax. Cal c. Cham. IRIS V. Lyc. Mag c. *Nat c. Nat m. Nat p.* NUX V. ROBIN. Sul. Sul a. (See Charcoal. Elm. Gum Arabic. Lime. Soda. See Diet H. Z.)

Alive, jumping sensation, CRO. Sang. Tarant C.

Biting, *Hell.* Mos. Stram.

Boring, *Agar. Ars.* Carbol a. *Nat s.* Sep.

Bruised feeling, *Asa.* Caust. *Mer prot. Nux v.* Lyc. Sul.

Bubling, Hydropho—As from Lime slaking, Caust.

Bulging pit, Cal c.

Burning, Æs. ARS. Cal p. CANTH. *Caust.*

Carb v. Cic. Dios. Lach. Mer c. *Mez.* PHO
Sul. Tereb.

— With intense thirst, Ars. Canth.

Clawing, COC. *Carbo an.* Lyc. Nux v. *Sul a.*
ZN.

Clutching, Bell. Cann I.

Coldness, Absinth. *Bovis.* Caps. CHIN. Elaps.
PHO. RHUS. Sul a—As if fall of cold water,
Kal c. Kreo—As if lump of ice lying in it,
Bovis.

Constriction, COC. Colo. CUP M. GRAP.
Nux v. Sul.

Cramp, Ant c. CUP M. COC. KAL C. Grap.
LYC. *Stan.*

Crawling, Lactuca. Pul.

Cutting, Bell. Cal c. *Coc.* DIOS. Kal c. Sep.

Distension, Arg n. ASA. Cal c. Caps. *Carb. v.*
CHIN. LYC. Mos.

Distress, anguish, Cann I *θ*. Dios *θ*. See
Gastralgia.

Drawing, *Bry.* Cham. *Cup m.* Ig.

Dyspepsia: HYDRAS 3x 5 grs. before meals.
Oenanth θ 10 drops after meals. *Ova l* 3x.
SANG 3x 5 grs. before meals. Strych 3x.
Kola. Nut 5 gr. tablets before meals. See
various symptoms of the stomach. See Diet.
C. R. S. See *Indigestion.*

Empty "gone" feeling: Carbo an. CIMI.
Hydras. Hydroct. Gel. IG. Lept. Pet. Pod.
Sep. Ustil. Verat a—With sinking faintness,
Dios. Dig. Pho. Tab—Not relieved by eat-
ing, Sep.

Eructation—belching: Aco. Amb. Arg n.
Carb v. Pho. Pul.

— Bitter, *Arn.* NUX V. *Pul.* Tart e.

— Burning, Iod. Lyc. Ph a.

— Loud, ARG N. *Con.* Mer bin. Pet. PLAT.

— Sour, Cham. *Lyc.* Nat c. Nat m. NAT P. *Nux v.* Sul. Sul a.

— Tasting—foul, *Mer.* Nux v. Sul—As of spoiled egg, *Arn.* Cham. Sul—Garlic, Mos.

Fermentation: Apo c. Cro. Grap.

Flatulence, Collin—See Distension.

Fluttering, Æs. *Cact. Nux v.* Xanth.

Fullness. See Distension.

Gastralgia, Pain in the Stomach: Abies n 1x. CANN I 1x trit. 5 gr. COCAINE 2x. *Coc.* DIOS θ 60 drops in hot sweetened water. EUCA. MANG 1x 5grs. before meals. Nux v. PASS θ 30 to 60 drops. Pul. Sul. ZN— Pains as from hunger, Nit a. Verat a—Pressure of food in the stomach, "as of a stone," Bry. Lyc. Nux v. Pul—Or "hard boiled egg," Abies n—Terrible pain, Arg n 2x in water. Atrop 2x—Especially after dinner, Arg n. Cedron. See Gastric Ulcer.

Gastritis: See Fever—Gastric.

Gastric catarrh, chronic, or subacute: Carbol a. *Chel.* HYDRAS 3x. Homar 3x. Lyc. *Pet. Pip m* θ 5 drops before meals. SANG 3x—Relief by eating, Lyc. See EUCALYP. See Diet R. and S. See various symptoms of the stomach.

Gastric ulcer: ARG N 2x in water. Ars. Atrop 2x. Bar c. Bism 1x, 10 grs, 3 hours. HYDRAS 3x. *Hydroct.* Mang 1x.

— Belching loud violent, ARG N.

— Burning pain—Black vomit, Ars. Kreo.

— Horrible pain—Bloody vomit, *Atrop.* Bell.

— Violent burning and retching, Canth.

— Yellow tongue and sour vomit, Kal bi.

— Hæmatemesis, Bell. Ipe. Ham. Kreo. Ice.

— Perforation. Opium for days.

Sixteen cases of ulceration of the stomach reported cured with Resorcin 5 grs, in an ounce of water, taken when the stomach is empty. It stops the pain at once. Controls the sensitiveness of the stomach, and enables it to retain food nicely. Rest in bed in severe cases is to be enjoined. Restrict the food to milk—predigested in some cases. "Ice cream diet exclusive will cure the disease." Food by suppository, or per rectum may effect a cure. See Food. (See Charcoal. EUCALYP.)

Gagging, Ant c. *Cina.* Cap m. Ipe.*Kreo.* Lob i. *Pod.*

Griping, COC. CUP M. Grap. Lyc. *Nux v. Pho.* SIL.

Gnawing, Am m. *Mer. Sep.* Stry.

Gurgling, Ana. Fl ac. Kal iod. Lob i—When drinking, Cina. *Cup m. Laur.* Thuj.

Hæmatemesis. See Vomiting—of blood.

Hardness, Ars. *Kreo.* Lept. Mer prot. Pul.

Hanging down relaxed, Stap.

Heartburn, Cal c. *Card θ. Caps.* Carb v. (See Charcoal). Con. DIOS θ. Iod. LYC. *Nat m.* Pip m θ. PHO—Constant, *Lob i.*

— During meals, Mer—Especially after meals, Carb v. *Lyc.* Nux v. *Pho.* Sep—From sugar, ZN—With drowsiness, Lyc. Pho—At night on turning in bed, Con.

Heat, *Aco.* Apis. Arg n. *Ars.* Canth. Nux v. Sep. *Tereb.*

Heaviness of food, as if undigested, *Abies n.* Bry. Lyc. *Nux v.* Pul.

Hiccough, Hyo. Ig—During meal, Mer— After meal, Cyc. Hyo. Mer. Verat v.

Hunger canine, Cal c. *Cina. Mer.* STAN. Sec.

Sul. *Stap*. ZN—Must eat often, Grap. IOD.
Lyc. Pet—Cannot wait for dinner, so faint,
Sep. *Sul*—Greedy, hasty eating, Coff. *Hep.*
Ig. Plat. Sep. *Sul.* ZN.

— Night hunger, Chin. Pho. Ph a—Wakens
up smothering and must eat for relief, Grap.

Indigestion: From overloading the stomach,
Ant c—From *ice cold* food or drink, *Ars.*
Bry. *Bellis p*—From rich fat food, Pet. *Pul-*
Lacto-pepsin, adult 10 to 20 grs; or rennet
wine adult, a wineglassful taken immediately after meals, is the approved mode of
treatment for *Indigestion, Dyspepsia, Liver
Complaint, Heart burn, Water brash.* Pep-
tic salt may be used in the place of salt at
the table to aid digestion.

Nausea: Apomo. IPE. *Kreo.* LOB I. Sil.
SYMPHORI 200. *Tab* 2x—Sudden deathly,
Ferr p. Dig.

—In the morning, *Dig.* Ip. *Nux v.* Sep. *Sil.*
Sul.

—From a drink of water, *Ham.* Nux v. *Pho.*
Verat a.

—From riding, *Coc.* Lyc.

—From *closing the eyes*, Therid; or *steadfast
gaze*, Therid.

—From smell of food, Colch.

—Felt in the throat, Coc. Ph a. Phyt.

—During pregnancy. See Female—Pregnancy.

Numbness: Aco. Castor.

Pulsation: See Throbbing.

Regurgitation: See Eructation,

Retching, Bell. *Cina*. HELL. IP. KREO.
Nux v. POD.

—In the morning, Cina.

—With cold sweat, Tart e. *Verat a.*

Spasm, Augus. Card.

Stitches, *Bry.* Cal c. *Chel. Kal c.* Nit a. RHUS. SEP.

Swelling, See Distension.

Throbbing, *Asa.* CACT. Glo. Nux v. OL. PUL. *Sep.* Tart e.

Tenderness, Bar c. *Bry.* Kal c. *Mer c.* Nat m. *Nux v.* Pho. Sil—With fever, *Aco. Bell.* Ox a ix. Sang—From coughing, Lyc. Stan. Verat a.

Tightness: Carb v. Chin. Lyc—As of a cord tied tightly around the waist, Arg n.

Trembling, Agar. *Arg n.* Carb v. *Cimi.* Nat m. RHUS.

Twisting, Kal c. *Nat m.* Pho. Plat.

Ulcer: See Gastric ulcer.

Vomiting: AMYG *θ.* Ant c. Apomo 200. *Cocaine 2x.* Codein ¼ gr in water. IPE. Iris min. IRIS V. *Lob i.* Pepo. SYMPHORI 200. TAB 2x. Tart c. VERAT A. Verat v.

—Easy without much nausea, Apom. Phyt— Incessant, MER C—With intense nausea, Amyg. Gambog. IPE. *Pepo. Symphori* 200.

—Violent straining, *Gambog.* Tart e. VERAT A. *Verat v*—With cramp, *Cup m*— With cold sweat, *Verat a.*

—Vomiting from any cause, *Cocaine* 2x. Codein ¼ gr. in water. Oil of Cloves 1 drop in water. " Ingluvin, adult 5 to 10 grs; repeat the dose in an hour if necessary. To *prevent recurrence* take a dose night and morning, or before meals."

—A baby that vomited almost constantly was cured by ½ gr of Pepsin placed upon its tongue.

(See Diet, C. D. E. Z—See Ice. Mustard.)

—In the morning, Amyg *θ*. Con. *Dig*. Ipe. *Lach*. *Nux v*. *Pepo*. Pul. *Symphori* 200—

—During menses, Grap.

—In the evening, *Kreo*. Pul.

—In pregnancy:—See Female—Pregnancy.

—In Typhoid: See Ice.

—Of Drunkards: See Alcoholism.

—From Chloroform: Saturate a cloth with vinegar and hold it to the nose, until return of consciousness, or after if necessary. This will prevent vomiting.

—From cancer or ulcer in stomach: See Gastric ulcer.

—Sympathetic, Bell. Hell. Kreo. (See Gagging.)

—Relieved by eating, Ig—Breakfast, Bovis—By sipping cold water, Cup m. Lob i.

—Black vomit, Arg n. ARS. Crotal. *Hyo. Ipe. Pho*. NUX V. Sec. *Verat a*.

—Black vomit from cancer or ulcer, Ars. Bacill. Condu. Thuj.
(Like coffee grounds, Con.)

—Bloody, *Aco. Arn*. Cinnamon *θ. Cocaine* 2x. *Ferr*. Ham. Hyo. IPE. *Pho*. Stan. Verat a.

—Bluish, Ars. Cup.

—Brown, Ars. Bism. Con. PB.

—Fæcal, Ars. Bell. *Bry* OP. PB. *Sul*.

—Food, Ars. *Bry*. FER P. *Mer*. Nat m. NUX V. *Pho*. Sul.

—Frothy, Aco. Pod. Verat a.

—Green, Aco. *Ars*. Eup per. IRIS VER. *Mer c*. NAT S. *Verat a*.

—Hot, Pod.

—Luminous, Pho—In streaks, Croton.

—Milk, *Apom*. Ars. Carb v. Kal bi. Lach.

Mer c. *Sam*—Curdled, Sabin. *Sul.* Tart e—
Breast Milk in thick curds, ÆTH.

—Mucus—Slime: Ant c. Arg n. *Bell. Dul.*
IP. Mer c. Pho. Phyt. Pod. PUL. *Sul.*
TART E. Tereb. VERAT A.

—Sour, Cal c. *Cham.* IRIS V. *Lyc. Nat p.*
Nux v. *Pho. Pul.* Sul.

—Sweet, Cup a. Kal bi. *Kreo.*

—Urinous, Op.

—Watery, *Bry.* Cal c. *Caust.* Bell. Bry. *Dros.*
ROBIN.

—White, *Æth.* Ars. Colch. *Mer c. Verat.*

—Worms, *Aco.* Cic. Sec.

—Yellow, Ars. Colo. Grat. KAL BI. Tereb—
Bright yellow, bitter, Kal bi.

Water brash (See Charcoal), Bism. CAL C.
Carb v. Grap. IRIS V. Nux v. Pul. SEP. Sul—
After eating, Sil. Sul—After drinking, Nit a.
Sep—Morning, Sul—Evening, Cyc—Night,
Carb v. Grap.

Things that Disagree :—(See Aggravation—
from food.)

Coffee, Cham. Ig. Nux v.

Tea, Chin Ferr.

Eggs, Ferr

Milk, Æth. *Cal c. Mer.* SIL. *Sul*—Vomited as
soon as swallowed, Apomo. Sul—Breast milk
vomited, Sil—In thick curds, *Æth.* (See
Diet G. H. Z. See Elm.)

Onions, Thuj.

Pastry, Pet. Pul.

Potatoes, Alu.

Sweets, Arg n. ZN.

The *simplest food* causes distress in the
stomach, *Carb v.* Hep—Even the smell of
food nauseates, *Colch.* Dig; or sight of it, Mos.

Water is disgusting, Ham. Pho—Causes gagging, Hep. Phos. Verat a; or hiccough, Ig; or pain in the chest, Thuj; or stomach pains, Apo c; or is immediately thrown up, *Ars.* Sil. Verat a; or vomited as soon as becomes warm in the stomach, *Pho.* Verat a.

Aversion to:—

Bread, *Kal c.* Lyc. NAT M. Nux v. *Sul*—Bread and butter, Cyc. *Sang.*

Butter, Carb v. Chin. *Mer.*

Coffee, Bry. *Nat c.* Nat m. NUX V. *Rhus.*

Fat, *Carb v.* Hep. NAT M. *Pet.* PUL. Sul.

Fish, Grap. ZN.

Meat, Cal c. Carb v. FERR. Ig. *Mur a. Nit a.* PUL. Sep. SIL. *Sul.*

Milk, Cal c. CINA. IG. *Nat c. Sep.* Sil. Sul—Mother's milk, Cina. *Mer.* Sil.

Pork, Colch.

Potatoes, Thuj.

Salt, *Grap.* Selen,

Sour things, Bell. Coc. FERR. *Sul.*

Sweets, *Caust. Grap.* Nit a. PHO. Sul.

Warm food, Bell. Ig. *Ferr.* PHO. *Sil.*

Water, Ham. Pho.

Disgust for food : Ip. Kal c. Nat m—Although hungry, Asa. Coc—Cannot bear the sight, Mos. Symphori; or smell, Dig. *Colch.* Symphori 200; or thought of food, Nat m.

Craving for:—

Beer, *Aco. Caust.* Nux v. Pet. *Sul.*

Bitter things, *Dig.* NAT M. Nux v.

Brandy, Ars. *Hep. Lach.* Sul.

Chalk, lime, clay, ALU. Calc c. *Nit a.* Nux v.

Charcoal, *Cic.* Con.

Cheese, Arg n.

Eggs, Cal c.

Fat, Nit a. Nux v.

Herring, smoked, *Nit a*. Verat a.

Milk, APIS. Ars. CAL C. *Mer. Rhus. Sil.*
Stap—Cold milk, Rhus.

Oysters, Apis. Lach. Rhus.

Pickles, Hep. Stap—See Sour.

Potatoes, raw, Ars. Cal c.

Rags, Alu.

Rice, dry, Alu.

Salt, Carb v. Cal c. NAT M. Verat a.

Smoked meat, Cal p.

Sour things—Acids: *Aco.* Ant c. ARN. *Chin.*
Hep. *Sul.*

Sweets, ARG N. *Chin.* Ip. *Kal c. Lyc*—Which
disagree, Arg n.

Tea grounds, Alu.

Uneatable things, Bry.

Wine, ACO. *Cal c.* Cic. Hep. Lach. *Sep.* STAP.

During meals, or when eating :—

Fullness, sudden, LYC—After eating a little,
Con. Nat m. Sul.

Food gulped up as soon as swallowed, Bism.
Pho. Mer—When partly swallowed returns,
Asa.

Heartburn, Mer c. Nat m.

Hiccough, Mer.

Spasm, Mag m. Mag p.

Stomach-ache, *Bar c.* Sep— Every mouthful
causes pain, *Cal p* 1x. *Nux m.* Stap.

Sweat, Carb v. Nat m. Nit a—In the face, *Ig.
Nat m*—About the head, Cham. Nux v—
Hot sweat, Cham.

Urging to stool, Ferr.

Vertigo, Am c. Sil.

Vomiting, sudden, Ars. Mer. *Rhus*—Without
any apparent cause, Mer.

After meals, or after eating :—

Belching — Eructation, ARG N. Ars. *Bry.* Nux v. Pul. *Sil.* Sul—Acrid, Nux m—Bitter, Bry. Chin—Loud, *Arg n.* Cal c—Sobbing, Cyc—Sour, Carb v.

Distension of the stomach, *Carb v.* CHINA. Lach. Lyc. Grap. NUX M.

Drowsiness, CHIN. Lach. *Lyc.* NUX M. *Nux v.* PHO. Sil. ZN.

Empty feeling, Verat a.

Face red, Lyc. Nux v. Sil—Red and hot, Nux v.

Faintness, Dig.

Flatulence, *Chin.* Carb v. Kal c. *Sul.*

Food lies heavy "like a stone," Æs. *Bry. Nux v.* Pul.

As if lodged in the chest, Abies n. Œnanth θ.

Hands hot, Lyc. *Pho.*

Head hot, Lyc. Nux v.

Headache, BISM. Carb v. Chin. Lyc. NUX M. *Nux v.* Rhus. *Sul.*

Heart burn, Am c. Con. Mang ıx. NAT M. PHO. Sil.

Heat, *Cal c.* Nux v. *Pho.* Viol t.

Hiccough, *Cyc.* HYO. *Mer.* Verat a.

Indolence, *Chin.* Lach. Nux v. *Pho.*

Pain in the stomach—Stomach ache, Ars. CHIN. *Cocaine* 2x. COC. *Mang* ıx. NUX V. ŒNOTH θ 20 drops after meals. *Pul.* Sul. ZN—Stitches, Verat a.

Stitches in the anus, Lyc. Nux v—In the bowels, Verat a.

Sweat, Nit a. Sul a—In the face, Cham. Viol t. (See During Meal.)

Vertigo, Lach. Nat m. *Nux v. Pul.* Sul.

STOOL.

Vomiting, ARS. FERR P. *Hyo. Ipe. Nux v.*
Pho. Sul. TAB 2x.

Water brash, Cal c. Sil. Sul.

Weakness, CHIN. DIG. Nit a. Sul. Thuj.

STOOL.—See Bowel.

STRABISMUS.—See Eye.

STRANGURY.—See Urinary Organs.

STRICTURE.—See the part.

STRUMA.—See Scrofula.

• **STUPOR.**—See Sleep. See the Affection—Cause.

STUTTERING.—See Speech.

STYE.—See Eye-lid.

SUB-INVOLUTION.—*Alet.* Sec. *Ustil. Ergot,*
hypoderm—See Female.

SUGAR.— *Wound dressing:* Keep the wound com-
pletely covered with pulverized sugar. "This is
equal to Iodoform."

Baby's sore mouth: Reduce granulated sugar by
moisture to a paste, and with the finger rub
this upon the sore surface several times a day.

Diabetes: A case reported cured by eating freely
of maple sugar.

Speedy purgative: "Sugar of milk, adult, 3 teaspoonfuls in half teacupful of hot milk, or hot
water, taken one hour before breakfast, will
move the bowels in two hours."

Universal antidote: Sugar in water, solution
thick and rich as can be swallowed; fill the
stomach. If the kind of poison taken is not
known, give white of egg and strong coffee
with the sugar. See Antidote.

SULPHUR.—*Lumbago, Sciatica, Rheumatism:*
Imbed the seat of pain in flowers of Sulphur,
and hold in place by compress.

Open Cancer: Dust it full of Sulphur, pulv.

Ague, Locomotor ataxia, Paralysis: Sulphur ointment to spine daily.

Guard against Colic, Cramps, Piles, Rheumatism, Cholera: Carry brimstone about the person.

Hay fever—Rose cold: Put 10 grs. of flowers of Sulphur into a vessel, saturate it with alcohol, and set fire to it, and inhale the fumes, during ten minutes, four times a day. Same for *Chronic Sore throat, Follicular Pharyngitis, Chronic Bronchitis, Chronic Catarrh, Consumption:* During first eight or ten days, irritation or cough, may increase, but afterwards the recovery will be rapid.

Pimples: Dust with Sulphur powder on going to bed.

SUMMER COMPLAINT--CHOLERA INFANTUM.—See Bowel.

SUNSTROKE.—Camp *0*. GLO 3x. Hyo. *Therid.* *Quinea hypoderm.* Inject water copiously into the bowels—Heat apoplexy, Chin. Hyo. *Nux v.*

SUPPOSITORY.—(B. and T.)

Anal—Rectal:—

For Constipation, Collinsonia. Hydrastis.

— Fissure, Iodoform.

— Fistula, Iodoform.

— Piles bleeding, Æsculus + Hamamelis. Hamamelis.

— — Non bleeding, Æsculus. Æsculus+ Hamamelis.

— — obstinate with constipation, Æs.+Collin -! Ham. Collinson.

— — Painful piles, Stramonium.

— Prostate gland enlarged, Iodoform.

— Pin worms, Santonine.

— PAIN, Opium.

Vaginal:

For Amenorrhœa, Arsenic.

— Aphthæ of os, Thuja.

— Bleeding, Arsenic—With burning, Arsenic.

— Bleeding granulations, Carbolic acid.

— Bleeding excrescences, Thuja.

— Cauliflower excrescences, Thuja.

— Cancer, Carbolic acid. Eucalyptus.

— Catarrh, Eucalyptus. Sanguinaria nit.

— Congestion and Inflammation, Belladon. Gelsem. Hamamel.

— — Follicular inflammation of vagina, Calendula.

— Endometritis, Cimicifuga, Gelsemium.

— Dysmenorrhœa, Cimicif. Iodoform. Opium.

— Erosion of mouth of cervix, Calendula.

— Induration and swelling of uterus and ovaries, Iodine.

— Leucorrhœa, Arsenic—Stringy, tenacious discharge, Hydrastis—Acrid, corroding the linen, Iodine.

— Polypus, Sanguinaria nit. Thuja.

— Prolapsus, Belladonna.

— Menorrhagia, Arsenic.

— *Threatening puerperal Fever*, heat, pain, tenderness, OPIUM.

— Tumors, erectile burning, Thuja.

SUPPURATION.—Arn. *Carbol ac.* Hep. Iod. Sil—Prolonged, Skook—Promotive, Hep—Preventive, IOD. *Pho. Pyrogen.* Sil. "Chamomile tea." (See Salicyl. Logwood.)

SURGICAL DRESSING. — See Wound. See Amputation.

SWEAT CURE.—See Lime—Sweat.
SWEAT.—

Only on *covered* parts, Thuj.

Only on under side, lying, Chin.

All over except the head, Rhus.

Bloody, Cal c. Crotal. *Lach.* NUX M. Nux v.

Cold, clammy, CUPRUM ARS 3x. *Ars.* Carb
v. *Mer.* Ph. a. Tab. Verat a—Cold and sour,
Hep. Lyc. Mer. Sul.

Oily, *Agar. Bry. Chin.* MER. Thuj.

Profuse, exhausting, Aco. PILO 2x—Day and
night especially, about the chest, Hep—
Without relief, Alo. Hep. *Mer.* Tart e—In
rheumatic fever, Bell. *Bry.* TART E—In
typhoid fever, Ars. Pho. Verat a.

Night Sweat:—(See Diet L.) AGARICIN 1x
trit 1 gr. Bacill 200. CHAM 0 5 drops in hot
water at bed time. China. CHINA ARS 2x.
Euca. Iod. Kal c. Nit a. Ph a. SIL. Sul. Thuj
—Cold night sweat, Dig. Lyc. Mer—Offensive,
Carbo an. Pso. Sil—Staining yellow, Carbo an.
Mer. Thuj—Preventing sleep, Ars. Mer. Verat
a—Driving from bed, Mer—Sweat, not during
sleep, but profuse immediately on waking,
Sam.

"A pinch of German Chamomile flowers
stirred in a cup of boiling water and taken at
bed time will cure night sweat in a week."

Morning sweat after waking, *Cal c.* Nit a. Pho.
Sul—Sour, Iod.

Local sweat: See Alcohol. Hot water.

Sweating Fever: See Fever—Sweating.

Color of Sweat:—

Greenish, Cup.

Red stain, Dul. Nux v.

Yellow, Carbo an. Grap. MER. *Rheum.* Stan.

J   289

Odor of Sweat:—
As of honey, Thuj.
—Spice, Rhod.
—Spoiled egg, Stap.
— Onion, Bovis. Lyc.
—Musk, Apis. Pul. Sam.
Musty, Nux v. Rhus. Stan.
Offensive, Bap. *Carbo an. Grap. Kal p. Kreo.*
   MER. SIL. *Sul.* See Locality.
Sour, Arn. BRY. Hep. Ipe. Mag c. MER.
   RHEUB. *Sep. Sil. Sul*—Hot and sour, Bell—
   Morning sour, Iod.
Urinous odor, Berb. Bovis. *Canth. Colo.* Grap.
   Lyc. *Nit a.*

SWOON.—Cann I. Mos.

SYCOSIS.—See Skin.

SYNCOPE.—See Fainting.

SYNOVITIS.—Apis. Bry. Carbol ac. Kali m.
Sticta. See Limb—Joint.

SYPHILIS.—Ars bro. Ars iod. Aur. Bacil 30-200.
Carbol a. Hoang. *Iris v.* KAL IOD. Kreo.
MER. PHYT. POD. *Tarant C.* "All forms
the one remedy." POD.
   Of infants, *Ars iod.* Bacill. KREO. Pod.
   Affecting the *skin* especially, Ars bro. *Ars iod.*
     Kal iod. Mer. Phyt. THUJ.
   — The Bones, AUR. Fl ac. KAL IOD. *Mer.*
     Mez. Pho. Still.
   — The Eyes, Ars iod. Kal iod. Mer.
   — The Nose, AUR. Kal bi. *Kal iod.* Kal m.
   — The Mouth and Throat, Fl ac. Hydras. Iod.
     Kal bi. *Kal iod. Mer.* Nit a PHYT θ—
     Cracks in corners of the mouth, Nit a.
   " Remedies for syphilis should be given, as a
     rule, in their lower attenuations. In ob-

stinate cases Kal iod may be given pure, 15
to 20 grs, 6 hours "

Bubo: Forming, Mer s. PHYT θ in. and ex.

— Indolent, Ars iod. *Mer iod.*

— Open—Treat as Chancre.

Chancroid—Simple Soft Chancre: Ars. Hep.
Jac. Kal bi. Mer. Ph a. Sil. Dust with Bism.
powder. Bism. 5 per cent in Lanolin; apply.
"Dust with Quinea powder every other day.
Cure in a week." Iodoform dressing, secured
by compress. See *Solar Cautery.*

True Chancre—Indurated Ulcer:—

— Recent uncomplicated, Mer 3x.

— Red edge, hard base, Mer 3x.

— Painful bleeding, Mer 3x. Nit a.

— Phagedenic, Mer c. 3x-30-200.

— Ichorous pus, Ars. Mer c 3x.

— Painless with Bubo, Mer iod, 3x.

— Gangrenous, Ars. Ars iod 3x. Mer c. 3x.

— Fungous growths, Nit a. Thuj.

Corroding discharges, Ars. Kreo. Nit a.

Dust the chancre with Calomel powder. Dress
with a mixture of Camphor gum 1 drachm,
Acetate of Lead 1 drachm, starch 2 ounces;
and over this place a pad of borated cotton,
saturated with olive oil, and keep it in place
by compress. "Apply Vienna paste; or still
better sulphuric acid mixed with vegetable
charcoal to make a half solid paste. This
converts the ulcer into a simple wound,
which will soon heal." "Cleanse with Castile soap and water, and upon the ulcer lay
a pledget of lint moistened with Calendula θ
1 part, to water 4 parts; change 3 times a
day; give Mer prot 1x, 2 grs every night
for a week, then every other night for two

TABES.

weeks, then twice a week, until the ulcer heals. Cure in from 6 to 8 weeks. If despite this treatment the chancre stands in *statu quo;* then touch the sore with ointment made of Nitrate of Mercury, mixed with 5 parts of simple cerate; or apply lightly Nitric acid; and give Mer c 2x trit, 3 times a day. If there should be a tendency to gangrene, give Ars iod 3x trit. in alternation with Mer c.'' (See *Solar Cautery.*)

TABES.—See Atrophy.

TAMPON.—See Alum. Borax. Glycerine. Vinegar.
"To preserve a sponge tent from offensive odor, charge it with a 5 per cent solution of the oil of cloves.''

TANNIN.—*Carbuncle:* Sprinkle on it Tannin powder, dry, as long as it will dissolve; wash off and apply fresh daily.

Abrasion, Excoriation, Sore Nipples, Tender piles, Tender feet: Tannic acid 4 ounces, glycerine 1 drachm, and water 2 drachms; mix: Apply daily.

Nasal Catarrh. Catarrhal affections of the throat, Relaxed sore throat, Elongated uvula: Tannin glycerole; use it as a gargle, and snuff it up the nostrils, until it drops back into the throat.

Otorrhœa. Deafness: Tannin glycerole; a few drops in the ear daily, retained by plug of cotton.

Dandruff: Cleanse the scalp with alcohol dilute, wipe dry, and rub on glycerole of Tannin, 20 grs. to the ounce, twice a week.

TAPE WORM.—See Worm.

TARTAR ON TEETH.—Lave with dilute vinegar. See Iodine.

TASTE.—See Mouth—Taste.

TEETH.—See Mouth—Teeth.

TEETHING.—See Mouth—Teething—See Infant.

TEMPERATURE.—Normal, 98.6°; dangerously high, 105°; usually fatal, 107°; collapse, 95°; dangerously low, 93°; usually fatal, 92°.

TENDERNESS.—See parts affected—See Myalgia.

TERROR.—See Mind—Night terror. See Sleep.

TESTES.—See Male.

TETANUS.—See Lockjaw.

TETTER.—See Skin—Herpes.

THIRST.—See Mouth—Thirst.

THROAT.—

Diphtheria:—(See *Chlorine.* Hydrogen. Kerosene. Thuja. *Turpentine.*)

Alcohol diluted one-half with water, a teaspoonful every hour; and gargle with the same.

"Iodine 1x and Salicyl acid 1x; 10 drops of each in ½ tumbler of water, a teaspoonful every ½ hour alternately, until better, then at longer intervals."

"For ten years have used only Carbolic acid 2x, with uniform success; dose 1 drop in water, every hour, gargle with the same."

"Bromine one per cent. solution in distilled water. Kept in a dark bottle in a dark place: Give from 1 to 3 drops in sweetened water, from a glass spoon, or wine glass, every hour; or if croupy, every ¼ hour. After evidence of improvement, reduce the doses, and extend the time between them,

but·not over two hours. The first three or
four doses of the Bromine, reduced the
pulse rate from 140 to 80. Complete restoration in three days."

"Pyrogen 6 in water, dose every hour or two,
gives very satisfactory results."

Kal bi 2x and Mer bin 2x, 5 grs. of each in ½
glass of water, taken alternately, a teaspoonful every ½ hour at first, then length-
ening the intervals as the case would admit, cured 140 cases in succession. Although in some cases the medicines simply
held the disease in check for several days,
yet the final triumph was sure.

"Oil of Turpentine The victor" : to a child
seven years old, 1 teaspoonful in a ½ teacup
of warm milk 12 hours."

Sulphur Treatment—"No failure" : Place a
teaspoonful of pulverized sulphur in a small
plate, and some water in another; then with
a *moistened* swab, apply the sulphur to the
fauces until a large portion of it has been
taken up; then give 3 grains of Sulphur in
toddy. This cures the case."

Reported 80 cures in succession with Sulphate
of Iron powder, blown upon the patches,
several times a day.

Brewer's yeast, a teaspoonful every 2 hours in
water or milk, shows a good record.

Borax, child 2 grs, 2 hours, adult 5 to 10 grs, 2
hours; only three deaths in 60 cases.

"Platt's Chlorides, diluted (1:1) with water,
applied by cloths saturated therewith, placed
over the nose and mouth, 10 minutes at a
time. Every hour, or half hour, or almost

constantly in desperate cases. Constitutes the only treatment needed."

"Pineapple juice, gargle and swallow *ad libitum*. It aids in the cure, is pleasant, refreshing, and does not interfere with the action of medicine."

Aching back and limbs, PHYT.

Beginning on the left side, Lach—Right, Lyc.

Black lips, cracked, Mur a.

Burning blisters in the throat, Canth.

Choking on waking, Lach. Naj.

Cold clammy sweat, Lach.

High fever, *Apis.* Bell. PHYT *θ. Pyrog.* Tarant C.

Hot scanty urine, Canth.

Nasal discharge, thin, corroding, Kali permang. Mur a.

Œdema of the neck and face, *Apis.* Ars.

Patch *gray*, Apis. Mer cya. Mur a. Phyt— Purple, Apis. Lach—Yellow, Kal bi.

Prostration extreme, Apis. Ars. Canth., Kal. permang. LACH. Mer cya. Mur a.

Putrid malignant type, Ars. BAP. KAL PERMANG 2x. Kal p 3x. Kali m. MER CYA 3x. *Mur a.* Nit a. Tarant C. Thuj— DIET nourishing; *Milk. Egg. Broth. Cream. Ice Cream.* Koumis.

Diphtheria developed upon the Skin, (*on an abraded surface, or on a sore*)*:* Apply Sulphate of Copper, 20 grs, to the ounce of water; or strong solution of Quinia; or Naphthalin.

Diphtheritic Croup:—Ars iod 2x. Kal bi 2x. "KAL BI 2x and SPONG 2x, ¼ hour alt." Kali m. Kal p—Choking on waking, Lach. Naj. (See EUCALYPT. *Iodine. Turpen.*)

Paralysis following diphtheria: Bap. Coc.
Gel θ. Kal p. NUX V. Sil. ZN p 3x.

Quinsy, Tonsilitis:—Apis. Bar c. *Bell.* Caps.
Guai θ drop doses on tablets. " *Ferr p. and
Kali m.*" Lach. Mer bin. MER C 3x. Pepper
grain tea gargle. Mustard seed tea gargle.
(See Hot water. Ice. Kerosene.)
— Gathering, Hep. Mer. (See Hot Water.
See Poultice.)
— Putrid, Am m. Ars. *Bap. Mer.*
— Ulcerative, Bapt. Hydroct. Mer. Phyt.

**Sore Throat in General—Catarrh of the
Throat:**—Aco. *Apis.* Bar c. *Bell.* Carbol a.
Gel. *Guai θ. Lach. Mer.* MER C 3x. Mullein
oil, 1 to 5 drops. Gargle with Pepper grain
tea or Capsicum θ dilute. Or gargle with
Mustard seed tea, or Sinapis θ dilute.

Chronic Sore Throat:—Fl ac. *Hep.* LACH.
LYC. Mer c. *Phyt* Sul.
— Soothed by swallowing, Cist. Ig.
— From public speaking, or singing—"Clergy-
man's sore throat." (See Diet A.) Arn.
Arum. Arg n. Rhus— With hoarseness,
Ferr p. PHO, low, in water, or on tablets.
(See Alcohol. Benzo. Ham. Ice. Ichthy.
Iodine. Kerosene. Lactic ac. Mustard.
Myrrh. Potash. Sulphur. Thuj.)

Ulceration of the Throat:—Hep. Kal bi. Lach.
Mer. Mur a. Nit a. Sul—Glistening, Lac c—
Putrid, AM C. Arum. AIL. Apis. BAP. Cist.
Crotal. *Hydroct.* LACH. *Mer.* Mur a. Nit a.

**Pains, Sensations and Conditions of the
Throat:**—
Aching, Lach.
Ball ascending, sense of: Asa. Con. Ig. Kalmi.

Lyc. PB—Descending by swallowing, and then returning, Lach. Rum c.

Burning, Am c. *Ars.* Arum. Bell. CANTH. CAPS. Lach. MER C. RHUS. *Sul*—Like fire, Æs. *Canth. Mez.* Phyt—Like pepper, Caps—As if scalded, Sang.

Burning stinging, Aco. APIS. Mer.

Blisters, Apis. Canth. *Rhus.*

Choking, nervous, Arg n. *Asa.* Bell. Cic. *Coc.* Mag p. PHYT. Val—Constant sense of choking, Phyt—On waking, *Lach.* Naj. Sep—From fright, Ig. (Induce sneezing.)

Coldness, Caust. Laur. *Verat a.*

Dryness, Alu. Bell. CIST. MER. Pho. *Phyt.* SANG. SUL. Stap—Especially in the morning on waking, *Ail.* Alu. NUX M. Phyt. Sang—Dry heat, Cham. Mos—Dry glistening, Pho—Painful dryness, Kalmi. *Lach.* Mer — Impeding deglutition, Bell. Hyo. Lach. Stram.

Enlargement, sense of: Hyper. *Lach. Phyt*—With burning, *Phyt.*

Gulping, Caust. Mag p—When walking against the wind, Con.

Gurgling sound, when drinking, Cup m. Lach. Laur.

Hawking (See Benzo), Kal c. Lach. Lyc. Pho. Sep—Constant, Arg n. Arum. Nat c—Violent, Nat c.

— Painful, Lach. Kal m.

— In cool damp weather, Dul.

— More in the morning, Arg n. *Arum.* Cist. Kal bi. Lach. *Nat m. Pet.* Pho. *Sep*—On walking, Lach.

— With choking, *Amb.* Lach — Gagging, Cal p.

— unable to raise the phlegm, Caust—Because
so tenacious, Am m. Arg n. *Kal c.*

— Phlegm easily raised in great quantities,
Arg m. Hep. Lob i.

— Mucus *bitter*, Arn. Cist. Tarant C—*Bloody*,
Fl ac. *Lyc.* Sep—*Cold*, Pho—Green, Ars.
Dros Colch—Geen, fetid tubercles, Mag c—
Hard lumps, Sil—Mouldy mass, Teucr—
Putrid, Angus—Salty, Ars. Mer. Nat s. Pho.
Sul—Soapy, Arum—Sour, Laur. Mag s. Pho
—Thick, ropy, Alu. *Hydras. Kal bi*—Yel-
low, Dros. Hydras. *Kal bi.* Rum c. Sil.

Heat in the throat, Cham. Ferr. Laur.

Itching, *Cist.* Sam. Spig.

Lump, or plug sense of, Alu. Nat m. PB.   See
Ball.

Nausea felt in the throat, Apis. Coc. Cyc. Ph a.

Narrowness, Constriction — Stricture: *Alu.*
Bell. Caust. *Lyc.* Nit a—Can only swallow
small morsels of food, Alu—Food clogs in
the throat, Alu. Kal c. Lyc—"Goes the
wrong way," Nat m—Descends with great
difficulty, Bap. Condu. PB—With pain between the shoulders, Kal c. *Rhus*—Food returns by the nose, Pet. Sil—Liquids so return, Bell. Lach. Mer.

Œdema of the Glottis: APIS. Ars. Sang—In ·
hale fumes of boiling vinegar.   Anoint
throat with Oil of Mustard.

Palate relaxed—Uvula elongated. See Mouth.

Paralysis of deglutition, Apis. Camp. GEL.
Kal bi. Sec.

— After diphtheria. See Diphtheria.

Pricking like a fishbone or splinter, Alu.
Arg n. Hep. Kal c. NIT A.

Rawness—Sense of: *Bar c. Bell.* Arg m.

Mag m. Mur a. *Stan*—When coughing, Arg m.

Relaxation. See Alum. Mustard.

Risings, Asa—Cold, Caust—Hot, Mer. Pho.

Scraping soreness, *Arg n.* Caust. Nux v. Pul.

Shooting pain, Amb. Gel—Into the ear when swallowing, KAL BI. Mer. Phyt.

Softness—Sense of—Like cotton, *Cist.* Pho.

Spasm, *Arg n.* BELL. IG. Nux v. Plat. STRAM.

Splinter—Sense of. See pricking.

Stinging, *Aco.* APIS Bell. IG. *Mer. Nit a.* Sep.

Stricture, *Alu. Bell* Cal c. Nat m. *Sul.* See Narrowness.

Stitches, Amb. Am m. Bry. HEP. IG. Kal bi. *Kal c.* Mer.

Suffocation, Bell. Hep. See Choking.

Tenderness to outside pressure, Ail. *Apis.* Bell. LACH.

Tickling, *Lach.* Nat a. RUM C. SANG—As from a crumb, Dros. Lach—As from a hair, Kal bi. Sil—Or thread, Val—Or loose skin, Thuj.

Tingling, Aco. Carb v. Lach.

Tonsillitis. See Quinsy.

Tonsils enlarged: Ars iod. Bar c. CAL IOD. Cal p. Kal m. *Nat m* 30. "Alum applied in stick form will speedily reduce the size."

Uvula relaxed: See Mouth—Purple uvula, Lach.

Valve—Sense of: Iod. Spo.

THRUSH.—See Mouth—Sore.

THUJA.—*Fig warts, Condylomata, Fungus growths, "Proud flesh:"* Thuja fl. ex. in. and ex. 3 times a day.

TIC DOULOUREUX.

Sloughing wound, Skin Cancer, Uterine Cancer, Gangrene:—Thuja fl. ex. on borated cotton, apply.

Itching anus, Vaginal itching, Itching ulcer, Syphilitic sore, Diphtheria: Thuja fl. ex. in. and ex.

Piles, Hydrocele: Inject Thuja fl. ex. pure, or dilute.

Ozæna: Thuja fl. ex. on cotton pledget; in one nostril for a few hours, then in the other.

TIC DOULOUREUX.—See Face—Neuralgia.

TINEA CAPITIS.—See Scalp—Favus.

TINGLING.—Aco—See the part affected.

TOBACCO, ANTIDOTE AND SUBSTITUTE.
—"Saturating tobacco with the juice of water cress, deprives it of all deleterious properties, without injuring its aroma"—"As a substitute for tobacco, smoke in pipe mullein leaves well dried in an oven; the mullein exhilarates and braces the nerves, and cures *bronchial* and *throat* affections."

TOBACCO HABIT.—For injuries resulting from the use of tobacco, especially heart affections, *Apoc.* Ars. *Aurum mur* 2x. Glo. *Ig.*

To produce disgust for tobacco take Plantago maj 6-30-200.

TOE.—See Limb—Leg (*foot*).

TONGUE.—See Mouth.

TONIC.—Aletris *fl.* Cinchona 1x 5 gr. before meals. Helon in 1x trit. Strychninum 3x trit. "Hensel's Tonicum" (B. & T.). Koumis. "There is no better tonic than Chamomile Tea." See Diet R. See Debility. See Prostration.

TONSILLITIS.—See Throat—Quinsy.

TOOTHACHE.—See Mouth—Teeth.

TOOTH EXTRACTION WITHOUT PAIN.—
Add together tincture of Cannabis Indica 1 part,
and water 3 parts; and in this solution soak cotton and apply it *around* the tooth to be drawn,
and *in* it if hollow; also warm the beaks of the
forceps, and dip them into the solution before
applying them. (See Chloroform. Ether.)

TRACHOMA.—See Eye-lids (*granular*.)

TRANCE.—Cann. I.

TRAUMATIC FEVER.—Aco. Arn. EUCA 1x.

TREMOR—TREMBLING.—See Nerve—Trembling.

TRICHINOSIS — TRICHINIASIS.—Ars 2x.
Apis. *Carbol a*. Ergot, hypoderm. Glycerine,
adult, ½ ounce, 4 times a day for 2 weeks.

TRISMUS.—See Lockjaw.

TUBERCULOSIS.—Bacill 30-200, one dose a
week. Pho. See Chest—Consumption.

TUMOR.—Ars bro. *Ars iod. Bacill* 200. Bar c.
CAL IOD. THUJ—From a hurt, Bellis p.
Cartilaginous, Cal fl. Cal p. Sil.
Fatty, Bar c.
Fibroid, Cal iod 1x. Sec 2x. Ustil 2x.—See
Female—Uterus.
Osseous—See Bone.
Ovarian, Apis. Thuj. Plat—See Female ovary.
Splenic, Ceanoth. See Spleen—Enlarge-
ment.
Pulsating, Bar c. Brom.
(See *Seaton*—See Clay. Iodine. Iodoform.
Ichthyol. Resorcin. Solar Cautery.)

TURPENTINE. — *Asthma*, *Croup*, *Cramp*,
Spasm, *Whooping Cough*, *Hæmorrhage from*

301

TWITCHING.

the Lungs. Inhale Spirits of Turpentine, from cloth or sponge. Protect the eyes from the smarting fumes.

Consumption:—Inhale fumes of Turpentine, five minutes at a time, several times a day.

Internal, deep-seated . pain:—Flannel cloths wrung out of hot water, and saturated with oil or Spirits of Turpentine, apply, and cover with warm compress.

Lockjaw from wound, prevented:—Pour hot Oil of Turpentine into the wound, and keep the wound saturated with Turpentine on cloth. The same for *Hospital gangrene.*

Diphtheria:—Burn in the room, near the patient, a mixture of Turpentine and Tar, in a pan, or deep dish. The fumes dissolve the false membrane, and cure the disease.

Fistula, and Fistulous Caries:—Inject essence of Turpentine, pure. "Grand success."

TWITCHING.—See Nerve.

TYMPANITIS.—See Abdomen—Bloat.

TYPHOID FEVER.—See Fever—Typhoid.

TYPHUS FEVER.—See Fever—Typhus.

TYPHLITIS. — See Abdomen — Appendicitis. Same treatment.

ULCER.—"CANTHARIS θ, 1 drop, 6 hours. No bandage, rapid cure." EUCA. *Syzygium,* powdered seed, 2 to 5 grs. daily.

Cutaneous, especially, CAL P 1x 5 grs for a child; 10 grs for adult, two or three times a day. No salve. "The greatest of all remedies for varicose ulcers, CARDU M θ 5 drops, 6 hours."

Internal ulcer especially, AURUM MUR 3x. HYDROCT.

Black, *Ars*. Carb v. Con. LACH. Mur a. Thuj.

Blue, Con. LACH. Sec. Sil.

Bleeding, Ars. *Carb v*. Hep. LACH. Mer. *Nit a. Pho*. Sul.

Bone-ulcer: Asa. AUR. Cal fl. Hep. Mer. Sil. Therid—See Bone—Caries.

Burning, ARS. Bell. CARB V. Hep. Mer. *Mez*. Rhus. Sec. *Sul*.

Cancerous. See Cancer.

Crusted, Ars. MEZ. Mur a. See Skin—Scab.

Deep "as if cut out with a punch," Kal bi.

Fetid—Putrid, Ars. Carb v. Grap. Lach. Pet. Sil—See Eucalyp. See Bone-ulcer.

Fistulous, Cal c. Cal fl. FL AC. Lyc. Nit a. *Pæon. Pho*. Sil 30-200. Sul. (See Fistula.)

Fungoid, *Ars*. Grap. Sul. THUJ.

Gangrenous, *Ars*. Asa. Kal p. *Pæon*. TARANT.

Glutinous, Grap.

Green, *Ars*. Aur. Mer. Rhus.

Hard, Grap. *Mer. Sil*.

Itching, Ars. Grap. Hep. *Ran b*. Rhus. Lyc. Sep. Sil. (See Thuj.)

Maggoty, Sil. Sul. Dust with Calomel powder.

Mercurial, Aur. Hep. Lyc. Nit a. Sil.

Pimply—surrounded by pimples, or boils, Cal p. *Hep*. Lach. Rhus.

Raw, Mer. Nit a.

Scrofulous, Cal c. CAL P ix. CIST. Sul. (See Scrofula.)

Sensitive, tender, *Ars*. HEP. Lach. Mer. Sul.

Spotted, Kreo. Lach. Mer. Sil.

Stinging, Grap. Hep. Mer. Nit a.

Syphilitic, Lach. Mer. Nit a. Phyt. (See Iodoform. Thuj.) See Syphilis.

Varicose—From broken vein, CARD θ. *Ham*. Sul.

Wart-ulcer, Cal c. *Nit a. Thuj.* (See Solar
Cautery.)

**Topical Treatment of Ulcers — Especially
Chronic Indolent Ulcers:—**

" Bread soaked in water is the best dressing."
Crude opium plaster. White lead paint.
Pine pitch ointment on old linen. (See Ace-
tan. Alcohol. Calendula. CARBOL A. *Clay.*
Charcoal. Ichthyl. Iodoform. Hydras. Lime.
Logwood. Potash. Salt. SILVER. THUJA.
Solar Cautery. Vinegar—See Ointment.)

URÆMIA.—CANTH. *Carbol a.* Op. PB. Pilo.
TEREB.

With dropsy, Apo c.

— Slow weak pulse, Dig.

— Spasms, Morph. hypodem. Chloroform
enema, as for Puerperal spasm—See Chloroform. Hot poultice over the loins. Hot
water enemas.

URETHRA.—See Urinary Organs.

URETHRAL FEVER.—Aco.

URINALYSIS.—

Albumen: Brown, or blood red hue, smoky; co-
agulates by heat, or nitric acid. Glacial acetic
acid, small piece dropped in, produces cloudi-
ness; Sulphuric acid gives a black deposit. In
Bright's Disease *casts* are found.

Sugar: Pale frothy, with odor of cider; attracts
flies: deep brown on being boiled with equal
quantity of Liquor Potassæ; deep green if
boiled with an alkaline solution of Bichromate
of Potash. Always present in Diabetes.

Bile: Dark green hue, stains yellow; is changed
to brown by touch of Nitric acid; Purple on
addition of Sulphuric acid and a little sugar;

yellow and turbid when agitated with a few
drops of Chloroform.

Phosphorus in excess: Pale yellow color, fetid
odor; earthy phosphates precipitated by heat,
or touch of Aqua Ammonia, but readily dissolved by Nitric acid. (Alkaloid phosphates,
as of Soda and Ammonia, are not thus precipitated.)

Urea in excess:—High color, strong urinous
odor.

Uric acid in excess:—High color, clear, throws
down a reddish sediment by touch of Hydro-
chloric acid.

Red sediment:—Indicates uric acid if crystalline,
otherwise urate of ammonia.

White Sediment:—Denotes phosphates if soluble
by heat; otherwise urate of ammonia.

Pink Sediment:—Denotes urate of soda and phos-
phate of ammonia.

"If the *foam* on urine shaken in a bottle *soon*
subsides, it contains *no sugar, or albumen.*"

"On a strip of white filtering paper drop a
drop of urine, heat the paper over a lamp
slowly and carefully, seeing that the urine
is *dried* without being browned by the flame.
Now if there is *no stain* on the paper there
is *no sugar* or albumen in the urine. If it
contains sugar the stain will be brown, or
yellow brown. If it contains albumen, the
stain will be yellow or reddish yellow."

URINARY ORGANS.—

Albuminuria : Ars. *Berb.* KALI M 2x. Kalmia.
Mer c. Pho. Pilo. *Tereb.*

Azoturia : Con. Gel. Nat m.

Ball—sense of—in the bladder, Lach.

Biting sensation in the urethra, Prun s. Teuc. Thuj.

Bright's Disease :—Apis. ARS. Euony 2x. Ferr. APO C θ 3 drops, 3 hours, in water. *Kali m* 1x, 5 drops, 5 hours. PB. Sabal s θ. *Tereb* 1x. Butter-milk. Skim-milk. Lime water. (See Diet O. V.)

—Bloat under the eye, Apis. ARS. Pho.

—Slow pulse, *Dig*. Kalmia.

—Skin pale, waxy, ARS. Apis.

—Tongue smooth, red, Apis. *Ars. Tereb.*

—Urine red and scanty, Aco. APIS. Berb. Mer— Dark red or bloody, Hep. TEREB—Fetid, *Mer*. Sep. Sul.

—Sediment of urine, red sand, *Lyc.* Pho. Sep— Snow white, Rhus—Containing cell *casts*, Ars. CANTH. Pho. PB. *Tereb*—Oil globules. Ars. Pho.

—Spasms, *Canth.* Tereb.

—Stupor, Canth.

Renal cirrhosis, PLUMBUM MET 6x trit.

Waxy kidney, Amyloid. Kal iod. Mer. *Nit a.* PH A. Sars. Sil.

Bruise-like pain in kidney, Arn. Berb. Eup per. Rhus.

Burning : Kidney, Cann. I. *Canth.* Bell. *Hep.* Hydras. Sul. *Tereb.* ZN.

—Bladder, BERB. *Colch.* Lach. Rhen. *Sep.*

—Urethra, Ars. *Cann s. Canth.* Mer. Sul.

—Urine, Borax. *Canth. Cann s* Mer.

Catarrh of the Bladder:—Ben a. CHIMAP θ, adult 5 to 10 drops in water, 3 hours. *Dul.* Eup pur. Lyc. *Pul.* "Rhus arom. θ adult 10 drops, 4 hours." SABAL S θ. *Solid v θ.* Sep. Sul. Tart e. VESICAR θ. (See Alum— *Resorcin.*)

Colic, renal "Kidney Colic" — Stone lodged :—Arnica in. and ex. Berb θ 5 drops on sugar, 5 minutes. Chimap u θ. DIOS θ 60 drops in hot sweetened water. *Nux v.* PASS θ 60 drops in hot water. Piper m θ 5 drops on sugar, 5 minutes. Pareira θ 5 drops in hot water, 10 minutes. Chloroform 10 drops on sugar, ¼ hour. *Opium suppository.* Morphia hypoderm. Hot fomentations. Hot sitz bath. See Pain—*Topical* treatment. (See Onion—Starch.)

—*Position to pass water:*—First lie down upon the stomach, then slowly rise on "all fours" and in this position urinate.

—*Preventive treatment:*—BURSA θ. Cal p. *Helon.* Lyc. Nux v. POD ix. Uran n. URTICA θ. Drink a tumbler full of hot water before breakfast daily. See Diet V.

Constriction, in bladder, Caps. Pul. Pho.

Contracted kidney, Clem.

Cramp, Kidney, *Kal iod.* Sul.

—Bladder, *Prun s.* ZN.

—Urethra, Chel. Pho.

Cutting, Kidney, *Canth* Clem. *Colo.* Mer. Nux v—Before urinating, Grap. Lyc.

—Bladder, Berb. *Canth.* Caps. *Kal c. Lyc.* Tereb.

—Urethra, CANTH. Berb. DIG. *Equis. Mer,* Nit a. PH A.

Chyluria: Berb. Ph a. Uva.

Cystitis: Aco. Apis. Bell. BERB. *Cann s.* CANTH. *Equis.* Piper m θ 10 drops. SABAL S θ. *Uva* θ. LITH C pure 3 gr doses. *Visicar* θ. Same remedies as for catarrh of the bladder—See Diet Q.

In exceedingly troublesome cases, introduce

within the urethra, ¼ gr. of Morphia sulph; follow next day with ⅛ gr. Male subject, apply Veratrum v ointment along under-side of penis. When pain of urination is intolerable inject, before passage, Cocaine 4 per cent. solution, 1 drachm.

— When the inflammation has been caused by an *injury*, Arn. Rhus. Ruta—*Fly-blister*, Camp θ—*Rheumatism*, Colch. Rhus.

— When the pains are especially, *burning*, Canth. Cann s—*Cutting*, Bell. Con—Sting-ing, Apis. Mer—Stitching, Aco. Lyc.

Diabetes—Glucosuria: "May find aid in ori-ficial surgery." Arg n. "ARS. and TERB." *Eucalyp.* fl. ex. 20 drops, 4 times a day. *Helon.* Kreo. PB. PHO A 1x. URAN N 1x 5 gr. doses. LACTIC ACID, 2 teaspoonfuls in a glass of water once a day. Eat nothing but meat, fish, eggs, and toasted bread. "Rhus aromat. adult 30 drops, 12 hours." Syzygium, powdered seed, 2 to 5 grs. 6 hours; or pulv. seeds, 1 ounce in hot water, 1 pint steep, when sufficiently infused add Glycerine, 1 ounce: Of this solution, adult take 1, tablespoonful 4 times a day. "In 10 days there will be no sugar in the urine." "Eat freely of maple sugar." "Subsist upon skim-milk exclusively, adult, 8 to 10 pints daily. Cure in 7 weeks." Gratify the thirst with water. See Diet. I. N. U.

Diuresis: Cann I. Gel. Kreo. Nat s. *Pilo 1x.* Pod. Pul. Sul—Urine pale, Gel. Nat m. Val—Loosing flesh, see Diabetes.

Drawing sensation in Kidney, *Clem.* Nux m. *Tereb.*

— Bladder, Dig. Cal p. Rhod.

— Urethra, Colch. Copai. Nat m. Pul. ZN.

Enuresis. See **Micturition**—Involuntary.

Fatty degeneration of Kidney, Ars. PHO.

Glucosuria: Aco. *Arg n* 200. Bell. Gel. Mag p.
Ph a. Spig. See Diabetes.

Gravel: BURSA θ. Cal c. Hep. Hydras. *Lyc.*
Nux v. PB. POD ıx. Ruta. Sars. Sep.
THLASP B θ 10 d, 3 h. *Uran n.* URTICA θ.
Drink a tumberful of hot water daily before
breakfast. See Colic, Renal. See Diet V—
See Urine—Sediment.

Hæmaturia: Ars. Bell. CANTH. *Merc. Mill.*
PHO. PB. THREB. Tart e.

Inflammation of the Kidney. See Nephritis.

— of Bladder, see Cystitis.

— of the Urethra, Aco. *Cann s Canth.* Mer.
Nux v.

Irritation of the Bladder: *Apis,Cann s.* Copai.
Eup pur. LIL T. Lith c. *Sabal s θ. Vesicar θ.*

— With Bloody dripping, Bell. Canth. Nux v.
Rhus.

— — Brick-red sediment, Arn. Pho. Pul.

— — Burning heat, Canth. Dig. Nux v.

— — Crampy pain, Canth.

— — Cutting flow, Con.

— — Dribbling, Arn. Bell.

— — Fetid urine, Benz a.

— — Gouty symptoms, Colch.

— — Interrupted flow, Con.

— — Pinching pain, Aco.

— — Red sand sediment, Lyc.

— — Stinging pain, Apis.

— — Stitching, Lyc.

— — Straining, Arn.

Itching in bladder or urethra, *Berb.* Cann s.
Canth. Copai. Pet. *Sul. Thuj.*

Jerking in bladder, Agar.
— Urethra, Nat c. Pho.
Numbness in bladder, Fl ac—Urethra, *Ced.*
Mag m. *Thuj.*

Pains, Painfulness, in general :—

— In kidney, *Alu.* BERB. *Cal p.* CANN I.
Cep. Mez. *Nux v.* Ox a. PB. Phyt. SOLID
V ix. ZN—*When* lifting, Cal p—Stooping,
Sul—Walking, Carb a. Nit a—Relieved by
flow of urine, Lyc. See the several kinds of
pain.
— In bladder, Bell. BERB. Cann s. Canth.
EQUIS. *Phyt*—Terrible pain on passing
urine, *Equis.* Pareir θ. Piper m θ. ("Inject
into urethra before micturition, Cocaine 4
per cent solution I drachm ")—Pain with
swelling and tenderness, EQUIS. Mer.
Sabal θ. See the several kinds of pain.
— In the urethra, Arg n. *Cann I.* Con. *Equis.*
Sars. From beer Thuj 30.
Paralysis of bladder: Ars. Bell. *Caust.* Cann s.
Hell. Hyo. Laur. PB. Sec. *Stram.*
Pinching in bladder, Mez. Sep.
— in urethra, Carb v. Lyc. Nat m.
Polypi of bladder: CAL C. Sang. *Stap. Thuj.*
Polyuria: See **Micturition.**
Pressure, sense of, in kidney, *Kal c. Ran s.*
Thuj. *Tereb.* ZN.
— Bladder, Con. Lach. LIL T. Nit a. SEP.
— Urethra, *Colch.* Lach. Pul. *Sul.* TEUC.
Pulsation, kidney, *Berb.* Chel. Kal iod.
— Bladder, Canth.
— Urethra, *Benz a.* Canth. *Copai.* Dul. *Mer.*
Softening of the kidney, Kal bi.
Smarting: Bladder, Eup per. Pho.

— Urethra, *Berb*. Borax. Cal fl. *Equis*. LIL T. ·
Sec. SUL.

Soreness of kidney, Benz a. Chel. Phyt. ZN.

— Bladder, *Cal p. Canth*. Lact a. Pul. TEREB.

— Urethra, *Canth. Carbo an. Nat m*. Mez.
Nit a.

Spasm of bladder, Ars. *Caps. Canth*. Clem.
Sep. *Tarant c*. Tereb.

Stinging kidney, *Bell*. Canth. Hep. *Kal c.
Ph a*. ZN.

— Bladder, *Canth. Lyc*. Sul. Tart e.

— Urethra, *Canth*. Lach. Mer.

Stitching kidney, BERB. Cann I. Mez. PB.
Sep. *Tarant c*.

Stone: See Gravel.

Strangury: APO C. CANTH. Camp. EUP
PUR. Cann s. Caps. Copai. *Mer c. Nux v.
Pul. Stap*. Tarant c—From fly blister, Camp *θ*.
(See Chloroform, Ice, Onion.) See Mictur-
ition. See Catheter.

Tenesmus. See **Micturition.**

Tension—Tightness of bladder, Eup per. Tart e.

Throbbing kidney, Canth—See Nephritis.

— Bladder, Canth.

Twitching kidney, Aco. Canth. Mang.

Ulceration. Bladder, Canth. Mer bin. Ran b.

— Urethra, Canth.

Worm—sense of—in bladder, Bell.

Micturition :—

Before the flow:

Pain in abdomen, Sul.

— Back, Lyc.

— Bladder, Lil t.

During the flow:

Escape of air from bladder, Sars.

Emission of prostatic fluid, Sabal *θ*. Thuj.

Colic, Aco. Verat a.

Gastralgia, Laur.

Spasm of bladder, Asa.

Stool involuntary, Mur a.

Smarting vulva, *Kreo*. Mer. Nat m.

Stoppage, sudden, Dios *θ*. Mag p—Very painful, Aco. Canth—Stoppage and starting *without* pain, CON. Clem.

Straining — Tenesmus: CANN I. CANTH. *Caps*. Lith c. *Mer c*. NUX V. PB. Pul. *Sars*. Viol t—From stricture—"thread stream"— *Chimap θ*. CLEM. Pet. Sul. Thuj—From enlarged prostate, Apis. Chimap *θ*. SABAL ix. Thuj—Unable to pass water without stool, Alu. Mur a; or without being on the knees, Pareir; or standing, feet apart, and bent forward, Thuj; or standing bent backward, ZN—No expulsive power, Hep.

Terrrible pains in passing water, Piper m *θ*. Pareira. Equis. Inject into bladder before passage Cocaine 4 per cent solution, I drachm.

At the close of the flow :

Cutting pains, Colch. Sars.

Dripping, Pic a. Thuj—Bloody, Hep. ZN.

Last drop lodges, Hep. Kal bi. Thuj—And burns, Clem.

After the flow :

Nausea, Dig. Nux v.

Shuddering, Plat.

Spasm of bladder, Asa.

Weakness, Nux v.

Scanty flow—Diminished secretion :

APIS. APOC. ARS. Equis. Eup pur. Hell. Lil t. *Mer*. PB. Sul. Tart e—No secretion, PB. Zing. See Dropsy.

Obstructed flow—Retention of urine : (See Ice. Chlorof. Onion. See Catheter.)

— In general, Aco. Bell. Camp. Sec

— In brain affection, Cic.

— In typhoid fever, *Ars.* Bell. HYO. Op. Stram. *ZN.*

— In child-bed, ACO. Ars.

— In new born babe, Aco. Benz a. Hyo.

— Painful, ACO. Bell. *Canth.* Croton.

— With straining, tenesmus, Apis. *Canth.* Cann s. Camp. Caps. Mer c— Flowing by drops, *Canth.* Bell. Kreo. Sabal θ.

Involuntary flow—Incontinence :

Ars. Bell. CAUST. *Eup pur.* Hyo. Nat m. PUL. Rhus. Sep—Paralytic, Nux v. Thuj.

—Dribbling day and night, *Arg n.* Bell. Caust. *Gel.* Pet. *Pod· Sabal s.* θ—Only by day, Ferr p.

—After great exertion, Amb.

—From having retained the urine a long time, Caust.

— A fall on the back, Hyper.

— Spine affecti· n, Nux v.

—When coughing, CAUST. Nat m. *Pul. Squil.* Verat a.

— Sneezing, Caust. Pul.

— Sitting, Pul.

— Standing, Bell. Pul.

— Walking, Cal c. Nat m.

— In typhoid fever, Bell. Hyo. Rhus.

— Incontinence when lying on the back, Kreo.

— During sleep— "Wetting the bed," *Antipyrine*, 1 gr. doses. Bell 1x. CAUST. *Canth·* 1x. EQUIS. Ferr. *Ph a.* 1x. PLANTAGO 1x. "Rhus arom. θ. 10 drops, 12 hours." Sabal 1x. SUL. Mullein oil, drop doses in

water. " Parrish's food, 1 teaspoonful twice
a day." "Prevent patient from lying on
the back, by wearing a sash with a large
knot at the back."

— Warty subject, Thuj—Urine fetid, Benz a.
Nit a—From worms, Cina.

— Boy, Nux v—Girl, Bell—Old man, Con—
Onanist, Ph a—In first sleep, Sep.

Frequent call to urinate — Polyuria : Apis.
Canth. GEL. Kreo. LIL T. Lith c. *Lyc. Ph a.*
PLANTAGO. SABAL S θ. Squil. *Tab* 2x —
Especially at night, Aco. *Borax. Kreo.* Lach.
Sil.

— Urgent calls, cannot wait, *Canth.* Caust.
KREO. Mag p. *Mer.* Nux v PET. *Thuj.*

— Must go at once or have pain, Ferr p—Pain
in the back, Berb. Con. LYC—Stitches in
bladder, Tart e.

Urine and Sediment — Condition, Color, Odor:—

Acrid, Borax. Caust. *Hep.* Iod. *Mer.*

Albuminous, MER C. Pho. Phyt. PB.

— Sediment, *Apo c.* Euony. Kal bi. *Mer c.*
PB. Pho. Phyt. Spart. *Tarant c.* (See Albuminuria.)

Blackish, Ars. Colo. *Lach.* Nat m. Verat a—
Containing black specks, Hell.

Blue, Nit a.

— Sediment, Prun s.

Bloody, *Bursa* θ. Cann I. CANTH. IPE.
MER C. Mill. PHO. PUL. Sabal θ. TEREB
—Pure blood, CINNAMO θ. Ham. IPE.
Mill. *Nit a. Sec.* TEREB—From a hurt,
ARN. Ham. *Hyper.* Mill—Strong drink,
Nux v—Suppressed piles, Nux v—Scurvy,
Nat m.

Brick-dust sediment, Arn. *China.* LYC. Nat m. PHO. *Pul.* Sep.

Brown urine, BENZ A. BRY. CHEL. *Colch.* Lach. MER. Nat m. NIT A. *Pho*

—Sediment, *Amb.* Æs.

Burning urine, Ars. BORAX. Caps. CANTH. MER. Pho. *Vesicar.*

Clay-like sediment, BERB. Pho. *Sul a.* Sep. ZN.

"Coffee ground" sediment, Hell.

Cold urine, Agar. Nit a.

Covered with scum, Arg n. Colo. MER C. Paris. *Pul.* PB—Green scum. Sep.

Dark urine, Aco. *Bry. Chel.* Equis. PB.

Fatty casts, in urine, Ars. Pho. Phyt.

Fetid urine, BENZ A. "*Boric acid* 10 to 20 grs, 3 hours." CAL C. *Colo. Dul. Guai. Mer.* NIT A. *PB. Pul.* SEP. SUL—Thick and fetid, Colo. Dul.

Frothy, *Lach. Lyc.* Spo.

Greenish, ARS. CAMP. *Cann I.* Chel. RHEU. Ruta. *Kal c.* Mag c. *Santo.*

Jelly-like sediment, BERB. Pho. Pul.

Mealy sediment, BERB. Sul. ZN.

Mucous, sediment, BERB. *Chimap θ.* Copai. DUL. Mer. *Nat m.* PUL. Sep—Mucus and pus, Pichi. Uva—Fetid mucus, Colo. Dul. Euca.

Odor of Cat urine, Borax. Viol t.

—Horse urine, Absinth. Nit a.

—Hartshorn, *Asa.* Carb v. Mos. *Nit a.*

—Violets, Nux m. *Tereb.*

—Sour, Amb. Mer.

Oily Pellicle.   Pet. Pul. Sul. Sumbul.

Pale urine, Cham. *Cann I.* GEL. Hyo. IG.

Nat m. *Val*—Pale, very copious, and skin hot, *Acet a.*

Pasty sediment. SEP.

Pink stain in the vessel, SEP.

Purulent sediment, Canth. Clem.

Rank urine, BENZ A. Nit a.

Red urine, ACO. Ant c. *Berb.* BRY. *Colch.* Hell. MER. Nux v. *Tereb*—Staining red, Hyo Lyc. Phyt.

—Sediment red, BERB. Grap. LYC. Mer. *Nat m. Pul.* SEP—Red sand, Dig. Lob i. LYC. Pho. Sil.

Sandy sediment, Am c. Benz a. BURSA *θ. Lyc.* Pichi. Sars. Skook. Stigm. URTICA *θ. Uva.*

—Sand and blood, *Thlasp b θ.*

White urine, Aur. CANN I. CON. Cyc. Hep. Mer. PHO, PH A—After standing, Cina,

—Sediment white, BERB. Colch. GRAP. *Hep. Pho.* PH A. RHUS. *Sep.* Spig. Spo—White sand, Am c.

Yellow, saffron hue, CHEL. *Lach.* RHEU. Spo. *Santo* ZN—Yellow stain, Chel.

—Sediment, *Bar c.* CHAM. *Lach.* Sep. ZN.

URTICARIA.—See Skin—Hives.

UTERUS.—See Female.

UVULA.—See Mouth—Palate.

VACCINE DISEASE.—Ars. Bacill 30-200. *Sil.* THUJA.

VARICOCELE.—See Male—Scrotum.

VARIOLA—VARIOLOID.—See Smallpox.

VEINS BROKEN.—See Skin—Varicocele.

VERATRUM VIRIDE.—*Deafness, Earache:*— Into an ½ ounce bottle put 7 drops of Verat v θ, and fill the bottle ½ full of glycerine, and then fill up the bottle with water; apply this in the ear.

Spine pain, from whatever cause:—Verat v ointment, 8 grs to the ounce of base; apply to seat of pain.

Inflamed Joints, Sprains, Bunions:—Verat ointment.

VERTIGO.—See Head.

VICARIOUS BLEEDING. — See Female — Menses.

VINEGAR.—*Paralysis, Spinal weakness, Involuntary passage of urine or stool, Asthma, Pains of various kinds in the body:*—Rub the spine thoroughly three times a day with *hot* vinegar; especially that point nearest the seat of ailment.

Milk Crust:—Cut off the hair closely, wash the scalp thoroughly with Castile soap, and apply twice a day pure cider vinegar diluted with water, one part to three. Use Ichthyol soap.

Nose bleed:—Plug nostrils with cotton saturated with dilute vinegar.

Bleeding wound, Bleeding lung, or nose:—Inhale the fumes of boiling vinegar. "*Nothing better.*"

Nasal Polypus:—Inject 5 drops of Acetic acid into it.

Influenza, Coryza:—Saturate a small pledget of cotton with vinegar and insert it into one nostril *loosely*, and after an hour remove it; and put one in the other nostril; thus alternate and cure.

Gonorrhœa:—Acetic acid inject: first a 1 per cent solution in lukewarm water, six or eight times a day; after a day or two increase the strength to 4 per cent. In desperate cases, shockingly neglected, or mistreated, apply

hot poultices for a day or two, before beginning
the Acet ac. treatment. "No treatment more
satisfactory."

Black specks in the skin of the face:—Wash the
face with vinegar, full strength on going to
bed. The same for *Ring-worm* and *Wart.*

Diseased gums, foul, spongy:—Use dilute vinegar
as a mouth wash.

Birth mark: Soak cotton in strong vinegar, and
apply under compress. "It peels off."

Ulcer:—Vinegar, 10 per cent solution in water,
use as a lavement, three times a day.

Burn or scald:—Apply vinegar, full strength,
until pain abates.

Corns:—Bind on bread crumbs or cotton, soaked
in vinegar, nightly.

Mad dog bite:—Lave wound with hot vinegar,
and wipe dry; then pour into it several drops
of Nitric acid. "This will prevent rabies."

Hæmorrhage from the womb:—A sponge or cloth
saturated with vinegar dilute, convey into the
womb, and retain it there a few seconds. Give
also gill doses of vinegar. "Nothing better."

Chronic gout—Enlarged joints:—Into a given
quantity of hot vinegar put as much salt as it
will dissolve; with this bathe the part, and
"*dry it in,*" by the fire, several times a day.

VISION.—See Eye—Light.

VOICE.—See Chest.

VOMITING.—See Stomach.

WAKEFULNESS.—See Sleep.

WARTS.—See Skin.

WASTING AWAY.—See Atrophy. See Consumption.

WATER BRASH.—See Stomach.

WATER STAGNANT, OR TURBID RENDERED INNOXIOUS.—See Lemon. See Alum.

WEAKNESS.—See Debility. Prostration. Tonic.

WEANING.—Mother: See Female. Breasts. See Belladonna.—Child: See Diet D. E. F. G. H. Z.

WEN.—See Benzo. Collodion.

"WETTING THE BED."—See Urinary Organs—Micturition—(*Involuntary flow*).

"WHITE SWELLING."—See Iodine. Potash. See Scrofular.

"WHITES."—See Female—Leucorrhœa.

WHITLOW.—See Limb—Arm—(*Hand*).

WHOOPING COUGH.—See Chest—Cough—(*Whooping*).

WOMB.—See Female—Uterus.

WORMS.—

Common large worm—(Lumbricoid): Absinth. CINA. "*Cina 2x and Ig 2x alt.*" CHENOPOD. Anth 2x. Child two or three years old, 3 to 5 drops, 3 times a day. This cures *all* complaints and derangements caused by worms. Santonine 2x trit 2 grs, 3 hours. This is a genuine specific for the round worm. "Santo 1x, 5 grs, 3 nights, and Podo 2x, 5 grs in the mornings."

"Santonine, to a child 5 to 7 years old, give in the evening after a light supper, 1 grain rubbed into sugar of milk and mixed with cream; next morning a dose of castor oil; repeat three times if necessary." "Terebinth oil, 5 to 10 drops in milk on an empty stomach, three mornings."

"Crumble some *green* vitriol on a stove, not
too hot; when it turns white, rub it down to
a fine powder; of this give to a child, from
5 to 7 years old, as much as would make the
bulk of a small pea, in syrup or molasses,
three mornings in succession, then wait
three, then give three, until nine doses are
given. This succeeds when all else fails."

Verminous diathesis—Slimy stool: Ant c. Mer c.
Stan.

Seat Worm—(Pin-worm—Thread-worm—Oxy-
uris) :— *Aco. Cina.* Ferr. Ig. Mer. Stan.
" *Cina and Ig. alt.*" *Indigo* 2x. Teucr 2x, 5
grs, 6 hours. "Lyc 30, twice a day for three
days, then Verat a three times a day for three
days, then Ipe three times a day for three days.
This does the work thoroughly." URTICA
U θ 3 drops on sugar at bed time, for three
days.

(See Chloroform. Lard. Salt—See Suppository.)

Tape Worm—(Tænia) : "Oil of Turpentine,
adult 3 teaspoonfuls in milk, combined with
½ ounce of Castor oil." "Chloroform on
sugar, one teaspoonful in the morning before
breakfast—having taken no supper the evening before—immediately after taking the
Chloroform take a dose of 'salts.' In an hour
the worm comes away entire." "Take a tablespoonful of gun powder in a cupful of sweet
milk, followed in ten minutes with an ounce
of Castor oil."

"Take one teaspoonful of Elixir of Vitriol
undiluted. One dose is enough."

"Right light diet for two days, and no
drink but lemonade; then put a pint of

hulled pumpkin seeds, well bruised, into a pint of hot water, rub the mass thoroughly together for a few minutes and strain it through a colander; and in the morning, fasting, take one-half of it, and the rest in an hour after; and in three hours after the last portion take a dose of Castor oil."
" Take *one ounce* of pumpkin seed, the shells having been removed; mash it up and make an emulsion with milk. Take this dose at bed time, after having fasted from breakfast. In the morning take a tablespoonful of Castor oil, abstaining from breakfast." " Eat two quarts of pumpkin seeds, hulled, during twenty-four hours, and eat nothing else; then take a full dose of Castor oil." " Eat the meat of a whole cocoanut, and drink the milk."

"Give drop doses of Male Fern, every four hours, and a dose of Mer c, night and morning, for several days."

"Give *Pomegranate fl. ex. fresh*, *one ounce* in a wine glassful of water in the morning before eating—having preceded it by a dose of Castor oil an hour previous—repeat this dose at intervals of an hour until *three ounces* have been taken This will cause the prompt expulsion of the whole worm."

"Give Rottlera tinct, two or three teaspoonfuls, after twelve hours' fasting. A dose of Castor oil may be given if no purgative action follow the taking of the medicine. This is a pleasant, safe and sure remedy."

Reported cure with *Filix m* 30, night and morning, for one week.

WORSE.

WORSE.—See Aggravation. See Pain. See the several affections and organs.

WOUND DRESSING.—(See Amputation Dressing)—

Crude opium plaster, size to cover an inch beyond the margin of the wound, press it on firmly, it will adhere for weeks. It is aseptic, sedative, and curative, heals by " first intention," prevents suppuration. The same for an indolent ulcer. (See *Acetan.* Alcohol Aloes. Arnica. Bism. *Calendula. Carbol a.* Eucalyp. Hot water. Ichthyol. Lead. Onion. Salicyl a. Sugar.)

Bleeding: See Alcohol. Alum. Chloroform. Hot water. *Iron. Vinegar.*

Contused: See Alcohol. Arnica. Calendula.

Gun-shot: See Alcohol. Calendula.

Incised wound: See Benzo. Calendula.

Painful: See *Aloes. Lead.* Onion—*Smoke of burning wool* — Pain after amputation, HYPER. Cep *θ*— Cold pain, Led—Pain in an old fracture or sprain, Ruta. SYMPH —Pain in an old scar, *Hyper.* Grap. I ach.

Poisoned wound: See Alcohol. Carbol a. ICH-THYOL. (See Bite)

Unhealthy wound: See Calendula. Carbol a. *Charcoal.* Chlorine. Chloral. *Clay.* Potash.

To keep wound open: See Elm.

Guard against lock-jaw: See Onion. Turpentine See Lock-jaw.

WRINKLES.—Rub them out with Lanolin.

WRIST.—See Limb—Arm (Hand).

YEAST.—*Purgative:*—A cupful of fresh yeast. It it pleasant, safe and sure.

Bowel obstruction: Inject yeast by the quart.

YELLOW FEVER.

Boil diathesis — "Crops of boils": Brewer's yeast, adult, a tablespoonful, twice a day for a week.

Colic: Yeast, adult, a teacupful; this banishes the pain directly.

Inflammation: Apply poultices made of Indian meal, boiled in yeast, and saturated with Laudanum. Apply them *hot*, and renew them as often as they become cool. In case of *threatened mortification internal:* Administer yeast, adult, a tablespoonful every 2 hours, and apply yeast poultice over the seat of inflammation.

YELLOW FEVER.—See Fever—Yellow.

ZINC.—*Ophthalmia:* Use eye-water made of Acetate of Zinc 2 grs, Sulphate of Morphia 2 grs, and water 1 ounce, mixed; drop a few drops into the eye several times a day.

Eye ointment made of Yellow Oxide of Mercury 2 grs, in Vaseline 1 ounce, is excellent for *Conjunctivitis and Granular lids.*

Sulphate of Hydrastis 2 grs, in distilled water 1 ounce, is also excellent for the same.

Opium 1 gr, in Rose water 1 ounce, a few drops in the eye several times a day, removes *inflammation.*

ABBREVIATIONS.

Abies n.	Abies nigra.
Acalyph.	Acalypha Indica.
Acet. a.	Acetic acid.
Aco.	Aconite.
Æs.	Æsculus hippocastanum.
Æth.	Æthusa.
Agar.	Agaricus.
Ail.	Ailanthus glandulosa.
Alet.	Aletris farinosa.
Alo.	Aloes.
Alu.	Alumina.
Amb.	Ambragrisea.
Ambros.	Ambrosia artemisifolia.
Am. c.	Ammonium carbonica.
Am. m.	Ammonium muriaticum.
Amyg.	Amygdala amara.
Amyl.	Amyl nitrite.
Ana.	Anacardium.
Anth.	Anthraxin.
Ant. c.	Antimonium crudum.
Apis.	Apis mellifica.
Apo. c.	Apocynum Cannabinum.
Apom.	Apomorphia.
Aral. r.	Aralia racemosa.
Arg. m.	Argentum metallicum.
Arg. n.	Argentum nitricum.
Arn.	Arnica.
Ars.	Arsenic.
Ars. bro.	Arsenicum bromicum.
Ars. iod.	Arsenicum iodatum.

ARUM.

Arum.	Arum triphyllum.
Asa.	Asafœtida.
Asar.	Asarum.
Aster.	Asterias rubens.
Atrop.	Atropinum.
Aur. bro.	Aurum bromicum.
Aur. m.	Aurum metallicum.
Aurum mur.	Aurum muriaticum.
Avena.	Avena sativa.

Bacill.	Bacillinum.
Bad.	Badiaga.
Bap.	Baptisia.
Bar. c.	Baryta carbonica.
Bar. iod.	Baryta iodatum.
Bar. m.	Baryta muriaticum.
Bell.	Belladonna.
Bellis p.	Bellis perennis.
Ben. a.	Benzoicum acidum.
Berb.	Berberis.
Bism.	Bismuth.
Blatta.	Blatta orientalis.
Bovis.	Bovista.
Brom.	Bromium.
Bry.	Bryonia alba.
Bufo.	Rana bufo.
Bursa.	Thlaspi bursa pastoris.

Cact.	Cactus grandiflorus.
Calad.	Caladium seguinum.
Cal. c.	Calcarea carbonicum.
Cal. fl.	Calcarea fluorica.
Cal. iod.	Calcarea iodata.
Cal. p.	Calcarea phosphorica.
Camp.	Camphora.
Cann I.	Cannabis Indica.

Cann. s.	Cannabis sativa.
Canth.	Cantharis.
Caps.	Capsicum.
Carb. a.	Carbo animalis.
Carb. v.	Carbo vegetabilis.
Carbol. a.	Carbolic acid.
Card.	Carduus marianus.
Caul.	Caulophyllum.
Caust.	Causticum.
Ceanoth.	Ceanothus Americanus.
Ced.	Cedron.
Cep.	Cepa.
Cham.	Chamomilla.
Chel.	Chelidonium majus.
Chenop.	Chenopodium anthelminticum.
Chimap.	Chimaphila.
Chin.	China.
Chin. ars.	Chininum arsenicum.
Chin. s.	Chininum sulphuricum.
Chion.	Chionanthus Virginica.
Cic.	Cicuta.
Cimi.	Cimicifuga.
Cina.	Cina.
Cinnamo.	Cinnamomum.
Cist.	Cistus Canadensis.
Cit. a.	Citric acid.
Coc.	Cocculus Indicus.
Coff.	Coffea cruda.
Colch.	Colchicum.
Coll.	Collinsonia.
Colo.	Colocynthis.
Com.	Commocladia dentata.
Con.	Conium.
Condu.	Condurango.
Coral.	Corallium rubrum.
Crat. ox.	Cratægus oxyacanthus.

CRO.

Cro.	Crocus.
Crotal.	Crotalus horridus.
Croton.	Croton tiglium.
Cup. a.	Cuprum aceticum.
Clem.	Clematis.
Cup. ars.	Cuprum arsenicum.
Cup. m.	Cuprum metallicum.
Cyc.	Cyclamen.
Cypr.	Cypripedium.
Dig.	Digitalis.
Diad.	Diadema aranea.
Dios.	Dioscorea villosa.
Doli.	Dolichos pruriens.
Dros.	Drosera.
Dul.	Dulcamara.
Epiph.	Epiphegus.
Equis.	Equisetum.
Euca.	Eucalyptus.
Euphor.	Euphorbium.
Euphr.	Euphrasia.
Eup. per.	Eupatorium perfoliatum.
Eup. pur.	Eupatorium purpureum.
Ferr. iod.	Ferrum iodatum.
Ferr. p.	Ferrum phosphoricum.
Ferr. pic	Ferrum picricum.
Fl. ac.	Fluoric acid.
Gambo.	Gambogia.
Gel.	Gelsemium.
Glon.	Glonoinum.
Grap.	Graphites.
Grat.	Gratiola officinalis.
Guai.	Guaiacum.

328

Ham.	Hamamelis.
Hec. l.	Hecla lava.
Hell.	Helleborus.
Helo. h.	Heloderma horridus.
Helon.	Helonias.
Hep.	Hepar sulphuris.
Hoang.	Hoang nan.
Hydras.	Hydrastis.
Hyo.	Hyoscyamus.
Hyper.	Hypericum.
Ig.	Ignatia.
Indig.	Indigo.
Iod.	Iodine.
Ipe.	Ipecacuanha.
Iris v.	Iris versicolor.
Jac.	Jacaranda.
Jug. r.	Juglans regia.
Kal. bi.	Kali bichromicum.
Kal. bro.	Kali bromicum.
Kal. iod.	Kali iodatum.
Kal. m.	Kali muriaticum.
Kal. p.	Kali phosphoricum.
Kal. s.	Kali sulphuricum.
Kalmia.	Kalmia latifolia.
Kreo.	Kreosotum.
Lach.	Lachesis.
Lact.	Lactuca.
Lac. a.	Lactic acid.
Lapp.	Lappa major.
Lat. m.	Latrodectus mactans.
Laur.	Laurocerasus.
Led.	Ledum palustre.

LIL. T.

Lil. t.	Lilium tigrinum.
Lith. bro.	Lithium bromicum.
Lith. c.	Lithium carbonicum.
Lith. lac.	Lithium lacticum.
Lob. i.	Lobelia inflata.
Lyc.	Lycopodium.

Mag. c.	Magnesia carbonica.
Mag. m,	Magnesia muriaticum.
Mag. p.	Magnesia phosphoricum.
Mag. pol. aust.	Magnetis polus australis.
Manc.	Mancinella.
Mang.	Manganum.
Meli.	Melilotus.
Mer.	Mercurius solubilis.
Mer. bin.	Mercurius biniodide.
Mer. c.	Mercurius corrosivus.
Mer. d.	Mercurius dulcis.
Mer. prot.	Mercurius protojodatus.
Mez.	Mezereum.
Mill.	Millefolium.
Mos.	Moschus.
Mur. a.	Muriatic acid.
Mygal.	Mygale lasidora.
Myosot.	Myosotis symphitifola.

Naj.	Naja tripudians.
Nap.	Naphthalin.
Nat. c.	Natrum carbonicum.
Nat. m.	Natrum muriaticum.
Nat. p.	Natrum phosphoricum.
Nat. s.	Natrum sulphuricum.
Nit. a.	Nitric acid.
Nitr.	Nitrum.
Nup. lut.	Nuphar luteum.

Nux. v.	Nux vomica.
Nux. m.	Nux moschata.

Œnanth.	Œnanthe crocata.
Œnoth.	Œnothera biennis.
Ol.	Oleander.
Oleum j.	Oleum jecoris aselli.
Onos.	Onosmodium Virginicum.
Op.	Opium.
Ova t.	Ova testa.
Ox. a.	Oxalic acid.

Pæon	Pæonia.
Pareir.	Pareira brava.
Paris.	Paris quadrifolia.
Paull.	Paullinia sorbilis.
Pass.	Passiflora incarnata.
Pet.	Petroleum.
Phell.	Phellandrium aquaticum.
Pho.	Phosphorus.
Ph. a.	Phosphoric acid.
Physos.	Physostigma.
Phyt.	Phytolacca.
Pic. a.	Picric acid.
Pilo.	Pilocarpine.
Pip. m.	Piper methysticum.
PB.	Plumbum.
Plant.	Plantago major.
Plat.	Platinum.
Pod.	Podophyllum.
Pothos f.	Pothos fœtida.
Pso.	Psorinum.
Ptelea.	Ptelea trifoliata.
Pul.	Pulsatilla.
Pyrogen.	Pyrogenium.

RAN. B.

Ran. b.	Ranunculus bulbosa.
Ran. s.	Ranunculus sceleratus.
Rheu.	Rheubarb.
Rhod.	Rhododendron.
Rhus aro.	Rhus aromatica.
Rhus.	Rhus toxicodendron.
Rob.	Robinia.
Rum. c.	Rumex crispus.
Ruta.	Ruta graveolens.
Sabad.	Sabadilla.
Sabal s.	Sabal serrulata.
Sabin.	Sabina.
Sali. ac.	Salicylic acid.
Sam.	Sambucus.
Sang.	Sanguinaria.
Sang. n.	Sanguinarina nitrica.
Sant.	Santonine.
Sars.	Sarsaparilla.
Scut.	Scuttellaria laterifolia.
Sec.	Secale cornutum.
Seneg.	Senega.
Sep.	Sepia.
Sil.	Silicea.
Silph.	Silphium.
Slag.	Slag.
Solid. v.	Solida virga-aura.
Solan. C.	Solanum Carolinense.
Spig.	Spigelia.
Spo.	Spongia tosta.
Squil.	Squilla.
Stan.	Stannum.
Stap.	Staphysagria.
Stict.	Sticta pulmonaria.
Stram.	Strammonium.
Strych.	Strychninum.

Sul.	Sulphur.
Sul. a.	Sulphuric acid.
Symph.	Symphitum.
Tab.	Tabacum.
Tarant. C.	Tarantula Cubensis.
Tart. c.	Tartar emetic.
Tarax.	Taraxacum.
Tell.	Tellurium.
Tereb.	Terebinthina.
Teucr.	Teucrium.
Therid.	Theridion.
Thuj.	Thuja occidentalis.
Trif. p.	Trifolium pratense.
Trill.	Trillium pendulum.
Uran. n.	Uranium nitricum.
Urti.	Urtica urens.
Ustil.	Ustilago maydis.
Uva.	Uva ursi.
Vaccin.	Vaccininum.
Val.	Valeriana.
Verat. a.	Veratrum album.
Verat. v.	Veratrum viride.
Vib. op.	Viburnum opulus.
Vib. pru.	Viburnum prunifolium.
Vinca m.	Vinca minor.
Viol. o.	Viola odorata.
Viol. t.	Viola tricolor.
Vis. a.	Viscum album.
Xanth.	Xanthoxylum.
Zing.	Zingibar.
ZN.	Zincum.
ZN. p.	Zincum phosphoratum
ZN. v.	Zincum valerianicum.

333

..The Medical Genius..

A Guide to the Cure.

BY

STACY JONES, M. D.

Respectfully Dedicated to all Those Who Prefer Curing Diseases to Contending About Dogmas.

Cloth.
328 pages.
8vo.
$2.00 net; by mail, $2.11.

By the Author of the Bee-Line Therapia.

———

WE know that the readers of the *Brief* will hail this practical work, giving hints and directions as to what should be done and *how to do it;* and if the purchaser of this work will apply the *sound common sense of the author* in its use, he will find it a perfect *vade mecum.* It contains a store of varied and valuable information such as *cannot be found in any other work.* The typographical appearance is *first-class,* and we congratulate the author on the manner of arrangement.—*St. Louis Medical Brief.*

———

BOERICKE & TAFEL, Publishers,

| Philadelphia, | New York, | Chicago, |
| Baltimore, | Pittsburgh, | Cincinnati. |

Boericke & Tafel,

Publishers of Homoeopathic and Other Medical Literature.

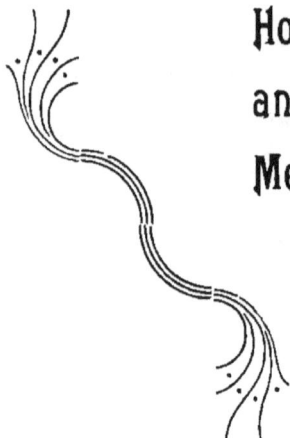

For Catalogue of books address
any of the Boericke & Tafel
Pharmacies as follows:

PHILADELPHIA—1011 Arch St.
PHILADELPHIA—111 South 13th St.
PHILADELPHIA—15 North 6th St.
NEW YORK—145 Grand St.
NEW YORK—15 West 42d St.
CHICAGO—44 East Madison St.
PITTSBURGH—627 Smithfield St.
BALTIMORE—228 North Howard St.
CINCINNATI—204 West 4th St.

Business Established in 1835.

MEDICAL WORKS

OF

DR. SAMUEL HAHNEMANN

PUBLISHED BY

BOERICKE & TAFEL,

PHILADELPHIA,   NEW YORK,   CHICAGO,
BALTIMORE,   PITTSBURGH,   CINCINNATI.

● ● ●

HAHNEMANN—*Organon of the Art of Healing. Aude Sapere. Fifth American Edition. Translated from the Fifth German Edition by C. Wesselhœft, M. D.* 244 pages. Large 8vo. Cloth, $1.75; *net*, $1.40; by mail, $1.55.

HAHNEMANN—*Organon of Medicine. Translated from the Fifth Edition, with an Appendix by R. E. Dudgeon, M. D.* 304 pages. 8vo. Cloth, $2.50 *net;* by mail, $2.63.

HAHNEMANN—*Materia Medica Pura. Translated from the Latest German Edition by R. E. Dudgeon, M. D., with Annotations by Richard Hughes, L. R. C. P. E.* Two volumes. 1427 pages. Royal 8vo. Cloth, price for the set, $10.00; *net*, $9.00; by mail. $9.64. Half morocco, $12.00; *net*, $10.80; by mail, $11.44.

HAHNEMANN—*The Chronic Diseases. Their Peculiar Nature and their Homœopathic Cure. Translated from the Second Enlarged German Edition of 1835, by Professor Louis H. Tafel, with Annotations by Richard Hughes, M. D. Edited by Pemberton Dudley, M. D.* Two volumes. 1600 pages. 8vo. Half morocco, $11.00 plus book expressage.

HAHNEMANN—*Defence of the Organon of Rational Medicine* and of his previous Homœopathic works against the attacks of Professor Hecker. An explanatory commentary on the Homœopathic system. Translated by R. E. Dudgeon, M. D. 130 pages. Cloth, $1.00 *net;* by mail, $1.05.

www.ingramcontent.com/pod-product-compliance
Lightning Source LLC
Chambersburg PA
CBHW021459210326
41599CB00012B/1062